SM 00007213
5-7-01
£3⁹

DP
(Rya).

611.710246
(Rya)

✓

ANATOMY *for*
DIAGNOSTIC IMAGING

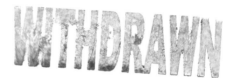

0702014478

Dedication

This book is dedicated to our husbands Tom Ryan and Billy Power and to our children Stephen and Ellen Ryan, and Barry and Jack Power.

ANATOMY *for* DIAGNOSTIC IMAGING

S.P. Ryan

MB, BCh, BAO, FRCSI, FFR, RCSI
Senior Fellow in Radiology, Children's Hospital and Medical Center,
Seattle, Washington
Presently Fellow in Interventional Radiology, Mayo Clinic, Minnesota,
Rochester, USA

M.M.J. McNicholas

MB, BCh, BAO, MRCPI, FRCR, FFR, RCSI
Senior Registrar, St Vincents Hospital, Dublin
and Lecturer in Radiology, University College, Dublin
Presently Fellow in Abdominal Imaging and Interventional Radiology,
Massachusetts General Hospital, Boston, Massachusetts, USA

WB Saunders Company Ltd
London, Philadelphia, Sydney, Tokyo, Toronto

W.B. Saunders
An imprint of Harcourt Publishers Limited

© 1994 W.B. Saunders Company Ltd.
© 2000 Harcourt Publishers Ltd.
Reprinted 1998
Reprinted 2000

A catalogue record for this book is available from the British Library.

ISBN 0 7020 1447 8

Edited, designed and typeset by Melanie Paton, Aldershot, Hampshire.
Printed and bound in the United Kingdom at the University Press, Cambridge.

CONTENTS

Preface		vii
Acknowledgements		viii
Chapter 1	**Head and Neck**	**1**
	The skull and facial bones	2
	The nasal cavity and paranasal sinuses	12
	The mandible and teeth	14
	The oral cavity and salivary glands	16
	The orbital contents	20
	The ear	24
	The pharynx and related spaces	26
	The nasopharynx and related spaces	27
	The larynx	31
	The thyroid and parathyroid glands	35
	The neck vessels	38
Chapter 2	**Central Nervous System**	**45**
	Cerebral hemispheres	46
	Cerebral cortex	46
	White matter	49
	Thalamus, hypothalamus and pineal gland	54
	Pituitary gland	55
	Limbic lobe	57
	Brainstem	58
	Cerebellum	60
	Ventrices, cisterns, CSF production and flow	62
	Subarachnoid cisterns	66
	Cerebrospinal fluid production and flow	67
	Meninges	68
	Arterial Supply	70
	Veins	77
	Cross-sectional anatomy	82
Chapter 3	**Spinal Column and its Contents**	**85**
	The vertebral column	86
	The joints of the vertebral column	95
	The ligaments of the vertebral column	96
	The intervertebral discs	97
	The blood supply of the vertebral column	98
	The spinal cord	98
	The spinal mcninges	100
	The blood supply of the spinal cord	101
Chapter 4	**The Thorax**	**105**
	The thoracic cage	106
	The diaphragm	109
	The pleura	113
	The trachea and bronchi	114
	The lungs	118
	Mediastinal divisions	124
	The heart	125
	The great vessels	133
	The oesophagus	135
	The thoracic duct and the mediastinal lymphatics	138
	The thymus	138

	The azygous system	138
	Important nerves of the mediastinum	139
	The mediastinum on the chest radiograph	139
	Cross-sectional anatomy	143
Chapter 5	**The Abdomen**	**147**
	Anterior abdominal wall	148
	Stomach	151
	Duodenum	157
	Small intestine	159
	Ileocaecal valve	161
	The vermiform appendix	162
	The large intestine	162
	Liver	167
	Biliary system	172
	Pancreas	176
	Spleen	180
	Portal venous system	182
	Kidneys	184
	The ureter	189
	Adrenal glands	190
	Abdominal aorta	192
	Inferior vena cava	195
	Veins of the posterior abdominal wall	196
	Lymphatic drainage of abdomen	197
	Peritoneal spaces of the abdomen	199
	Cross-sectional anatomy of the abdomen	201
Chapter 6	**The Pelvis**	**205**
	The bony pelvis, muscles and ligaments	206
	The pelvic floor	209
	The sigmoid colon, rectum and anal canal	212
	The blood vessels, lymphatics and nerves	214
	The lower urinary tract	217
	The male reproductive organs	221
	The female reproductive tract	225
	Cross-sectional anatomy	232
Chapter 7	**The Upper Limb**	**235**
	The bones	236
	The joints	243
	The muscles	248
	The arterial supply	251
	The venous supply	252
Chapter 8	**The Lower Limb**	**253**
	The bones	254
	The joints	261
	The muscles	268
	The arteries	271
	The veins	274
Chapter 9	**The Breast**	**275**
	General anatomy of the breast	276
	Radiology of the breast	277
	Age changes in the breast	277
Further reading		**279**
Index		**282**

PREFACE

As radiology registrars preparing for Part I of our fellow-ship examinations, we found that there was no single book that provided all the information we required to attempt both the oral examination and the multiple-choice question paper. In an attempt to cross-reference pure anatomy with the radiological features of each organ or system, we found ourselves surrounded by a small mountain of anatomy books and atlases on one hand, and another pile of radiology books on the other. We felt that there was a great need for a single book that covered both traditional anatomy and all its radiological aspects in all the imaging modalities. We hope that this book will save students some of the trouble and the time previously required to amass sufficient information from different sources to attain a competent knowledge of radiological anatomy.

With the rapid growth of imaging, especially the cross-sectional imaging modalities, a knowledge of cross-sectional anatomy is essential for anyone who comes into regular contact with imaging in their clinical practice.

This is an anatomy book aimed at those people who wish to improve their understanding of radiological imaging. We feel that it will be helpful not only to radiologists and radiographers in training, but also to surgeons and physicians who request radiological examinations. An understanding of the radiological anatomy will assist in their understanding of pathological findings together with the significance of these findings.

With more emphasis now being put on living anatomy in undergraduate training, and since most medical students will be given some teaching in radiology as part of their curriculum, this book should also be of interest to undergraduate medical students.

ACKNOWLEDGEMENTS

Amassing illustrative and radiological material for a book such as this is not an easy task, and would not have been possible without the help and enthusiasm of several people. We were extremely fortunate to have the approval of Professor J.B. Coakley, Professor Emeritus of Anatomy at University College Hospital, Dublin, to use many of his excellent line drawings. These have been appreciated by generations of medical students.

Professor J. Mc Nulty of St James' Hospital, Dublin, provided the initial encouragement and advice that launched us on this project. A large proportion of the radiological material came from the collections of Consultant Radiologists at St Vincent's Hospital, Dublin, particularly those of Professor D. MacErlaine and Dr J. Griffin. Dr J. Toland, Consultant Neuroradiologist at Beamont Hospital, Dublin, contributed most of the cerebral angiograms and plain skull films.

We would like to thank Senior Radiographer Elizabeth Darcy, St Vincent's Hospital, Dublin, for her enthusiastic help and expertise in obtaining many of the CT films.

The following physicians also donated material for reproduction: Dr A. Owens; Dr B. Hourihane; Dr J. Masterson; Dr J. Molloy; Dr G. Wilson; Dr D. O'Halpin; Dr C. Mc Creery; Dr B. Murphy; Dr T. Mahon; Dr J. Stack; Dr D. O'Connell.

Fig. 4.8 is reproduced with permission from Ellis, H. (1983) *Clinical Anatomy*, 7th Edn, Fig. 14, p. 22. Blackwell Scientific Publications, Oxford.

Figs 3.17 and 3.18 are reproduced with permission from Grainger, R.G. and Allison, D.J. (1992) *Diagnostic Radiology —an Anglo-American Textbook of Imaging*, Vol. 3, 2nd Edn, Figs 87.21 and 87.22, p. 1812. Churchill Livingstone, Edinburgh.

Figs 7.1, 7.4, 7.6, 8.1 and 8.2 are reproduced with permission from Dean, M.R.E. (1987) *Basic Anatomy and Physiology for Radiographers*, 2nd Edn., Figs 73, 74, 76, 85 and 87. Blackwell Scientific Publications, Oxford.

Figs 8.9, 8.10, 8.16, 8.17 and 8.18 are adapted with permission from Williams, P.L., Warwick, R., Dyson, M. and Bannister, L.H. (1989) *Gray's Anatomy — Descriptive and Applied*, 37 Edn., Figs 4.74, 4.75, 6.94, 6.95, 6.102, 6.128 and 6.129. Churchill Livingstone, Edinburgh.

CHAPTER 1 *HEAD AND NECK*

The skull and facial bones

The nasal cavity and paranasal sinuses

The mandible and teeth

The oral cavity and salivary glands

The orbital contents

The ear

The pharynx and related spaces

The nasopharynx and related spaces

The larynx

The thyroid and parathyroid glands

The neck vessels

THE SKULL AND FACIAL BONES

The skull consists of the calvarium, facial bones and mandible. The calvarium is the brain case and comprises the skull vault and skull base. The bones of the calvarium and face are joined at immovable fibrous joints, except for the temporomandibular joint, which is a movable cartilaginous joint.

THE SKULL VAULT (Figs 1.1–1.4)

The skull vault is made up of several flat bones, joined at sutures, which can be recognized on skull radiographs. The bones consist of the diploic space — a cancellous layer containing vascular spaces — sandwiched between the inner and outer tables of cortical bone.

The paired parietal bones form much of the side and the roof of the skull and are joined at the sagittal suture.

Fig. 1.1 Lateral view of skull.

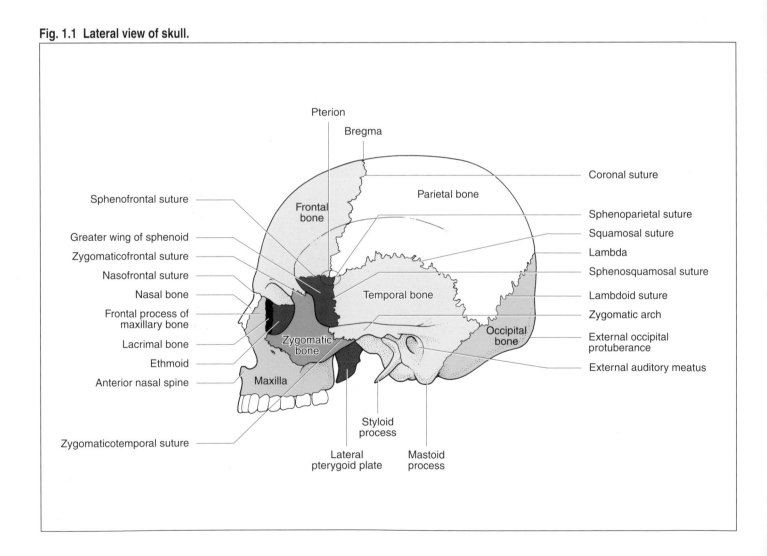

The frontal bone forms the front of the skull vault and is joined to the parietal bones at the coronal suture. The junction of coronal and sagittal sutures is known as the *bregma*. The occipital bone forms the back of the skull vault and is joined to the parietal bones at the lambdoid suture. The lambdoid and sagittal sutures join at a point known as the *lambda*.

The greater wing of sphenoid and the squamous part of the temporal bone form the side of the skull vault below the frontal and parietal bones. The sutures formed here are: (i) the sphenosquamosal suture between the sphenoid and temporal bones; (ii) the sphenofrontal and sphenoparietal sutures between greater wing of sphenoid and frontal and parietal bones; and (iii) the squamosal suture between temporal and parietal bones. The sphenofrontal, sphenoparietal and squamosal sutures form a continuous curved line on the lateral skull radiograph (see **Fig. 1.1**). The centre of the approximately 'H'-shaped intersection of these sutures is termed the *pterion* and provides a surface marking for the anterior branch of the middle meningeal artery on the lateral skull radiograph.

Fig. 1.2 Frontal view of skull.

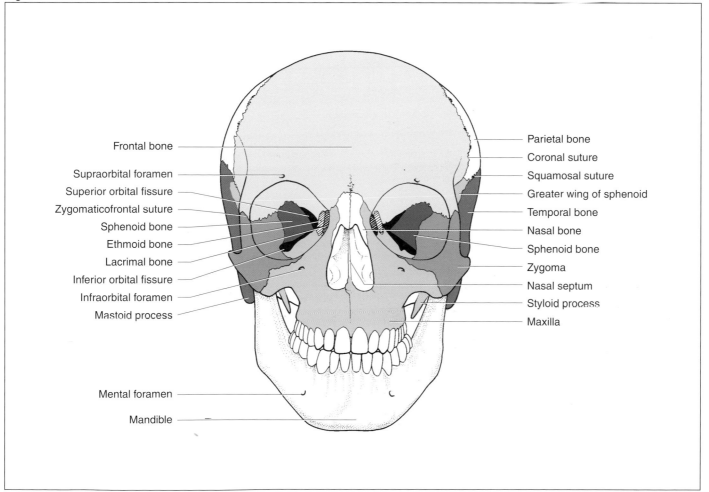

Frontal bone

Supraorbital foramen

Superior orbital fissure

Zygomaticofrontal suture

Sphenoid bone

Ethmoid bone

Lacrimal bone

Inferior orbital fissure

Infraorbital foramen

Mastoid process

Mental foramen

Mandible

Parietal bone

Coronal suture

Squamosal suture

Greater wing of sphenoid

Temporal bone

Nasal bone

Sphenoid bone

Zygoma

Nasal septum

Styloid process

Maxilla

Fig. 1.3 Lateral skull radiograph.

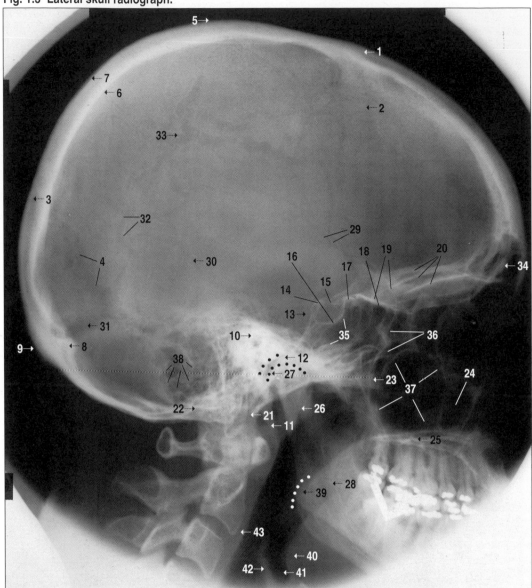

BONY LANDMARKS
1. Bregma
2. Coronal suture
3. Lambda
4. Lambdoid suture
5. Vertex
6. Inner skull table
7. Outer skull table
8. Inner occipital protruberance
9. Outer occipital protruberance
10. External auditory meatus
11. Styloid process
12. Clivus
13. Dorsum sellae
14. Posterior clinoid process
15. Anterior clinoid process
16. Pituitary fossa (sella turcica)
17. Tuberculum sellae
18. Planum sphenoidale
19. Greater wings of sphenoid
20. Undulating floor of anterior cranial fossa (roof of orbit)
21. Anterior limit of foramen magnum
22. Posterior limit of foramen magnum
23. Posterior wall of maxillary sinus
24. Malar process of maxilla
25. Hard palate
26. Neck of mandible
27. Temporomandibular joint
28. Condylar canal

VASCULAR MARKINGS
29. Middle meningeal vessels: anterior branches
30. Middle meningeal vessels: posterior branches
31. Transverse sinus
32. Diploic vein
33. Diploic venous confluence: parietal star

SINUSES / AIR CELLS
34. Frontal sinus
35. Sphenoid sinus
36. Posterior ethmoidal cells
37. Maxillary sinus
38. Mastoid air cells

SOFT TISSUES
39. Soft palate
40. Base of tongue
41. Vallecula
42. Epiglottis
43. Prevertebral soft tissues

Fig. 1.4 OF20 skull radiograph.

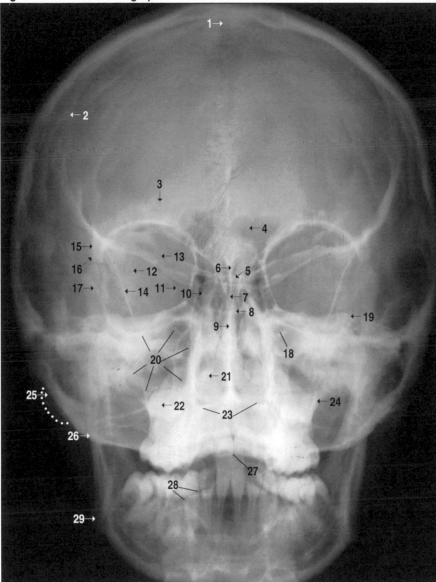

1. Sagittal suture
2. Coronal suture
3. Lambdoid suture
4. Frontal sinus
5. Planum sphenoidale
6. Crista galli
7. Perpendicular plate of ethmoid
8. Floor of pituitary fossa
9. Nasal septum
10. Ethmoid air cells
11. Superior orbital fissure
12. Greater wing of sphenoid
13. Lesser wing of sphenoid
14. Innominate line
15. Zygomatic process of frontal bone
16. Zygomaticofrontal suture
17. Frontal process of zygomatic bone
18. Foramen rotundum
19. Petrous ridge
20. Maxillary sinus
21. Inferior nasal turbinate
22. Unerupted third molar
23. Hard palate
24. Lateral wall of maxillary sinus
25. Mastoid process
26. Occipital bone
27. Dens of atlas
28. Atlantoaxial joint

THE SKULL BASE (Figs 1.5 and 1.6)

The inner aspect of the skull base is made up of the following bones from anterior to posterior:

■ The orbital plates of the frontal bone with the cribriform plate of the ethmoid bone and crista galli in the midline;

■ The sphenoid bone with its lesser wings anteriorly, the greater wings posteriorly, and body with the elevated sella turcica in the midline;

■ Part of the squamous temporal bone and the petrous temporal bone; and

■ The occipital bone.

INDIVIDUAL BONES OF THE SKULL BASE

The orbital plates of the skull base are thin and irregular and separate the anterior cranial fossa from the orbital cavity.

The cribriform plate of the ethmoid bone is a thin, depressed bone separating the anterior cranial fossa from the nasal cavity. It has a superior perpendicular projection, the crista galli, which is continuous below with the nasal septum on the frontal skull radiograph (see **Fig. 1.4**).

The sphenoid bone consists of a body and greater and lesser wings, which curve laterally from the body and join

Fig. 1.5 Skull base: internal aspect.

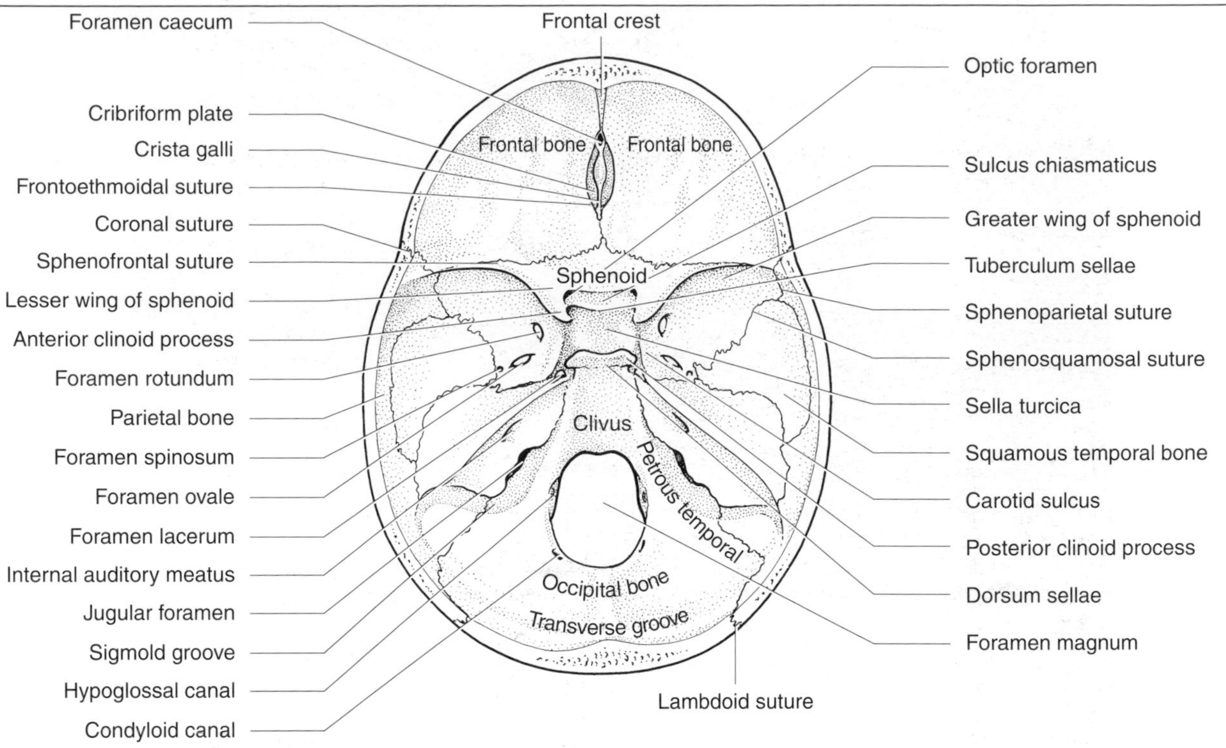
Foramen caecum
Frontal crest
Optic foramen
Cribriform plate
Crista galli
Frontal bone
Frontal bone
Sulcus chiasmaticus
Frontoethmoidal suture
Coronal suture
Greater wing of sphenoid
Sphenofrontal suture
Tuberculum sellae
Sphenoid
Lesser wing of sphenoid
Sphenoparietal suture
Anterior clinoid process
Sphenosquamosal suture
Foramen rotundum
Sella turcica
Parietal bone
Clivus
Foramen spinosum
Squamous temporal bone
Petrous temporal
Foramen ovale
Carotid sulcus
Foramen lacerum
Posterior clinoid process
Internal auditory meatus
Occipital bone
Dorsum sellae
Jugular foramen
Transverse groove
Foramen magnum
Sigmold groove
Hypoglossal canal
Lambdoid suture
Condyloid canal

at the sharply posteriorly angulated sphenoid ridge. The body houses the sphenoid sinuses and is grooved laterally by the carotid sulcus in which the cavernous sinus and carotid artery run. The sphenoid bone has a deep fossa superiorly (**Fig. 1.7**; see **Fig. 2.11**) known as the ***sella turcica*** or ***pituitary fossa,*** which houses the pituitary gland. On the anterior part of the sella is a prominence known as the ***tuberculum sella;*** anterior to this is a groove called the ***sulcus chiasmaticus,*** which leads to the optic canal on each side. The optic chiasm lies in this sulcus. Two bony projections on either side of the front of the sella are called the ***anterior clinoid processes.*** The posterior part of the sella is called the ***dorsum sellae*** and this is continuous posteriorly with the ***clivus***. Two posterior projections of the dorsum sellae form the ***posterior clinoid processes.*** The floor of the sella is formed by a thin bone known as the ***lamina dura***, which may be eroded by raised intracranial pressure or tumours of the pituitary.

The temporal bone consists of four parts:

- A flat ***squamous*** part, which forms part of the vault and part of the skull base;
- A pyramidal ***petrous*** part, which houses the middle and inner ears and forms part of the skull base;
- An aerated ***mastoid*** part; and
- An inferior projection known as the ***styloid process.***

The ***zygomatic process*** projects from the outer side of the squamous temporal bone and is continuous with the zygomatic arch.

The curved occipital bone forms part of the skull vault and posterior part of the skull base. It has the ***foramen magnum*** in the midline through which the cranial cavity is continuous with the spinal canal. Anterolaterally it is continuous with the posterior part of the petrous bones on each side, and anterior to the foramen magnum it forms the clivus. The clivus is continuous anteriorly with the dorsum sellae. Thus the occipital bone articulates with both the temporal and sphenoid bones.

CRANIAL FOSSAE (see **Fig. 1.5**)

The anterior cranial fossa is limited posteriorly by the sphenoid ridge and anterior clinoid processes and supports the frontal lobes of the brain.

The middle cranial fossa is limited anteriorly by the sphenoid ridge and anterior clinoid processes. Its posterior boundary is formed laterally by the petrous ridges and in the midline by the posterior clinoid processes and dorsum sellae. It contains the temporal lobes of the brain, the pituitary gland and most of the foramina of the skull base.

The posterior cranial fossa is the largest and deepest fossa. Anteriorly it is limited by the dorsum sellae and the petrous ridge, and it is demarcated posteriorly on the skull radiograph by the groove for the transverse sinus. It contains the cerebellum posteriorly and anteriorly the pons and medulla lie on the clivus and are continuous, through the foramen magnum, with the spinal cord.

Fig. 1.6 SMV view of skull.

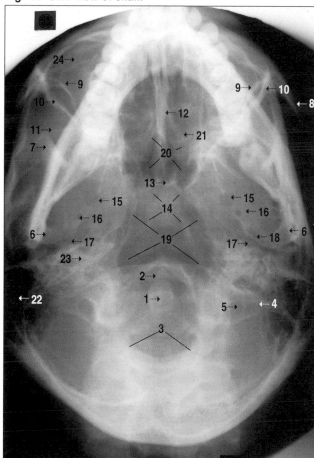

BONY LANDMARKS
1. Odontoid process of C1
2. Anterior arch of C1
3. Posterior limit of foramen magnum
4. Transverse process of C1
5. Foramen transversarium of C1
6. Condylar process of mandible
7. Coronoid process of mandible
8. Zygomatic arch
9. Posterior wall of maxillary sinus
10. Lateral boundary of orbit
11. Lesser wing of sphenoid: anterior limit of middle cranial fossa
12. Nasal septum
13. Posterior limit of hard palate
14. Clivus

FORAMINA AND CANALS
15. Foramen ovale
16. Foramen spinosum
17. Carotid canal
18. Bony part of eustachian tube

AIR SPACE AND SINUSES
19. Air in nasopharynx
20. Sphenoid sinus
21. Ethmoid air cells
22. Mastoid air cells
23. Pneumatization in petrous bone
24. Maxillary sinus

Fig. 1.7 Pituitary fossa: lateral view.

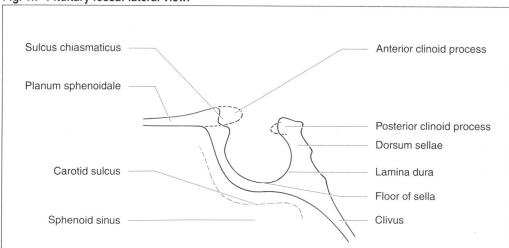

FORAMINA OF THE SKULL BASE
(see **Fig. 1.5**)

The *optic canals* run from the sulcus chiasmaticus anterior to the tuberculum sellae, anterolaterally to the orbital apex. They transmit the optic nerves and ophthalmic arteries. Owing to their oblique course, a special radiographic projection — the optic foramen view — is required for their visualization.

The *superior orbital fissure* is a triangular defect between the greater and lesser wings of sphenoid. It transmits the first (orbital) division of the fifth, and the third, fourth and sixth cranial nerves along with the superior orbital vein and a branch of the middle meningeal artery from the middle cranial fossa to the orbital apex. This fissure is best seen on the occipitofrontal view (see **Fig. 1.4**).

The *foramen rotundum* is posterior to the superior orbital fissure in the greater wing of sphenoid. It runs from the middle cranial fossa to the pterygopalatine fossa and transmits the second (maxillary) division of the fifth cranial nerve. It is seen on the occipitofrontal view of the skull with 20–25° caudal angulation (see **Fig. 1.4**), and also on occipitomental views.

The *foramen ovale* is posterolateral to the foramen rotundum in the greater wing of sphenoid. It runs from the middle cranial fossa to the infratemporal fossa and transmits the third (mandibular) division of the fifth cranial nerve and the accessory meningeal artery. This foramen is best seen on the submentovertical (SMV) projection for the base of skull (see **Fig. 1.6**).

The *foramen spinosum*, posterolateral to the foramen rotundum, is a small foramen and transmits the middle meningeal artery from the infratemporal to the middle cranial fossa. It is best seen on the SMV skull projection.

The *foramen lacerum* is a ragged bony canal posteromedial to the foramen ovale at the apex of the petrous bone. The internal carotid artery passes through its posterior wall, having emerged from the carotid canal (which runs in the petrous bone), before turning upwards to run in the carotid sulcus. This foramen can be seen on the SMV skull projection.

The *internal auditory meatus and canal* run from the posterior cranial fossa through the posterior wall of the petrous bone into the inner ear; they transmit the seventh and eighth cranial nerves and internal auditory artery. These are best seen on a straight AP view of the skull when they are projected over the orbits. Tomography in the coronal plane improves their visualization.

The *jugular foramen* is an irregular opening situated at the posterior end of the junction of the occipital and petrous bones. It runs downward and medially from the posterior cranial fossa, and transmits the internal jugular vein and ninth, tenth and eleventh cranial nerves. It also transmits the inferior petrosal sinus (which drains into the internal jugular vein), and ascending occipital and pharyngeal arterial branches. Special radiographic projections are required for its visualization because of its course.

The *hypoglossal canal* is anterior to the foramen magnum and medial to the jugular fossa and transmits the twelfth (hypoglossal) cranial nerve. It requires a special projection for radiographic visualization.

The *foramen magnum* runs from the posterior cranial fossa to the spinal canal and transmits the medulla oblongata, which is continuous with the spinal cord, along with the vertebral and spinal arteries and veins and the spinal root of the eleventh cranial nerve. This is best seen on the SMV projection.

RADIOLOGICAL FEATURES OF THE SKULL BASE AND VAULT

Plain films

Several projections are required for a full assessment of the skull vault. The standard projections are lateral, OF20° and Townes projections. The SMV view is used to assess the skull base and demonstrates most of the foramina. The *pituitary fossa* is visible on OF20 (occipitofrontal view with 20° caudal angulation), FO30 (fronto-occipital projection with 30° caudal angulation) and SMV views, but the lateral view is the most frequently used for its assessment. On this view its dimensions are 11–16 mm in length and 8–12 mm in depth. The dorsum sellae should have well-defined margins anteriorly and posteriorly.

Pneumatization of the sphenoid sinus may be rudimentary, presellar, sellar (extending under the entire sella), or extensive when it involves the dorsum. The third type (sellar) is the most usual. The degree of pneumatization has implications for trans-sphenoidal pituitary surgery.

Elongation of the pituitary fossa with a prominent sulcus chiasmaticus is variously known as a 'J-shaped', 'omega' or 'hour-glass' sella and is a normal variant in 5% of children.

The *middle meningeal vessels* form a prominent groove on the inner table of the skull vault running superiorly from the foramen spinosum across the squamous temporal bone before dividing into anterior and posterior branches.

The *diploic markings* are larger irregular less well defined venous channels running in the diploic space. They are very variable in appearance but a stellate confluence is often seen on the parietal bone on the lateral skull radiograph.

The *dural sinuses* are wide channels that groove the inner table. The transverse sinuses are readily seen on the Townes projection running from the region of the internal occipital protruberance laterally towards the mastoids before curving down to become the sigmoid sinuses, which run into the internal jugular vein.

The *supraorbital artery* grooves the outer table of the frontal bone as it runs superiorly from the orbit on the OF skull projection, and the *superficial temporal artery* grooves the outer table of the temporal and parietal bones, running superiorly from the region of the external auditory meatus on the lateral projection.

The *arachnoid granulation pits* are small irregular impressions on the inner table related to the superior sagittal sinus.

The major *sutures* sutures have been described. The *metopic suture* between the two halves of the frontal bone normally disappears by 2 years of age but persists into adulthood in approximately 10% of people, and may be incomplete. The *spheno-occipital synchondrosis* is the suture between the anterior part of the occipital bone and the sphenoid body. This usually fuses at puberty but may persist into adulthood and be mistaken for a fracture of the skull base on the lateral skull radiograph.

Wormian bones are small bony islands that may be seen in suture lines and at sutural junctions, particularly in relation to the lambdoid suture.

The *thickness of the skull vault* is not uniform. The parietal convexities may be markedly thinned and appear radiolucent. Also, marked focal thickening may be seen particularly in the region of the frontal bone in the normal person. The inner and outer tables are thickened at the internal and external occipital protruberances. The external protuberance and muscular attachments of the occipital bone may be very prominent in the male skull.

Cross-sectional imaging

Computed tomography (CT) provides excellent visualization of the skull base and foramina when narrow high-resolution images are obtained. MRI with narrow section thickness slices is excellent for demonstration of the soft-tissue contents of the foramina, in particular the cranial nerves. The plane of imaging can be chosen to demonstrate the structure of interest, for example imaging in several planes is necessary to demonstrate the course of the facial nerve through the skull base from its entry into the internal auditory canal to its exit through the stylomastoid foramen.

THE NEONATAL AND GROWING SKULL

At birth there may be overlapping of the cranial bones due to moulding; this disappears over several days. The diploic space is not developed, vascular markings are not visible and the sinuses are not aerated. The sutures are straight lines, the fontanelles are open and wormian bones may be seen. The skull vault is approximately eight times the size of the facial bones on the lateral skull radiograph.

The posterior fontanelle closes by 6–8 months of age and the anterior fontanelle is usually closed by 15–18 months. Two pairs of lateral fontanelles close in the second or third month. By 6 months the sutures have narrowed to 3 mm or less. They begin to interlock in the first year and have begun to assume the serrated appearance of the adult sutures at 2 years of age. By this time the diploic space has begun to develop and the middle meningeal and convolutional markings start to appear. The convolutional markings may be very prominent but become less so after the age of 10 years and eventually disappear in early adulthood.

The fastest period of growth of the skull vault is the first year, and adult proportions are almost attained by the age of 7 years. Growth of the facial bones is more rapid than that of the skull vault, being fastest during the first 7 years with a further growth spurt at puberty. Thereafter growth is slower until the facial bones occupy a similar volume to the cranium.

In old age the cranium becomes thinner, and the maxilla and mandible shrink with the loss of dentition and the resorption of the alveolar processes.

CALCIFICATION ON THE SKULL RADIOGRAPH IN THE NORMAL PERSON (see also Chapter 2)

The *pineal gland* is a midline structure situated behind the third ventricle and is calcified in 50% of adults over 20 years and in most elderly subjects. Before CT was widely available, shift of the calcified pineal by more than 3 mm was regarded as an important sign of intracranial pathology. Meticulous radiographic positioning is required to assess any shift accurately as even the slightest degree of rotation invalidates the measurements.

The *habenular commissure*, just anterior to the pineal gland, often calcifies in association with it in a reverse 'C' shape.

The *glomus of the choroid plexus* in the atria of the lateral ventricles is frequently calcified. The degree of calcification is variable, but calcification is usually symmetrical and bilateral.

Dural calcification may occur anywhere but is frequently seen in the falx and tentorium cerebelli. The *petroclinoid* and *interclinoid ligaments* are dural reflections that run from the petrous apex to the dorsum sellae and between the anterior and posterior clinoid processes. These may also calcify — especially in the elderly.

The *arachnoid granulations* may also calcify, usually close to the vault along the line of the superior longitudinal venous sinus.

The *basal ganglia* and *dentate nucleus* may show punctate calcification in asymptomatic individuals, again this is more frequent with increasing age.

The *internal carotid artery* may be calcified in the elderly — especially in the region of the siphon.

The *lens of the eye* may be calcified in the elderly.

THE FACIAL BONES (see Fig. 1.2)

Several bones contribute to the bony skeleton of the face including the mandible, which forms the only freely mobile joint of the skull. The maxillae, zygomata and mandible contribute most to the shape of the face, and the orbits, nose and paranasal sinuses form bony cavities contained by the facial skeleton. The individual components of the face will be described separately with reference to their radiological assessment.

THE ZYGOMA

This forms the eminence of the cheek and is also known as the malar bone. It is a thin bony bar that articulates with the frontal, maxillary and temporal bones at the zygomatico-frontal, zygomaticomaxillary and zygomaticotemporal

sutures. Its anterior end reinforces the lateral and inferior margins of the orbital rim. The zygoma forms the lateral boundary of the *temporal fossa* above, and the *infratemporal fossa* below.

The zygoma is prone to trauma and may be assessed radiologically on the OM projection (**Fig. 1.8**) and on modified Towne's and SMV views where the rest of the skull is shielded and a low exposure is used.

THE BONY ORBIT (Fig. 1.9)

The orbit is a four-sided pyramidal bony cavity whose skeleton is contributed to by several bones of the skull. The base of the pyramid is open and points anteriorly to form the orbital rim. Lateral, superior, medial and inferior walls converge posteromedially to an *apex* onto which

Fig. 1.8 OM skull radiograph.

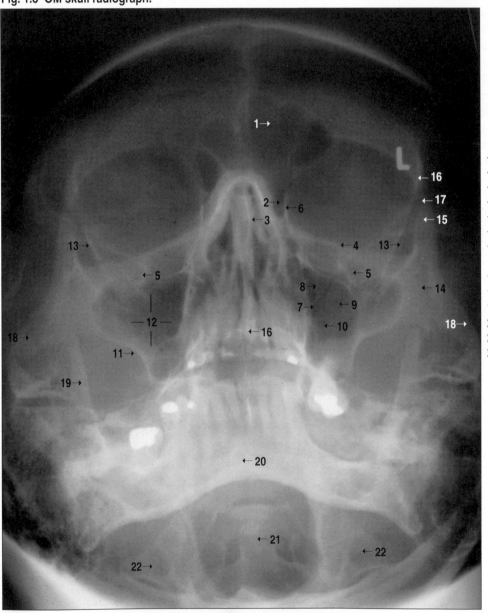

1. Frontal sinus
2. Ethmoid sinus
3. Nasal septum
4. Inferior orbital rim
5. Infraorbital foramen
6. Lamina papyracea (medial wall of orbit)
7. Superior orbital fissure
8. Lesser wing of sphenoid
9. Greater wing of sphenoid
10. Maxillary sinus
11. Lateral wall of maxillary sinus
12. Maxillary sinus
13. Innominate line
14. Malar process of maxilla
15. Frontal process of zygoma
16. Zygomatic process of frontal bone
17. Zygomaticofrontal suture
18. Zygomatic arch
19. Coronoid process of mandible
20. Body of mandible
21. Odontoid process of C2
22. Transverse process and foramen transversarium of C1

the *optic foramen* opens, transmitting the *optic nerve* and *ophthalmic artery* from the *optic canal.*

The lateral orbital wall is strong and is formed by the zygomatic bone in front, and the greater wing of sphenoid behind. It separates the orbital cavity from the temporal fossa.

The superior wall, or roof, is thin and undulating and separates the orbit from the anterior cranial fossa. It is formed by the orbital plate of the frontal bone in front, and the lesser wing of sphenoid behind.

The medial orbital wall is a thin bone contributed to by maxillary, lacrimal and ethmoid bones; it separates the orbit from the nasal cavity, ethmoid air cells and anterior part of sphenoid. The bone between the orbit and ethmoids is paper-thin and is known as the *lamina papyracea.*

The inferior wall, or floor, is formed by the orbital process of the maxillary bone, separating the orbit from the cavity of the maxillary sinus. The orbital process of the maxillary bone also extends superomedially to contribute to the medial part of the orbital rim.

The orbit has a superolateral depression for the *lacrimal gland,* and a medial groove for the *lacrimal sac* and its *duct.* It also bears the optic foramen, two fissures, and a groove in its floor to house the infraorbital nerve.

The *superior orbital fissure* is a triangular slit between the greater and lesser wings of sphenoid (converging lateral and superior walls of the pyramid). Its medial end is wider than its lateral end and is very close to the optic foramen in the apex of the cavity. It transmits the first division of the fifth, and the third, fourth and sixth cranial nerves, as well as the ophthalmic veins and a branch of the middle meningeal artery. The middle meningeal artery may communicate with the ophthalmic artery, forming one of the anastomotic connections between internal and external carotid systems.

The *inferior orbital fissure* is a slit between the lateral and inferior walls of the orbit as they converge on the apex. It runs downward and laterally, and its posteromedial end is close to the medial end of the superior fissure. In its posterior part, it forms an opening between the orbit and the pterygopalatine fossa, and more anteriorly it forms an opening between the orbital cavity and the infratemporal fossa. It transmits the infraorbital nerve, which is a branch of the maxillary division of the fifth cranial nerve after it has passed from the middle cranial fossa into the pterygopalatine fossa via the foramen rotundum. It also transmits the infraorbital artery, a branch of the maxillary artery.

The *infraorbital groove* runs from the inferior orbital fissure in the floor of the orbit before dipping down to become the infraorbital canal. The nerve emerges from the canal onto the anterior surface of the maxillary bone through the infraorbital foramen.

The *periorbita* is a fibrous covering that lines the bony cavity of the orbit. It is continuous with the dura through

Fig. 1.9 Bony orbit.

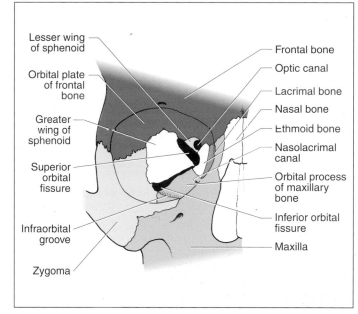

Lesser wing of sphenoid
Orbital plate of frontal bone
Greater wing of sphenoid
Superior orbital fissure
Infraorbital groove
Zygoma
Frontal bone
Optic canal
Lacrimal bone
Nasal bone
Ethmoid bone
Nasolacrimal canal
Orbital process of maxillary bone
Inferior orbital fissure
Maxilla

the optic canal and superior orbital fissure. It closes over the inferior orbital fissure, separating the orbit from the infratemporal and pterygopalatine fossae.

RADIOLOGY OF THE BONY ORBIT

Plain films

The orbits may be assessed on OF20 and OM projections (see **Figs 1.4** and **1.8**). Asymmetry between the superior orbital fissures is common. The fissure separates the greater wing of sphenoid (above) from the lesser wing (below).

A straight line is seen running through the orbit from the superolateral part of the rim inferiorly and medially. This is caused by the X-ray beam hitting the curving greater wing of sphenoid at a tangent and it is known as the *innominate line.*

Owing to its oblique course through the skull base, a specially angulated radiographic projection is required to demonstrate each optic foramen. The dimensions of the foramen should not vary by more than 1 mm. There may, however, be a separate opening for the ophthalmic artery below the foramen, or the foramen may have a keyhole configuration if the foramina are not completely separate.

The infraorbital foramen is seen on the OF20 and OM views and the floor of the orbit is best seen on the OM (see **Fig. 1.8**) and OM30 projections.

Computed tomography

The bony orbit and its soft-tissue contents are demonstrated very well by CT (see **Fig. 1.23**). Axial or coronal images may be obtained. Coronal imaging with reconstruction in the mid-sagittal plane of the orbit shows the floor of the orbit and is useful for the assessment of trauma where a fracture is suspected. MRI is more valuable for demonstration of the soft-tissue contents of the orbit than the bone.

THE NASAL CAVITY AND PARANASAL SINUSES (Figs 1.10 and 1.11)

The nasal cavity is a passage from the external nose anteriorly to the nasopharynx posteriorly. The frontal, ethmoid, sphenoid and maxillary sinuses form the paired paranasal sinuses and are situated around, and drain into, the nasal cavity. The entire complex is lined by mucus-secreting epithelium.

THE NASAL CAVITY

This is divided in two by the nasal septum in the sagittal plane. Its floor is the roof of the oral cavity and is formed by the palatine process of the maxilla, with the palatine bone posteriorly. The lateral walls of the cavity are formed by contributions from the maxillary, palatine, lacrimal and ethmoid bones. These walls bear three curved extensions known as *turbinates* or *conchae*, which divide the cavity into inferior, middle and superior *meati* — each lying beneath the turbinate of the corresponding name. The space above the superior turbinate is the *sphenoethmoidal recess*.

- The sphenoid air cells drain into the sphenoethmoidal recess;
- The posterior group of ethmoidal air cells drain into the superior meatus;
- The anterior ethmoidal air cells, maxillary sinus and frontal sinus drain into the middle meatus; and
- The nasolacrimal duct opens into the inferior meatus draining the lacrimal secretions.

THE PARANASAL SINUSES

The frontal sinuses

These lie between the inner and outer tables of the frontal bone above the nose and medial part of the orbits; they vary greatly in size and are often asymmetrical. They may extend into the orbital plate of the frontal bone.

The ethmoid sinuses

These consist of a labyrinth of bony cavities or cells situated between the medial walls of the orbit and the lateral walls of the upper nasal cavity.

The sphenoid sinuses

These paired cavities in the body of the sphenoid are often incompletely separated from each other and may be subdivided further into smaller bony cells. They are so closely related to the ethmoid air cell anteriorly that it may be difficult to distinguish a boundary. The anatomical relationships of the sphenoid sinus are of considerable importance. The sella turcica, bearing the pituitary gland with the optic chiasm anteriorly, is superior. The cavernous sinus and contents run along its lateral walls. The floor of the sphenoid sinus forms the roof of the nasopharynx.

The maxillary sinuses

The maxillary sinuses, or antra, are the largest of the paranasal sinuses. They are sometimes described as having a body and four processes.

The processes comprise: (i) the *orbital process*, which extends superomedially to contribute to the medial rim of

Fig. 1.10 Paranasal sinuses: coronal section through maxillary and ethmoid sinuses.

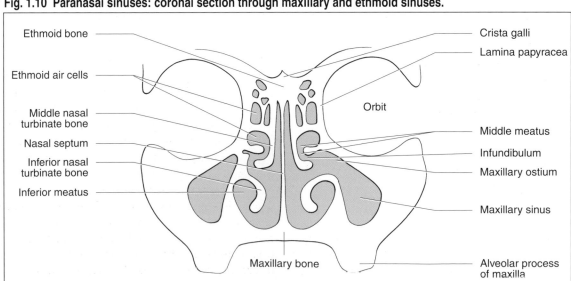

Ethmoid bone
Ethmoid air cells
Middle nasal turbinate bone
Nasal septum
Inferior nasal turbinate bone
Inferior meatus

Crista galli
Lamina papyracea
Orbit
Middle meatus
Infundibulum
Maxillary ostium
Maxillary sinus
Alveolar process of maxilla

Maxillary bone

Fig. 1.11 CT scan of the sinuses: coronal view.

1. Nasal septum
2. Maxillary sinus
3. Sphenoid sinus
4. Superior nasal turbinate
5. Middle nasal turbinate
6. Inferior nasal turbinate
7. Sphenoethmoidal recess
8. Superior meatus
9. Middle meatus
10. Inferior meatus
11. Region of maxillary ostium
12. Anterior clinoid process
13. Roof of sphenoid sinus
14. Apex of orbit
15. Superior orbital fissure
16. Posterior part of inferior orbital fissure
17. Temporal fossa and temporalis muscle (continuous inferiorly with the infratemporal fossa)
18. Zygomatic process of maxilla
19. Alveolar process of maxilla
20. Hard palate
21. Squamoos temporal bone
22. Temporal lobe

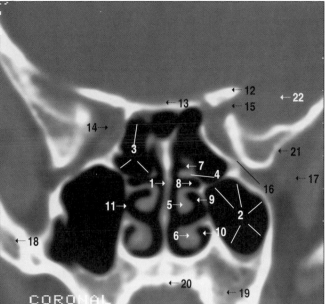

the orbit; (ii) the *zygomatic process*, which is continuous with the zygomatic arch; (iii) the *alveolar process*, which bears the teeth; and (iv) the *palatine process*, which forms the roof of the mouth and floor of the nasal cavity.

The body of the maxilla is roughly pyramidal in shape with its apex projecting superomedially between the orbit and nasal cavity. It houses the maxillary sinus. It has an anterior surface that is directed downward and laterally and forms part of the contour of the cheek. It has a curved infratemporal or posterior surface and this also forms the anterior wall of the infratemporal fossa. Its orbital or superior surface is smooth and triangular and separates the sinus from the orbital cavity. The nasal or medial surface forms the lateral wall of the lower part of the nasal cavity onto whose middle meatus the sinus drains. The medial wall of the sinus is continued superiorly as a bony projection known as the *uncinate process*. The maxillary *ostium* opens superiorly into the *infundibulum*, which is the channel between the infero-medial aspect of the orbit laterally and the uncinate process medially. The region of the ostium, infundibulum and middle meatus is important clinically and is known as the *ostiomeatal complex.*

RADIOLOGY OF THE NASAL CAVITY AND PARANASAL SINUSES

Plain films
The frontal sinuses are not visible on the skull radiograph until the age of 2 years and achieve adult proportions at the age of 14 years. Asymmetry is common and one or

both may fail to develop. Absence of both may be associated with persistence of the metopic suture between the two halves of the frontal bone. Development of the ethmoids occurs at a similar rate to the frontal sinuses.

Pneumatization of the sphenoid sinus commences at 3 years of age and may extend into the greater wings of sphenoid or clinoid processes. Failure of pneumatization is rare.

The maxillary sinuses are the first to appear and are visible radiologically from a few weeks after birth. They continue to grow and develop throughout childhood. The tooth-bearing alveolar process does not begin to develop until the age of 6 years. Full pneumatization of the maxillary sinus is not achieved until there has been complete eruption of the permanent dentition in early adulthood.

Computed tomography
CT scanning in either axial or coronal planes provides excellent visualization of the paranasal sinuses (see **Fig. 1.11**). Particular attention is paid to the region of the ostiomeatal complex, where the maxillary, frontal and anterior ethmoidal sinuses drain, and the sphenoethmoid recess and superior meatus, onto which the sphenoid and posterior ethmoid sinuses drain. The pneumatized sinuses should contain nothing but air.

MRI is surprisingly good at demonstrating the sinuses since the bony septa, which have no signal themselves, are lined by high-signal mucosa. The bone is seen as a low-intensity structure sandwiched between high-intensity mucosal layers. Air is also of low signal intensity.

THE MANDIBLE AND TEETH

THE MANDIBLE (Fig. 1.12; see Fig. 1.15)

The mandible is composed of two halves that are united at the *symphysis menti.* Each half comprises a horizontal body and a vertical ramus joined at the *angle* of the mandible. The ramus has two superior projections — the *coronoid process* anteriorly and the *condylar process* posteriorly — separated by the *mandibular notch*. The coronoid process gives attachment to the temporalis muscle, and the condylar process (or head of mandible) articulates with the base of the skull at the temporomandibular joint. The body of the mandible bears the *alveolar border* with its 16 tooth sockets.

The *mandibular canal* runs in the ramus and body of the bone, transmitting the inferior alveolar vessels and nerve (branches of the maxillary vessels and nerve). Its proximal opening is the *mandibular foramen* and is on the inner surface of the upper ramus, and its distal opening is the *mental foramen* on the external surface of the body below and between the two premolars.

THE TEMPOROMANDIBULAR JOINT (Fig. 1.13)

This is a synovial joint between the condyle of the mandible and the temporal bone. The temporal articular surface consists of a fossa posteriorly, the *temporomandibular fossa*, and an prominence anteriorly, the *articular tubercle*. The head of the mandible sits in the fossa at rest and glides anteriorly onto the articular tubercle when fully open.

Fig. 1.12 Mandible: inner aspect.

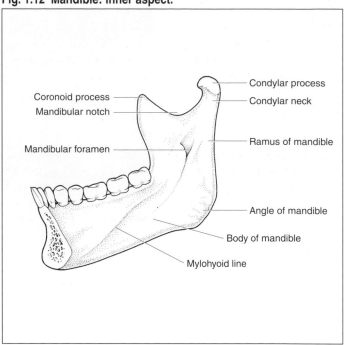

The articular surfaces are covered with fibrous cartilage. In addition, a fibrocartilaginous disc divides the joint into separate upper and lower compartments, each lined by a synovial membrane. The disc is described as having *anterior* and *posterior bands* with a *thin zone* in the middle and is attached to the joint capsule. The anterior band is also attached to the lateral pterygoid muscle. The posterior band is attached to the temporal bone. No communication between joint compartments is possible unless the disc is damaged.

Fig. 1.13 Temporomandibular joint.

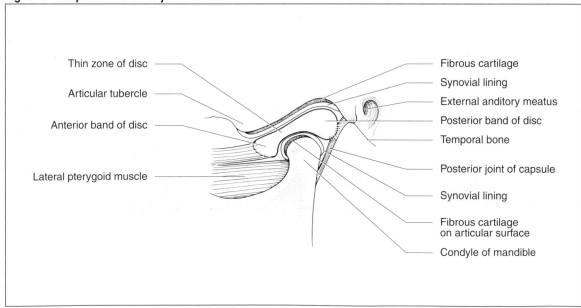

THE TEETH — NOMENCLATURE AND ANATOMY (Fig. 1.14)

There are 20 deciduous or milk teeth, and these are replaced in the adult by 32 permanent teeth. The complement of teeth in each quadrant is as follows:

- In the child: two incisors, one canine, two molars; and
- In the adult: two incisors, one canine, two premolars, three molars.

The teeth are referred to by their position in each of the four quadrants. The relevant quadrant is designated by two arms of a cross, and the tooth by its position relative to the midline. The permanent teeth are referred to by number and the milk teeth by capital letter. Thus the second right lower premolar in the adult is designated 5⌐, and the second left upper molar in a child's milk dentition is designated ⌐E .

Each tooth is has its own *root* embedded in a separate socket. The *neck* of the tooth is covered by the firm fibrous tissue of the gum and this is covered by the mucous membrane of the mouth. The exposed intraoral part of the tooth is the *crown*, and this is covered by enamel, which is the hardest and most radiopaque substance in the body. The remainder of the tooth is composed mostly of dentine, which is of a radiographic density similar to compact bone. A radiolucent *pulp cavity* occupies the middle of the tooth and is continuous with the *root canal*, which transmits the nerves and vessels from the supporting bone. The root and neck of the tooth

are surrounded by the *periodontal membrane*, which forms a radiolucent line around them on the radiograph. A dense white line of bone surrounds this and is known as the *lamina dura.* This surrounds the root of each tooth and is continuous with the lamina dura of the adjacent teeth around the margin of the alveolar crest.

Fig. 1.14 The structure of teeth.

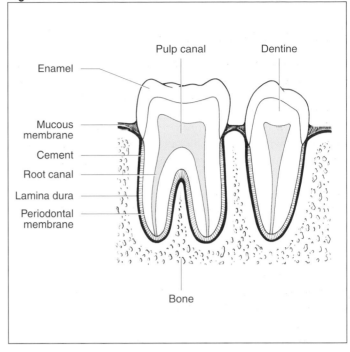

Fig. 1.15 Orthopantomogram. The third molars have been extracted.

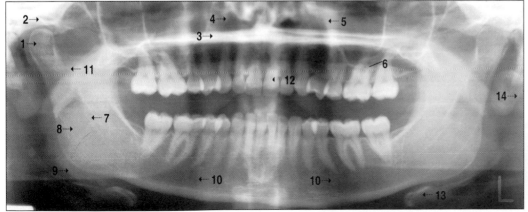

1. Condylar process of mandible
2. Temporomandibular fossa
3. Hard palate
4. Maxillary sinus
5. Medial wall of maxillary sinus
6. Floor of maxillary sinus
7. Condylar canal
8. Ramus of mandible
9. Angle of mandible
10. Body of mandible
11. Condylar notch
12. Upper left incisor
13. Hyoid bone (projected laterally)
14. Ear lobe

RADIOLOGY OF THE MANDIBLE AND TEETH (Figs 1.15 and 1.16)

Plain films

The mandible may be seen on the OF, OF20, OM, OM30 and lateral projections. Special oblique views may be required to show the rami if a fracture is suspected. There are also special views for the temporomandibular joints, and a full radiographic study of these includes images of both joints with the mouth open and closed. The teeth can be radiographed on small films placed close up against them inside the mouth, and provide excellent detail.

The symphysis menti fuses at 2 years of age. Eruption of the milk dentition is normally complete by this time. The permanent dentition develops in the mandible and maxilla during childhood and can be identified radiographically. Most has calcified by 3 years of age. The roots of the milk teeth are resorbed as the permanent teeth erupt. The first permanent molar erupts at 6 years of age, and all the permanent dentition is present by the age of 12 or 13 years except the third molar (wisdom tooth), which does not appear until early adulthood.

The mandibular canal and mandibular and mental foramina may be identified on radiographs of the mandible.

Cross-sectional imaging

High-resolution CT may be performed alone or after arthrography. MRI is excellent for the demonstration of the internal joint anatomy. The anterior and posterior bands and the thin zone of the disc are identifiable, as are the disc attachments.

Orthopantomography

The *orthopantomogram* (see **Fig. 1.15**) gives a panoramic image of both dental arches, as well as the mandible, temporomandibular joints and the lower maxilla. This study is obtained using special equipment that moves around the patient's face as the radiograph is being taken, mapping out the lower face and jaw in a straight line.

Arthrography

Arthrography of the temporomandibular joint may also be performed where radiopaque contrast is injected directly into the synovial spaces under radiographic control. Contrast should not pass from one synovial compartment to the other (see **Fig 1.13**).

THE ORAL CAVITY AND SALIVARY GLANDS

THE ORAL CAVITY (Fig. 1.17)

This forms a passage from the lips to the oropharynx. It is largely filled by the tongue and teeth and is lined by a mucous membrane. The parotid gland opens onto its lateral wall, and the submandibular and sublingual glands open onto its floor. The roof is formed by the hard palate anteriorly and the soft palate posteriorly. The soft palate is a mobile flap that hangs posteroinferiorly at rest, separating the oro- and nasopharynx. Two muscles insert into it from the lateral wall of the pharynx — the *levator* and *tensor veli palatini*. These elevate the soft palate during swallowing to prevent reflux into the nose. The *uvula* hangs from the middle of the soft palate, and two pairs of muscles run from its base to the tongue and pharynx — the *palatoglossus* and *palatopharyngeus*. These muscles and their overlying mucosa form the anterior and posterior *fauces* in whose concavity the *palatine tonsils* lie.

The muscles of the tongue form two groups. The *intrinsic* group are arranged in various planes and alter the shape of the tongue. The *extrinsic* group are paired muscles that move the tongue and have attachments outside it. The *genioglossus* arises from the inner surface of the symphysis menti and fans out to form the ventral surface of the tongue. Its inferior fibres form a tendon that attaches to the hyoid bone. The *hyoglossus* and *chondro-glossus* are thin sheets of muscle arising from the hyoid bone and inserting into the side of the tongue. The *stylo-glossus* passes from the styloid process to the side of the tongue. A median *raphe* divides the tongue into two halves.

The floor of the mouth is formed by other muscles that also support the tongue. The most important is the *mylohyoid* muscle, which is slung from the *mylohyoid line* on the inner surface of the mandible to the hyoid bone on either side.

The inferior fibres of *genioglossus* pass from the hyoid to the symphysis above the mylohyoid, and the *anterior belly of digastric* passes from the hyoid to the symphysis below the mylohyoid. The *stylohyoid* is lateral, passing from the styloid process to the hyoid. The *posterior belly of digastric* runs from the mastoid process to the lateral aspect of the hyoid bone. The *anterior belly* runs from here to the base of the anterior part of the mandible.

Lymphatic drainage of the oral cavity is to the submental and submandibular nodes, and to the retropharyngeal and deep cervical nodes.

Fig. 1.16 Occlusal radiograph of the teeth.

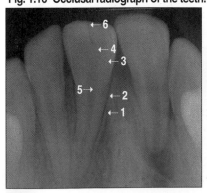

1. Lamina dura of bone
2. Periodontal membrane (radiolucent line between the lamina dura and tooth margin)
3. Dentine
4. Pulp chamber
5. Root canal
6. Enamel

Fig. 1.17 Floor of mouth: coronal section.

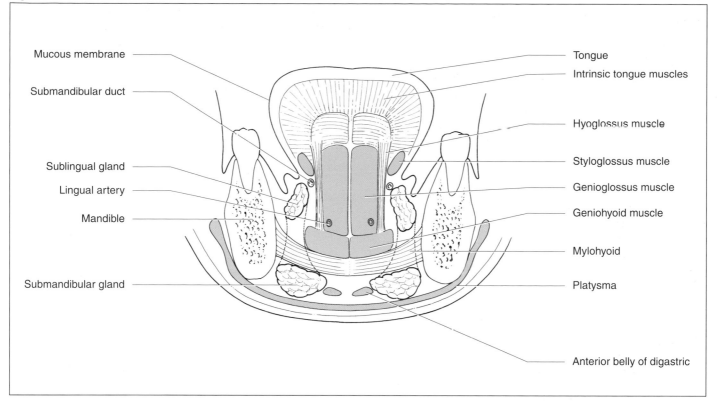

RADIOLOGY OF THE ORAL CAVITY

Since the oral cavity is amenable to direct vision, radiological assessment is not often required. However, in the case of infiltrating pathology such as tumours, cross-sectional imaging using CT or magnetic resonance imaging (MRI) is very useful. The hard and soft palate, palatine fossa, and extrinsic muscles of the tongue may be identified using both modalities, as may the maxilla, mandible, hyoid bone and surrounding structures.

MRI has inherently better soft-tissue contrast than CT and can image in coronal and sagittal as well as axial planes. There is no artefact from the mandible or dental amalgam and thus MR images are superior to CT in this area.

THE SALIVARY GLANDS

These exocrine glands are situated symmetrically around the oral cavity and produce saliva.

The parotid gland (Figs 1.18 and 1.19a, b)
This is the largest of the salivary glands and lies behind the angle of the jaw and in front of the ear. It is moulded against the adjacent bones and muscles. The gland has a smaller deep part and a larger superficial part, both parts of which are continuous around the posterior aspect of the ramus of the mandible via the *isthmus*.

The deep part of the gland extends medially to the carotid sheath and lateral wall of pharynx, separated from these by the styloid process and muscles. The superficial part lies anterior to the tragus of the ear, and is moulded to the mastoid process and sternomastoid muscle posteriorly, and to the posterior ramus of mandible and masseter muscle anteriorly. It has an anteroinferior extension, or tail, which wraps around the angle of the mandible.

The terminal part of the external carotid artery runs through the isthmus, dividing into superficial temporal and maxillary branches within the substance of the gland, and the confluence of the veins of the same name form the posterior facial vein just superficial to the artery. The facial nerve, having emerged from the stylomastoid foramen, runs through the deep part of the gland via the isthmus to the superficial part within which it branches into its five terminal divisions. It passes superficial to the artery and vein in the isthmus.

The parotid duct (*Stensen's duct*) begins as the confluence of two ducts in the superficial part of the gland and runs anteriorly deep to the gland. It arches over the masseter muscle before turning medially to pierce buccinator

Fig. 1.18 Parotid gland: (a) lateral view; (b) transverse section.

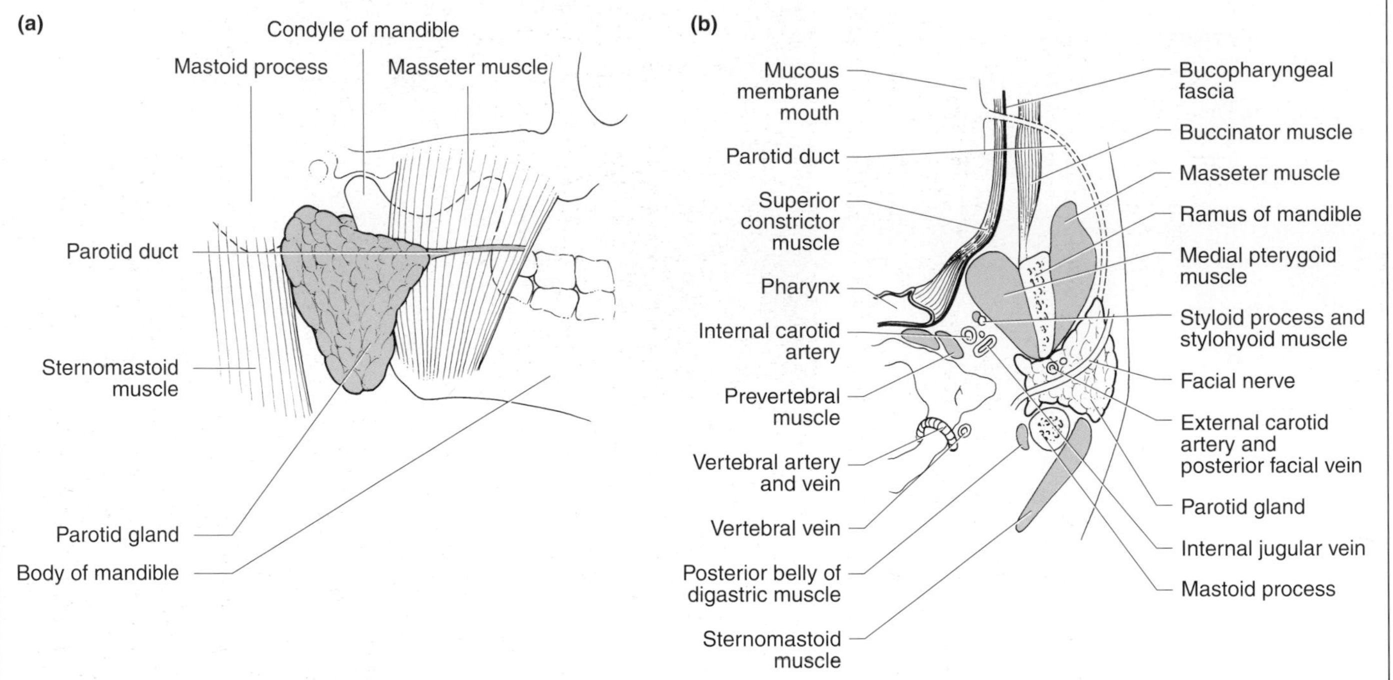

and drain into the mouth opposite the second upper molar. The duct is approximately 5 cm long.

The submandibular gland (Fig. 1.19c)

This gland lies in the floor of the mouth medial to the angle of the mandible. It has a lower superficial lobe continuous with a smaller deep lobe above around the posterior border of the mylohyoid muscle.

The submandibular duct is about 5 cm long, and commences as a confluence of several ducts in the superficial (lower) lobe. From here it runs superiorly through the deep (upper) lobe before running forward in the floor of the mouth to open at the side of the frenulum of the tongue.

The sublingual gland

This small gland lies submucosally just anterior to the deep lobe of the submandibular gland and drains via several ducts directly into the floor of the mouth.

RADIOLOGY OF THE SALIVARY GLANDS

Sialography (Fig. 1.19)

The ducts of the parotid and submandibular glands may be cannulated and injected with radiopaque con-

trast to outline the ductal system. The ducts of the parotid gland arch around the mandible because of the way in which the gland is moulded to the adjacent structures. This is best seen on the AP view. The parotid duct is seen on the lateral view. The submandibular gland and duct system may be seen on the lateral projection. The ducts of the sublingual gland are not amenable to canalization.

Cross-sectional imaging

CT (see **Figs 1.28** and **1.35**) and MRI are of particular value for tumours of the gland, to assess involvement of surrounding structures. CT may be performed after sialography to improve visualization of the ducts.

High-resolution MR images may actually demonstrate the facial nerve within the parotid gland. It is of slightly lower intensity than the surrounding gland on T1-weighted images.

Ultrasound

This may be performed through the skin or intraorally with high-frequency transducers.

Fig. 1.19 Sialography: (a) AP view of parotid gland; (b) lateral view of parotid gland; (c) lateral view of submandibular gland. Note how the duct and its branches are moulded around the ramus of the mandible.

(a)

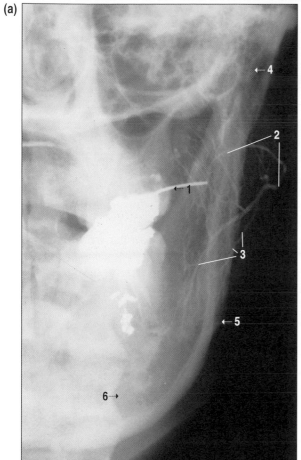

(c)

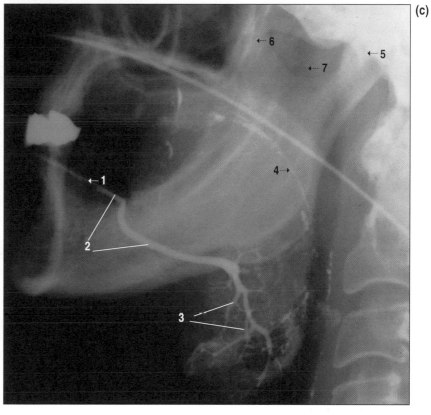

(b)

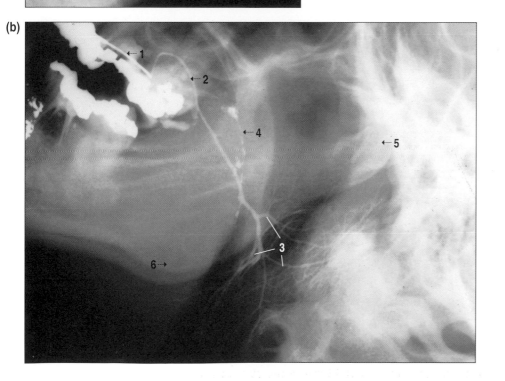

(a)
1. Cannula in parotid duct
2. Parotid duct (Stensen's)
3. Normal branching ductules
4. Condylar process of mandible
5. Angle of mandible
6. Body of mandible

(b)
1. Cannula in parotid duct orifice
2. Parotid duct
3. Secondary ductules
4. Contrast on surface of tongue
5. Condylar process of mandible
6. Angle of mandible

(c)
1. Cannula in orifice of
   submandibular duct
2. Submandibular duct
3. Secondary ductules
4. Contrast on superior surface
   of tongue
5. Condylar process of mandible
6. Coronoid process of mandible
7. Condylar notch

THE ORBITAL CONTENTS (Fig. 1.20)

The orbit contains the lacrimal gland, the globe, the extraocular muscles (including levator palpebrae), the optic nerve and the ophthalmic vessels. The whole is embedded in fat. The orbit is limited anteriorly by the *orbital septum.* This is a thin layer of fascia that extends from the orbital rim to the superior and inferior tarsal plates, separating the orbital contents from the eyelids. A fascial layer, the *periorbita*, lines the bony cavity of the orbit and this is continuous with the dura mater of the brain through the superior orbital fissure and optic canal.

The *globe* of the eye is composed of a transparent anterior part covered by the *cornea*, and an opaque posterior part covered by the *sclera*. These are joined at the corneoscleral junction known as the *limbus*. The anterior and posterior extremities of the globe are known as the anterior and posterior *poles*. The mid-coronal plane of the globe is the *equator*. A further layer of fascia, *Tenon's capsule*, covers the sclera from the limbus to the exit of the optic nerve from the eye. This fascial layer fuses with the fascia of the extrinsic ocular muscles at their insertions. Anteriorly, a mucous membrane known as the *conjunctiva* covers the anterior aspect of the eye. It is reflected from the inner surface of the eyelids and fuses with the limbus.

There are six extrinsic ocular muscles that insert into the sclera. The four rectus muscles, the *superior, inferior,* *medial* and *lateral rectus,* arise from a common tendinous ring called the *annulus of Zinn.* This is attached to the lower border of the superior orbital fissure. These muscles insert into the corresponding aspects of the globe, anterior to its equator. The *superior oblique* arises from the sphenoid bone superomedial to the optic foramen. It passes through a tendinous ring, the *trochlea*, which is attached to the frontal bone in the superolateral part of the orbit acting as a pulley. It then passes posteriorly to insert into the upper outer surface of the globe, posterior to the equator. The inferior oblique arises from the anterior part of the floor of the orbit and inserts into the lower outer part of the globe, behind the equator.

The *levator palpebrae superioris* is also within the anterior fascial limit of the orbit, arising from the inferior surface of the lesser wing of sphenoid (see **Fig. 1.9**), and inserting into the tarsal plate of the upper eyelid behind the orbital septum.

The arterial supply of the orbit is from the *ophthalmic artery.* This enters the orbit through the optic canal and gives off the *central retinal artery*, which runs in the optic nerve into the back of the eye. It supplies the orbital contents and its anterior branches anastomose with branches of the external carotid in the eyelids.

The venous drainage of the orbit is through the *superior and inferior ophthalmic veins* into the *cavernous sinus.* The superior ophthalmic vein anastomoses with the *angular vein*, which drains the periorbital skin, and thus

Fig. 1.20 Orbit: sagittal section.

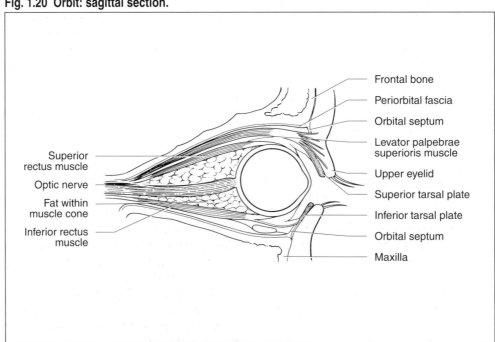

Superior rectus muscle

Optic nerve

Fat within muscle cone

Inferior rectus muscle

Frontal bone

Periorbital fascia

Orbital septum

Levator palpebrae superioris muscle

Upper eyelid

Superior tarsal plate

Inferior tarsal plate

Orbital septum

Maxilla

Fig. 1.21 Eye: internal anatomy.

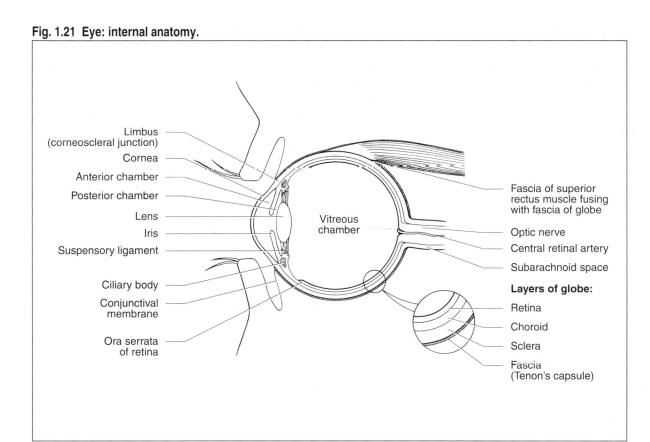

provides a possible pathway for infection causing potentially lethal cavernous sinus thrombosis.

The optic nerve is a direct extension of the brain. It is myelinated, and has external coverings of dura, arachnoid and pia forming its own subarachnoid space continuous with that of the brain. It is 4 mm thick and has four parts. The *intraocular part* begins at the optic disc. The *intraorbital part* runs posteriorly within the muscle cone formed by the four recti and is lax to allow movement of the globe. The *intracanalicular part* lies in the narrow optic canal with the ophthalmic artery, and the *intracranial part* is between the intracranial opening of the optic canal and the optic chiasm.

INTERNAL ANATOMY AND COVERINGS OF THE EYE (**Fig. 1.21**)

The globe of the eye is composed of three layers. The outermost layer consists of the tough white *sclera* posteriorly and the transparent *cornea* anteriorly. The junction of the sclera and cornea is called the *limbus*.

The middle layer is a vascular layer known as the *uveal tract*. It consists of *choroid* posteriorly, and the *ciliary body* and *iris* anteriorly. The ciliary body is a fibrous ring continuous with both the choroid and iris, and gives rise to the *ciliary muscle*, which alters the shape of the lens of the eye, allowing accommodation.

The innermost layer is the *retina*, which contains the rods and cones. The retina ends anteriorly a short distance behind the ciliary body, and its anterior limit is known as the *ora serata*. Posteriorly, nerve fibres converge to form the optic nerve at the *optic disc*. The nerve pierces both the choroid and sclera as it passes posteriorly. The sclera is continuous with the dural covering of the optic nerve. The *macula*, which has the greatest concentration of cones and is responsible for central vision, lies temporal to the optic disc.

The *anterior segment* of the eye is that part anterior to the lens. It is divided into two chambers. The *anterior chamber* is between the cornea and iris, and the *posterior chamber* is between the iris and lens. The two chambers are filled with *aqueous humour* and are continuous through the aperture of the iris (the *pupil).*

The *posterior segment* is behind the lens and is filled with a gelatinous fluid known as the *vitreous body.* The outer part of the vitreous is condensed to form the so-called *vitreous* or *hyaline membrane*. A potential space exists between the vitreous and the retina known as the *subhyaloid space*. Fluid or blood may accumulate in this space in pathological conditions.

RADIOLOGY OF THE ORBIT AND EYE (Figs 1.22 and 1.23)

Plain films

The orbital margins may be assessed by plain radiography and are well seen on OF20, OM and OM30 views of the facial bones. The floor of the orbit is undulating and not well defined. Lateral radiography of the anterior part of the eye may be performed on small dental films using a low exposure and demonstrates the cornea and eyelids. Tomography may be required to assess the floor of the orbit for trauma.

Ultrasound

Ultrasound of the eye using high-frequency transducers (5–20 MHz) can demonstrate its internal anatomy (**Fig. 1.22**). The higher-frequency transducer visualizes the anterior segment and the lower-frequency transducers (5–10 MHz) image the posterior segment. Scans may be performed in any plane but are usually obtained in

Fig. 1.22 Ultrasound of eye: (a) transverse image showing posterior structures; (b) longitudinal image showing anterior structures.

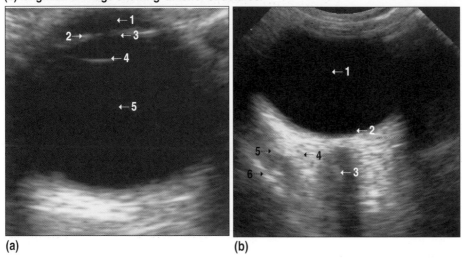

(a)

(a)
1. Anterior chamber of anterior segment
2. Iris
3. Anterior aspect of lens
4. Posterior aspect of lens
5. Posterior chamber

(b)
1. Vitreous in posterior segment of eye
2. Retinal surface
3. Optic nerve
4. Retrobulbar fat
5. Lateral rectus muscle
6. Lateral wall of bony orbit

(b)

Fig. 1.23 CT scan of orbit: axial section through optic nerve.

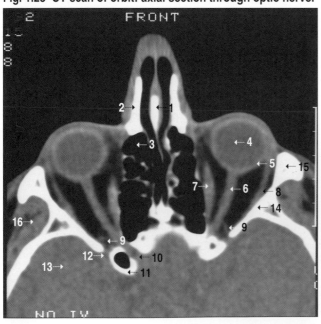

1. Nasal septum
2. Nasal bone
3. Ethmoid air cells
4. Globe of left eye
5. Sclera
6. Optic nerve
7. Medial rectus muscle
8. Lateral rectus muscle
9. Superior ophthalmic vein
10. Optic canal
11. Anterior clinoid process (pneumatized)
12. Superior orbital fissure
13. Middle cranial fossa
14. Greater wing of sphenoid
15. Frontal process of zygomatic bone
16. Temporal fossa/temporalis muscle

transverse (axial) and longitudinal (sagittal) planes. The aqueous and vitreous chambers are anechoic spaces. The cornea and lens are echogenic and easily defined. The inner walls of the eye — the choroid, retina and sclera — are not distinguishable from each other and are seen as a line of low-amplitude echoes. The retrobulbar fat is also echogenic, and the extraocular muscles and optic nerve appear as echo-free structures within it.

Computed tomography

CT is an excellent modality for the demonstration of the extraocular contents of the orbit (**Fig. 1.23**). The lacrimal gland, extraocular muscles, globe, optic nerve and superior ophthalmic vein are routinely seen on sections obtained at 4 mm intervals. Thinner sections give even better detail. The bony walls of the orbit are demonstrated, and the foramina of the orbit and related anatomy are assessed readily. Coronal images may also be obtained and demonstrate the extraocular muscles and the optic nerve.

Magnetic resonance imaging

MRI of the orbit demonstrates the soft tissues of the orbit. It may be performed in any plane. It is of particular value in demonstrating the optic nerve, allowing excellent visualization of the entire nerve including the intracanicular segment on vertical oblique images along the nerve's long axis. On coronal images the third, fourth, sixth and first division of sixth nerves can be seen just below the anterior clinoid process. Much of the internal anatomy of the eye can also be distinguished, as can the orbital septum, extraocular muscles, nerves and vessels.

THE LACRIMAL APPARATUS (Fig. 1.24)

This consists of the *lacrimal gland*, which lies in the superolateral part of the orbit and produces the tears, and the lacrimal *canaliculi*, *lacrimal sac* and *nasolacrimal duct*, which drain the secretions to the nose.

The lacrimal gland lies lateral to the levator palpebrae. This muscle grooves the gland, dividing it into an almond-sized *orbital lobe* posteriorly, and a smaller *palpebral lobe*, which extends anteriorly under the lateral part of the upper eyelid. The orbital lobe lies in a bony depression called the *lacrimal fossa*. The gland secretes tears into the space between the upper eyelid and eye (the *upper fornix*) through several small ducts.

On the medial margins of each eyelid are openings known as the *lacrimal puncta.* Tears drain through these openings into the superior and inferior lacrimal canaliculi. The canaliculi drain into the lacrimal sac, which is situated in a bony groove in the medial wall of the orbit but outside the fascial plane, which limits the orbit proper. This drains via the nasolacrimal duct, which runs in its own bony canal to the inferior meatus of the nasal cavity.

RADIOLOGY OF THE LACRIMAL GLAND

Dacrocystography

The canaliculi may be cannulated and injected with radiopaque contrast to outline the drainage system of the lacrimal apparatus.

Computed tomography and magnetic resonance imaging

These imaging techniques may be used to study the lacrimal gland and orbital contents. The bony canal of the nasolacrimal duct may be identified on axial and coronal CT images.

Fig. 1.24 Lacrimal apparatus: coronal section.

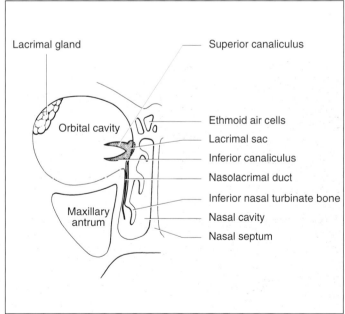

THE EAR (Figs 1.25 and 1.26)

THE EXTERNAL EAR

The external ear consists of the *pinna* and the *external auditory meatus.* The external meatus is 3.5 cm long, and runs medially to the ear drum or *tympanic membrane.* The outer part of the canal is cartilaginous and the medial two-thirds is bony. The entire canal is lined by skin.

THE MIDDLE EAR

The middle ear is a slit-like cavity housed in the petrous bone. It lies between the tympanic membrane laterally and inner ear medially.

It has an upper part, which is recessed superiorly into the petrous bone and is known as the *epitympanic recess* or *attic* since it lies at a higher level than the tympanic membrane. The roof of the cavity is formed by a thin layer of bone called the *tegmen tympani*, separating it from the middle cranial fossa and temporal lobe of the brain. The attic communicates with the mastoid air cells through a narrow posterior opening called the *aditus ad antrum.* This is of importance as infection may spread from the middle ear to the mastoid air cells, which are related posteriorly to the sigmoid sinus and cerebellum in the posterior cranial fossa (see **Fig. 1.26**).

The lower part of the middle ear contains the *ossicles*, and is continuous inferiorly with the *eustachian tube*, which opens into the lateral wall of the nasopharynx. This tube is 3.5 cm long, bony at first, and cartilaginous in its lower portion.

The floor of the middle ear is a thin plate of bone separating the cavity from the bulb of the jugular vein.

The lateral wall of the cavity is the tympanic membrane and the ring of bone to which it is attached.

The medial wall of the middle ear also forms the lateral wall of the inner ear, and its middle ear surface is shaped by the contents of the inner ear. The lateral semicircular canal causes a prominence in the wall superiorly. Below this is a bulge caused by the cochlea called the *promontory*. The *oval window*, into which the base of the stapes inserts, is above and behind the promontory. The *round window*, covered by a membrane, is below and behind. The bony canal of the third part of the facial nerve also causes a prominence on the medial wall of the cavity. This runs from front to back, between the prominence of the lateral semicircular canal and the promontory, before turning down in the posterior wall of the cavity to emerge through the stylomastoid foramen (fourth part).

The ossicles traverse the middle ear cavity. The *malleus* has a handle that is attached to the tympanic membrane, and a rounded head that articulates with the body of the *incus* at the *incudomallear joint*. This joint is orientated superiorly and projects into the epitympanic recess. The incus has a long process that articulates with

Fig. 1.25 Ear: coronal section showing outer, middle and inner ear.

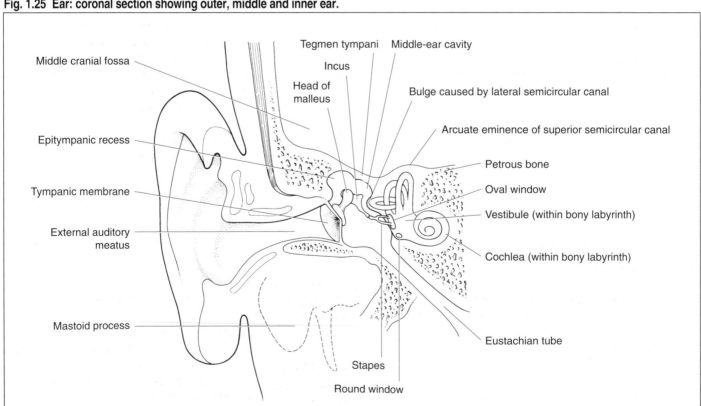

the head of the *stapes*, the base of which is firmly fixed in the oval window.

THE INNER EAR

This is a membranous labyrinth of fluid-filled sacs concerned with hearing and balance. It is housed in a protective labyrinth of dense bone and lies in the petrous bone medial to the middle ear. It consists of a *vestibule*, which communicates posteriorly with the three *semicircular canals*, and anteriorly with the spiral *cochlea*. The bony covering of the lateral semicircular canal bulges into the medial wall of the middle-ear cavity and that of the superior semicircular canal forms the *arcuate eminence* on the superior aspect of the petrous bone.

THE INTERNAL AUDITORY MEATUS

This bony canal is about 1 cm long and transmits the seventh and eighth cranial nerves from the posterior cranial fossa. Its lateral extent is separated from the inner ear by a perforated plate of bone. A crest on this bone, the *crista falciformis*, divides the canal into upper and lower compartments. The upper compartment contains the facial nerve and the superior vestibular branch of the eighth cranial nerve, and the lower compartment contains the acoustic and inferior vestibular branches of the eighth cranial nerve. The vestibular and acoustic nerves pass through the perforated plate of bone into the inner ear, and the facial nerve turns anteriorly through the anterior wall of the lateral part of the canal into its own bony canal. The first part of the facial nerve runs in the internal auditory meatus. The second part runs anteriorly from this in its bony canal, then curves laterally and posteriorly around the cochlea to the anterior part of the medial wall of the middle-ear cavity. This U-bend around the cochlea is known as the *genu* of the nerve. The third and fourth parts have been described (see p. 24).

The posterior lip of the medial end of the internal auditory meatus is called the *porus acousticus* and is normally sharply defined. It may be eroded by pathology in this region.

CROSS-SECTIONAL ANATOMY (see **Fig. 1.26**)

On high cuts through the petrous bone, the two limbs of the superior semicircular canal may be seen as two round bony defects.

At lower levels, the vestibule, with the horizontal semicircular canal projecting posteriorly in an arc, are seen. The entire horizontal semicircular canal may be seen as it lies in the plane of section. The internal auditory canal is seen medially, running laterally from the posterior cranial fossa to the cochlea. The vestibule is posterolateral. The posterior semicircular canal projects posteriorly from the vestibule. The malleus and incus are seen laterally in the epitympanic recess. The bony canal of the facial nerve passes from front to back, medial to the middle ear cavity, lateral to the vestibule and just below the level of the horizontal semicircular canal.

A slightly lower level passes through the external auditory canal and middle-ear cavity. The ossicles are seen traversing the middle-ear cavity. The basal turn of the cochlea is seen anteriorly. The lower part of the posterior semicircular canal and vestibule are posterolateral. The facial nerve in its bony canal may be seen in cross-section as a circular structure laterally running down to the stylomastoid foramen.

RADIOLOGY OF THE MIDDLE AND INNER EAR

Plain films

The internal acoustic meati and parts of the bony labyrinth of the inner ear may be identified on a straight OF skull projection. The dimensions of the internal acoustic meati, which may be measured from tomographic images, are of importance since pathology may cause bony erosion with consequent widening. The height is measured at the point of greatest diameter, and the two sides should not vary by more than 1 mm. The length is measured from the porus acousticus to the lateral extent, and the two sides should not vary by more than 2 mm. The porus acousticus should be sharply defined. The anterior wall of the medial extent of the internal auditory meatus merges with the petrous bone and is not well defined radiologically.

Plain tomography

Tomography is required for anatomical detail of the middle and inner ear, and numerous projections may be employed to display different parts to advantage. Coronal tomography in the plane of the vestibule demonstrates the internal acoustic meatus and semicircular canals, and tomography through the cochlear plane demonstrates the cochlea and middle-ear cavity.

Computed tomography

The more widespread availability of high-resolution CT has reduced the importance of plain tomography. Images may obtained in both axial and coronal planes. The internal auditory meati are readily assessed (see **Fig. 1.26**), and the extent of any pathology and its relationship to other important intracranial structures may be determined. High-resolution scanning of the temporal bone can image the cochlea, vestibule, semicircular canals, ossicles and bony canal of the facial nerve in axial or coronal planes. *CT air meatography* allows detection of very small lesions in the region of the internal auditory meatus. This technique involves the injection of a small volume of air into the subarachnoid space, which, when allowed to rise to the cerebellopontine angle cistern, delineates the seventh and eighth cranial nerves.

Magnetic resonance imaging
MRI may also be used to study the contents of the tempo-ral bone and has the advantage of being able to image in any plane. Coronal images demonstrate the contents of the internal auditory canal to advantage, showing the facial and cochlear nerves separated by a signal void caused by the falciform crest. These are best seen on T1-weighted images as relatively high-intensity structures on a low-intensity bony background. The cochlea and vestibule may also be identified. These are fluid-filled and of high signal intensity (and thus easier to see) on T2-weighted images.

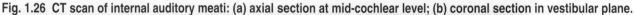

Fig. 1.26 CT scan of internal auditory meati: (a) axial section at mid-cochlear level; (b) coronal section in vestibular plane.

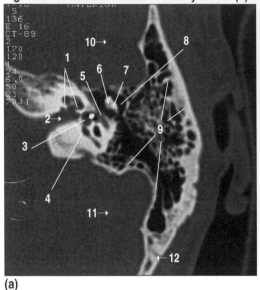
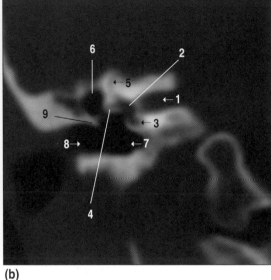

(a) 1. Cochlear turns
2. Internal auditory meatus
3. Vestibule
4. Posterior semicircular canal
5. Facial nerve in its bony canal
6. Malleus
7. Incus
8. Epitympanic recess
9. Mastoid air cells
10. Middle cranial fossa
11. Posterior cranial fossa
12. Lambdoid suture

(b) 1. Internal auditory meatus
2. Vestibule
3. Basal turn of cochlea
4. Lateral semicircular canal
5. Superior semicircular canal
6. Epitympanic recess
7. Middle ear cavity
8. External auditory meatus
9. Scutum (separating external auditory meatus and epitympanic recess)

(a)   (b)

THE PHARYNX AND RELATED SPACES (Fig. 1.27)

The pharynx is a muscular tube extending from the base of the skull to the level of C6 where it is continuous with the oesophagus. It lies behind, and communicates with, the nasal and oral cavities, providing a common entrance to the respiratory and gastrointestinal tracts.

The pharynx has three coats. Innermost is the mucous coat, which is continuous with the mucosa of the oral and nasal cavities. The submucous layer is the *pharyngobasilar fascia,* and forms a thick fibrous coat, which gives the pharynx its shape. It is attached superiorly to the base of the skull and is continuous with the fibrous material filling the foramen lacerum. It is pierced only by the eustachian tube. The outermost coat is formed by the three *constrictor muscles.* These fan out laterally from their anterior attachments to insert into a posterior raphe, which is attached superiorly to the base of the skull anterior to the foramen magnum, and is continuous with the oesophagus inferiorly.

The superior pharyngeal constrictor is attached anteriorly to the inferior extension of the medial pterygoid plate (the *pterygoid hamulus*), and to a raphe joining this to the inner surface of the mandible. The middle constrictor muscle is attached anteriorly to the hyoid bone and lower part of the stylohyoid ligament. Its upper fibres overlap the superior constrictor muscle superficially. The inferior constrictor muscle attaches anteriorly to cricoid and thyroid cartilages and overlaps the inferior part of the middle constrictor. Its lowermost fibres are horizontally orientated and merge with the circular fibres of the oesophagus. The muscles are covered by loose *buccopharyngeal fascia*, which is continuous with the fascia covering the buccinator muscle.

The pharynx lies behind the nasal and oral cavities and the larynx and is divided accordingly into the naso-pharynx, oropharynx, and hypo- or laryngopharynx. Posteriorly it lies on the upper cervical vertebrae and their prevertebral muscles.

Fig. 1.27 Pharynx: sagittal section.

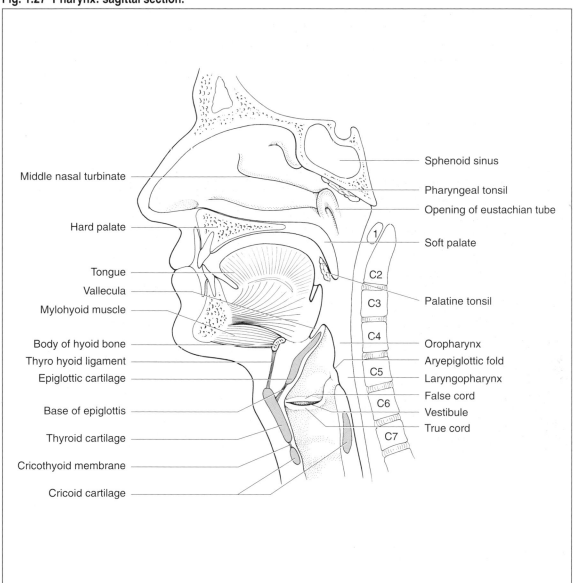

THE NASOPHARYNX AND RELATED SPACES (Figs 1.28–1.30)

The nasopharynx

The *nasopharynx* is that part of the pharynx between the posterior choanae and the lower limit of the soft palate. It communicates anteriorly with the nasal cavity, and inferiorly with the oropharynx. The roof of the nasopharynx is bound to the inferior surface of the sphenoid and clivus by the pharyngobasilar fascia. It has the parapharyngeal space and the deep soft tissues of the infratemporal space laterally. Posteriorly it lies on the upper cervical vertebrae and longus collis and capitus, and posterolaterally the styloid muscles separate it from the carotid sheath.

The eustachian tube opens onto the lateral wall of the nasopharynx on either side, piercing the pharyngobasilar fascia. This opening has a posterior ridge formed by the cartilaginous end of the tube known as the *torus tubarius.* Behind these ridges are the paired *lateral pharyngeal recesses,* also known as the *fossae of Rosenmueller.*

The muscular layer of the nasopharynx is formed by the superior pharyngeal constrictor. The palatal muscles arise from the base of the skull on either side of the eustachian tube. The *levator veli palatini* accompanies the eustachian tube, piercing the pharyngobasilar fascia before inserting into the posterior part of the soft palate. The *tensor veli palatini* runs around the nasopharynx, and hooks around the pterygoid hamulus before inserting into the membranous part of the soft palate. These

Fig. 1.28 CT scan of nasopharynx: axial section.

1. Nasopharyngeal space
2. Prevertebral muscle
3. Lateral pharyngeal recess
4. Cartilaginous end of eustachian tube
5. Opening of eustachian tube
6. Torus tubarius
7. Pterygoid bone
8. Medial pterygoid plate
9. Medial pterygoid muscle
10. Lateral pterygoid plate
11. Lateral pterygoid muscle
12. Parapharyngeal space

13. Styloid process
14. Internal carotid artery
15. Internal jugular vein
16. Parotid gland
17. Ramus of mandible
18. Infratemporal space
19. Coronoid process of mandible and masseter muscle
20. Zygoma
21. Maxillary sinus
22. Polyp in left maxillary sinus
23. Nasal bone
24. Nasal septum

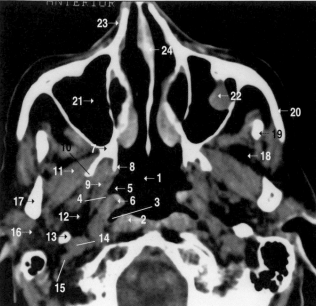

muscles, along with those in the palatopharyngeal arch elevate the soft palate, closing it against a muscular ridge in the superior constrictor muscle (known as the Passavant ridge) during deglutition thereby isolating the nasopharynx from the oropharynx.

Lymphoid tissue lines the nasopharynx, and this is prominent superiorly where it forms the *adenoids*.

The lymphatic drainage of the nasopharynx and related spaces is to the jugular chain of lymph nodes, especially the jugulodigastric node, which lies at the angle of the mandible.

Spaces related to the nasopharynx

The *parapharyngeal space* is a slit-like space just lateral to the nasopharynx extending down from the base of the skull. The space is bounded by the buccopharyngeal

Fig. 1.29 Nasopharynx: axial section.

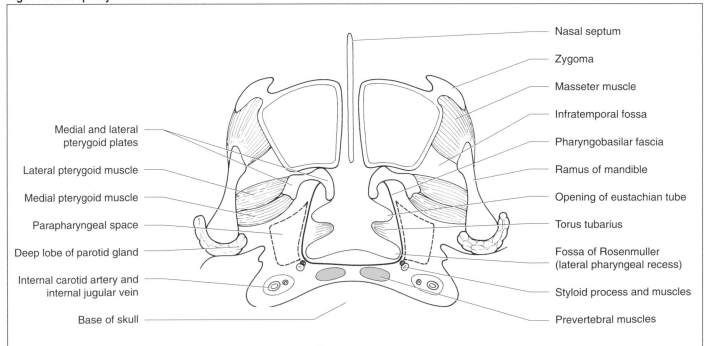

Nasal septum

Zygoma

Masseter muscle

Infratemporal fossa

Pharyngobasilar fascia

Ramus of mandible

Opening of eustachian tube

Torus tubarius

Fossa of Rosenmuller (lateral pharyngeal recess)

Styloid process and muscles

Prevertebral muscles

Medial and lateral pterygoid plates

Lateral pterygoid muscle

Medial pterygoid muscle

Parapharyngeal space

Deep lobe of parotid gland

Internal carotid artery and internal jugular vein

Base of skull

fascia. This fascial plane separates the pharyngeal muscles from the muscles of mastication (the pterygoids and the deep part of the temporalis muscle). It is loosely applied to allow movement and contains branches of the external carotid artery, pharyngeal veins and mandibular nerve. Posteriorly, it is separated from the carotid sheath by the styloid process and its muscles, and the deep part of the parotid gland lies laterally.

The *infratemporal space* (**Fig. 1.30**) lies lateral to the nasopharynx and paranasopharyngeal space behind the posterior wall of the maxilla. It extends from the base of the skull to the hyoid bone, and contains the pterygoid muscles. It is continuous superiorly with the temporal fossa through the gap between the zygomatic arch and the side of the skull. Medial to this, the roof is formed by the inferior surface of the middle cranial fossa and is pierced by the foramen ovale and foramen spinosum. Laterally, the space is bounded by the zygomatic arch, temporalis muscle, ascending ramus of mandible and its coronoid process. Medially, the space is limited by the lateral pterygoid plate and nasopharynx. The space lies anterior to the deep part of the parotid, the styloid process and its muscles, and the carotid artery and jugular vein.

The anteromedial limit of the infratemporal space is formed by the junction of the lateral pterygoid plate with the posteromedial limit of the maxilla superiorly and posterior border of the perpendicular plate of the palate

inferiorly. The anterior and medial walls of the space meet inferiorly, but are separated superiorly by the *pterygomaxillary fissure* where the pterygoid plates diverge from the posterior wall of the maxilla.

The *pterygopalatine fossa* is a medial depression of the pterygomaxillary fissure lying just below the apex of the orbit between the pterygoid process and the posterior maxilla. Its medial margin is the perpendicular plate of the palatine bone. It is important as it connects several spaces and may facilitate the spread of pathology between them. It communicates superiorly with the orbit through the posterior part of the inferior orbital fissure. The foramen rotundum opens into it superiorly, connecting it with the middle cranial fossa. Laterally it communicates freely with the infratemporal fossa. Medially the space communicates with the nasal cavity via the *sphenopalatine foramen* in the perpendicular plate of the palatine bone, and with the oral cavity through the *greater palatine canal*, which runs inferiorly between the palatine bone and the maxilla. The fossa contains the maxillary division of the fifth cranial nerve, which runs through the foramen rotundum and into the orbit via the inferior orbital fissure. It also contains the pterygopalatine segment of the maxillary artery, which makes a characteristic loop and gives off branches to the middle cranial and infratemporal fossae and to the nasal cavity, palate and pharynx.

Fig. 1.30 Infratemporal fossa: axial section.

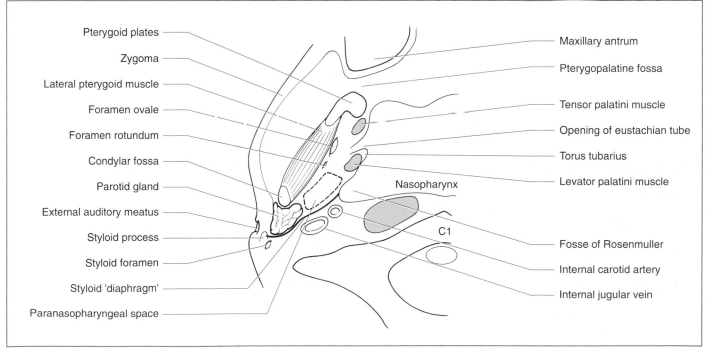

Pterygoid plates
Zygoma
Lateral pterygoid muscle
Foramen ovale
Foramen rotundum
Condylar fossa
Parotid gland
External auditory meatus
Styloid process
Styloid foramen
Styloid 'diaphragm'
Paranasopharyngeal space

Maxillary antrum
Pterygopalatine fossa
Tensor palatini muscle
Opening of eustachian tube
Torus tubarius
Levator palatini muscle
Nasopharynx
C1
Fosse of Rosenmuller
Internal carotid artery
Internal jugular vein

THE OROPHARYNX AND LARYNGO-PHARYNX

The oropharynx is the part of the pharynx that extends from the lower part of the soft palate to the epiglottis. It is continuous through the posterior fauces with the oral cavity and with the laryngopharynx below. It is lined by mucosa that is continuous with that of the oral cavity and nasopharynx. Its submucosal layer is continuous with the pharyngobasilar fascia above, and its muscular layer has contributions from the superior constrictor, some of the tongue muscles, and levator and tensor veli palatini.

The laryngopharynx is the part of the pharynx that lies behind the larynx. It extends from the level of the epiglottis to the level of C6 where it continues as the oesophagus. The upper laryngopharynx is moulded around the proximal part of the larynx forming two deep recesses on either side known as the *piriform fossae*. During deglutition, the epiglottis stands erect and conducts fluid and solid boluses along the piriform fossae from the oropharynx to the oesophagus, avoiding the entrance to the larynx.

CROSS-SECTIONAL ANATOMY OF THE NASOPHARYNX (see **Figs 1.28** and **1.29**)

At the level of the upper nasopharynx, the paired lateral pharyngeal recesses or fossae of Rosenmueller are posterolateral with the torus tubarius anteriorly. The entrance to the eustachian tube forms a recess anterior to the torus on either side. The medial and lateral pterygoid plates and their muscles are anterolateral to the nasopharynx. The lateral pterygoid muscle extends across the infratemporal space to the condyle and neck of the mandible. The parapharyngeal space is posterior to the infratemporal space lying anterior to the carotid vessels and the styloid process and its muscles. The deep part of the parotid gland is lateral to the parapharyngeal space. The prevertebral muscles and upper cervical spine are posterior. Anteriorly are seen the maxillary antra, with the nasal cavity between.

Fig. 1.31 Lateral radiograph of the neck: soft-tissue view showing pharynx and larynx.

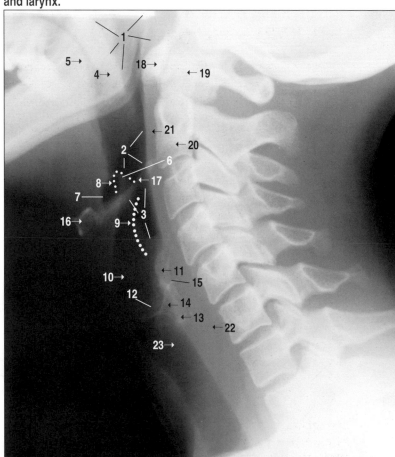

1. Nasopharynx
2. Oropharynx
3. Laryngopharynx
4. Soft palate
5. Tongue
6. Epiglottis
7. Base of tongue
8. Vallecula
9. Aryepiglottic fold
10. Ventricle
11. Irregular calcification in superior cornu of thyroid cartilage
12. Calcification in lamina of thyroid cartilage
13. Inferior cornu of thyroid cartilage
14. Cricoid cartilage
15. Calcification in arytenoid cartilage
16. Body of hyoid bone
17. Greater cornu of hyoid bone
18. Anterior arch of C1
19. Odontoid process of C2
20. Body of C2
21. Prevertebral space
22. Prevertebral space
23. Trachea

RADIOLOGY OF THE PHARYNX (Figs 1.31 and 1.32)

Plain films

Lateral views of the skull and neck demonstrate the soft-tissue outlines of the pharynx and lateral tomography gives improved separation of the soft-tissue planes.

The posterior wall of the pharynx forms a soft-tissue shadow curving posteroinferiorly below the body of the sphenoid and anterior to the cervical vertebrae. This soft-tissue shadow thins as it passes down anterior to the upper cervical vertebrae, measuring 3 mm anterior to C4. Below this the wall is thicker but should not exceed the AP diameter of the cervical vertebrae. In the child, lymphoid tissue results in a relatively thicker posterior wall, measuring up to 5 mm anterior to C4, and up to 12 mm anterior to C6. The lymphoid tissue in the upper posterior part of the nasopharynx (adenoids) may cause a large soft-tissue shadow. It tends to swell down towards the soft palate in young children and may be continuous with the pharyngeal tonsils on the lateral walls of the oropharynx and the lingual tonsils on the posterior surface of the tongue, forming a ring of lymphoid tissue known as Waldeyer's ring.

The base of the tongue and the epiglottis, forming the anterior surface of the oropharynx, are also identifiable on the lateral radiograph.

The posterior and lateral walls of the nasopharynx may be identified on the basal skull projection and the piriform fossae of the laryngopharynx are seen on AP views of the neck.

Pharyngography

This may be performed by outlining the walls of the nasopharynx and its lateral recesses with contrast but is rarely performed now with the availability of cross-sectional imaging modalities.

Cross-sectional imaging

CT and MRI provide excellent detail of the pharynx, its fascial planes and its related spaces (see **Fig. 1.28**). Pathology in this region tends to cause asymmetry, which is readily detected. Images are usually obtained in the axial plane and a good understanding of the cross-sectional anatomy is therefore required.

Coronal images may also be obtained by both modalities but are easier to obtain using MRI as this may be performed without moving the patient. Pathology, especially carcinoma, of the nasopharynx spreads along the fascial planes and may extend intracranially through the many foramina described. For this reason, imaging in both axial and coronal planes is necessary to evaluate the base of the skull. CT yields excellent axial images of the base of the skull and provides good detail. MRI is less useful in this situation as the bones are not well seen. Both CT and MRI demonstrate the muscles and soft-tissue planes and the examinations are complementary.

THE LARYNX (Figs 1.31–1.35)

The larynx forms the entrance to the airway and is responsible for voice production. It extends from the base of the tongue to the trachea, lying anterior to the third to sixth cervical vertebrae. It lies between the great vessels of the neck and is covered anteriorly by the strap muscles of the neck, fascia and skin. It is lined by mucosa, which is continuous with that of the pharynx above and trachea below. Its framework is composed of three single and three paired cartilages, which articulate with each other and are joined by muscles, folds and connective tissue.

The anchor cartilage of the larynx is the *cricoid cartilage.* This is shaped like a signet ring, with a flat, wide lamina posteriorly and an arch anteriorly. It is joined to the thyroid cartilage above by the *cricothyroid membrane,* and to the trachea below by the *cricotracheal membrane.* The paired pyramidal *arytenoid cartilages* sit on the superolateral margin of the signet posteriorly. These bear anteroinferior vocal processes, which give rise to the *vocal ligaments* of the true vocal cords.

The *thyroid cartilage* forms the anterior and lateral boundary of the larynx. It is formed by a pair of laminae, which are joined anteriorly forming an angle and are separated above to form the *superior thyroid notch.* The posterior part of the laminae have upper and lower projections known as the *superior* and *inferior horns* or

Fig. 1.32 AP tomogram of the larynx.

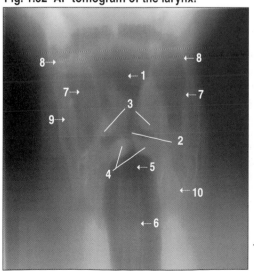

1. Vestibule
2. Ventricle
3. False cords
4. True cords (in phonation)
5. Infraglottic larynx
6. Trachea
7. Piriform fossae (sinuses)
8. Greater cornu of hyoid bone
9. Thyroid cartilage
10. Cricoid cartilage

cornua. The inferior horns project down posterolaterally to articulate with the signet of the cricoid cartilage. The vocal ligaments are attached to the inner surface of the thyroid cartilage near its lower margin.

The *epiglottis* is a leaf-shaped cartilage whose narrow base or *petiole* is attached to the inner surface of the thyroid cartilage at the same point as the anterior extremity

Fig. 1.33 Larynx: (a) sagittal section showing cartilages; (b) coronal section.

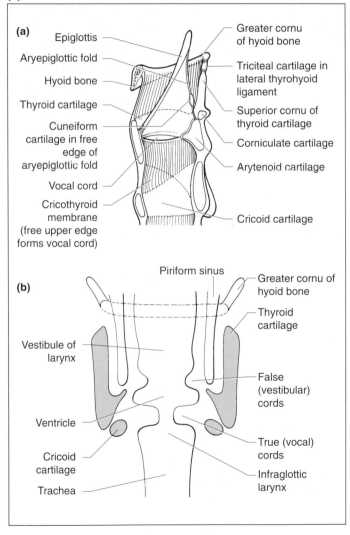

of the vocal cords. It projects up behind the base of the tongue and directs boluses laterally into the piriform fossae during deglutition, thus protecting the larynx. A pair of mucosal folds pass laterally from the epiglottis to the pharyngeal wall called the *pharyngeal folds.* Three mucosal folds pass from the anterior surface of the epiglottis to the base of the tongue — namely, a central and two lateral folds. These form paired recesses between the base of the tongue and the epiglottis known as the *valleculae.* A further pair of mucosal folds pass from the lateral margin of the epiglottis posteriorly to the arytenoid cartilages separating the larynx from the piriform fossae. These are the *aryepiglottic folds*, which, together with the epiglottis, define the entrance to the larynx.

Two further pairs of cartilages lie in the aryepiglottic folds. The *cornicular cartilages* sit on top of the arytenoid cartilages, and the *cuneiform cartilages* lie immediately laterally in the free margin of the fold.

The cavity of the larynx is divided into three parts by upper and lower pairs of mucosal folds. The upper pair of folds are the *vestibular* or *false cords.* The space between the laryngeal entrance and the false cords is known as the *vestibule* of the larynx. The lower pair of folds are the *true cords* and contain the vocal ligaments, which are responsible for voice production. The space between the false and true vocal cords is the *laryngeal ventricle.* This space may extend anterosuperiorly, forming a small pouch known as the *saccule* of the larynx. The term *glottis* refers to the true vocal cords and the triangular space between them when open (*rima glottidis*). The lowest part of the larynx is the *infraglottic larynx*, which lies between the true cords and the trachea. It is elliptical in cross-section superiorly, and circular inferiorly as it merges with the trachea.

The entire larynx is slung from the hyoid bone by the *thyrohyoid membrane and ligaments*. Anteriorly the thyrohyoid membrane arises from an oblique line on the thyroid cartilage and inserts into the inferior part of the hyoid bone. A midline thickening forms the thyrohyoid ligament. The thickened posterior part of the same membrane passes from the superior horns of the thyroid cartilage to the greater horns of the hyoid bone, forming the lateral thyrohyoid ligaments. The hyoid bone, in turn, is attached to the mandible, tongue and styloid process, and to the pharynx by the middle pharyngeal constrictor.

CROSS-SECTIONAL ANATOMY OF THE LARYNX (Figs 1.34 and 1.35)

Supraglottic level (Figs 1.34a and 1.35a)

The larynx is anterior to the piriform sinuses, separated from them by the aryepiglottic folds. At a higher level, the thyroid cartilage and the hyoid bone, with its greater horns laterally, may be seen. The epiglottis, pharyngo-epiglottic folds, valleculae and base of tongue may also be identified posterior to the hyoid bone. The sterno-cleidomastoid muscles are seen posterolaterally with the carotid and internal jugular vessels medial to them.

Glottic level (Figs 1.34b and 1.35b)

A complete ring of cartilage is seen at this level — the thyroid cartilage anteriorly and the lamina of the cricoid and arytenoid cartilages posteriorly. The vocal processes of the arytenoids may be identified giving attachment to the vocal ligaments and defining the level of the glottis.

The anterior fusion of the vocal cords is known as the *anterior commissure* and is very thin when the cords are abducted. Similarly, the *posterior commissure*, which is seen between the arytenoids, is thin in abduction of the cords. Both commissures may appear thickened during adduction of the cords (phonation). The larynx is elliptical in shape at the level of the true cords and triangular at the level of the false cords, which are at a slightly higher level. Here the false cords form the lateral wall of the larynx, and the aryepiglottic folds form the posterior wall. The thyroid cartilage is anterior. The *paralaryngeal space* is between the larynx and the thyroid cartilage.

Infraglottic level (Figs 1.34c and 1.35c)

Just below the cords, the larynx is elliptical. The lamina of the cricoid is posterior, with the cricothyroid membrane anterior. The inferior thyroid horns and part of the thyroid lamina are posterior and lateral to the cricoid. At a lower level, the larynx is more circular and the cricoid forms a complete ring. Part of the lobes of thyroid gland may be seen laterally, with the neck vessels situated posterolaterally. The external jugular vein may be seen anterior to the sternocleidomastoid muscle.

Fig. 1.34 Larynx: (a) axial section, supraglottic level; (b) axial section, glottic level; (c) axial section, infraglottic level.

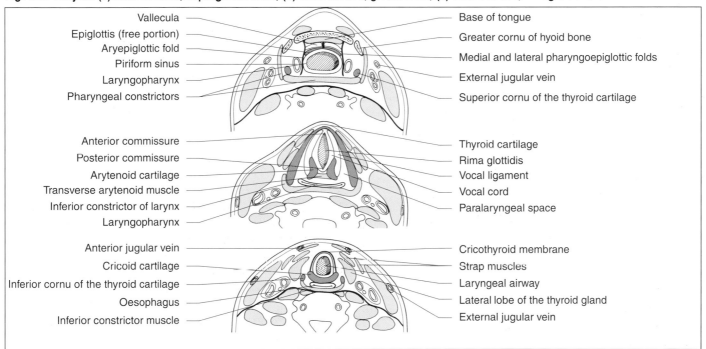

Fig. 1.35 CT scan of the larynx/neck: (a) supraglottic level; (b) glottic level; (c) infraglottic level. Compare with Fig. 1.34.

(a)
1. Base of tongue
2. Medial pharyngoepiglottic fold
3. Lateral pharyngoepiglottic fold
4. Vallecula
5. Epiglottis
6. Laryngopharynx
7. Pharyngeal constrictor muscle
8. Greater cornu of hyoid bone
9. Tip of piriform sinus (the sinus is separated from the laryngopharynx on lower cuts by the aryepiglottic fold)

10. Internal carotid artery
11. Internal jugular vein
12. Sternomastoid muscle
13. External jugular vein
14. Submandibular gland
15. Platysma muscle
16. Subcutaneous fat
17. Prevertebral muscle
18. Foramen transversarium

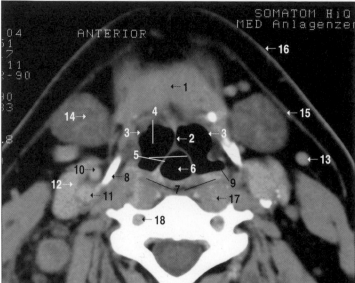

(b) Scan obtained during rapid infusion of contrast. (There is a pathological abscess in the left sternomastoid muscle.)

1. Thyroid cartilage
2. Cricoid cartilage
3. Vocal process of arytenoid cartilage
4. Vocal cord
5. Anterior commissure

6. Laryngopharynx
7. Upper pole of thyroid gland
8. Anterior jugular vein
9. Strap muscles
10. Sternomastoid muscle
11. Internal jugular vein
12. Common carotid artery
13. External jugular vein
14. Prevertebral muscle
15. Abscess in sternomastoid muscle

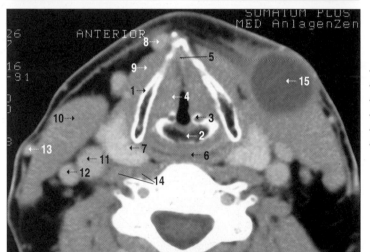

(c) Scan obtained during rapid infusion of intravenous contrast.

1. Cricoid cartilage
2. Cricothyroid membrane
3. Right lobe of thyroid gland
4. Left lobe of thyroid gland

5. Oesophagus (collapsed)
6. Prevertebral muscles
7. Common carotid artery
8. Internal jugular vein
9. Sternomastoid muscle
10. External jugular vein
11. Anterior jugular veins

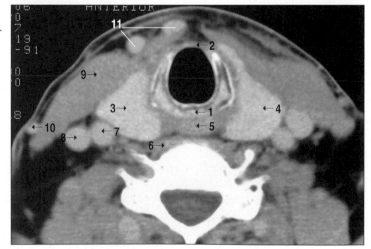

RADIOLOGY OF THE LARYNX (Fig. 1.35; see Figs 1.31 and 1.32)

Plain radiography

This is a relatively simple method of demonstrating the anatomy of the larynx.

Lateral views are the most useful as the larynx is not obscured by overlying bone. The air in the pharynx and larynx provides intrinsic contrast with the soft-tissue walls and mucosal folds (see **Fig. 1.31**).

On the lateral view, the hyoid bone and cartilages of the larynx are seen. The thyroid, cricoid and arytenoid cartilages are composed of hyaline cartilage and may calcify or undergo true ossification. Calcification is often irregular but may be homogeneous with a dense cortex and less-dense medulla. The other cartilages are composed of yellow elastic fibrocartilage and do not calcify. The lateral thyrohyoid ligaments may contain *triciteal cartilages*, which can calcify and should not be mistaken for foreign bodies. The base of the tongue, vallecula, epiglottis, aryepiglottic folds, and true and false cords may be identified. The vestibule, ventricle and infraglottic larynx are those spaces above, between and below the cords.

Tomography

This is useful in the AP plane when overlying bony densities are blurred to allow better detail (see **Fig. 1.32**). The true and false cords and laryngeal ventricle are best seen in this view. The piriform fossae are seen on either side of the proximal larynx, between it and the thyroid cartilage. Symmetry of the soft-tissue planes is important.

Xeroradiography

This method uses an electrochemical method of film processing to further enhance contrast between the tissues, whereas in contrast laryngography the inner walls of the larynx are outlined by a contrast agent and any irregularity of the mucosa is readily seen. Both are performed in lateral and AP planes.

Computed tomography and magnetic resonance imaging

Cross-sectional imaging using CT (see **Fig. 1.35**) or MRI provides excellent anatomical detail of the larynx and surrounding structures. Scans are usually obtained in the axial plane but, with MRI, sagittal and coronal imaging is also possible.

The cartilages are of low density on CT unless calcified, which occurs increasingly with age. They are of high signal intensity on MRI as they contain fatty marrow. The mucosa of the subglottic larynx and the anterior commissure should be not be thicker than 1 mm on MR images. The true cords (ligament) are of low signal intensity and the false cords (fat-containing) are of high signal intensity.

THE THYROID AND PARATHYROID GLANDS

THE THYROID GLAND (Figs 1.35, 1.36a, b and 1.37)

The thyroid gland consists of two lateral *lobes* joined by a midline *isthmus*, and lies anterior and lateral to the trachea. The lobes are approximately 4 cm in height and extend from the thyroid cartilage of the trachea superiorly to the sixth tracheal ring inferiorly. They are described as having upper and lower *poles*. The lobes are often asymmetrical, with the right being larger than the left. The isthmus is draped across the second to fourth tracheal rings at the level of C6. The gland is invested in the *pretracheal fascia*. This fascial layer also invests the larynx and trachea, and the pharynx and oesophagus. The deep surface of the gland lies on these structures. Posterolaterally are the neck vessels, invested in their own fascia, the *carotid sheath*. Behind these, on either side, are the prevertebral muscles and their fasciae.

Anterior to the gland are the strap muscles of the neck and the sternomastoid muscles invested in an outer layer of fascia. Superficially, the *anterior jugular vein* runs in the midline, and the *external jugular vein* runs inferiorly on either side. The *parathyroid glands* lie close to the deep surface of the gland.

CROSS-SECTIONAL ANATOMY (Fig. 1.36b)

At the level of C6, the gland appears as two triangles of tissue draped across the trachea by the connecting isthmus. Each triangular lobe measures approximately 3 cm in depth by 2 cm in width and has a convex anterior surface. The strap muscles of the neck, sternomastoid and the jugular veins are anterior. The posterolateral surface is related to the carotid sheath. The posteromedial surface lies on the trachea and oesophagus and may be interposed between them.

Blood supply and lymph drainage

Two constant pairs of arteries supply the thyroid gland. The *superior thyroid artery* is the first branch of the external carotid and supplies the upper pole. The *inferior thyroid artery* arises from the thyrocervical trunk, which is a branch of the subclavian artery. This passes behind the carotid sheath to gain access to the deep part of the gland. Both arteries anastomose freely with each other. A variable third artery, the *thyroidea ima,* may arise from the brachiocephalic artery or the aortic arch and ascends anterior to the trachea to join in the anastomotic plexus.

Fig. 1.36 Thyroid gland: (a) gross anatomy; (b) axial section. (Courtesy of Prof. JB Coakley.)

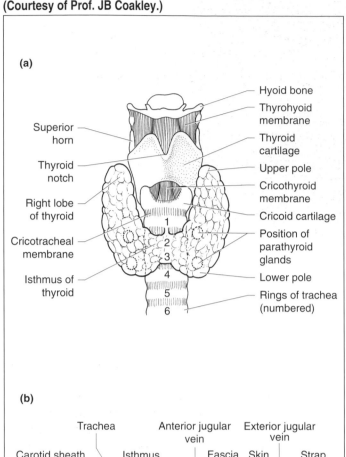

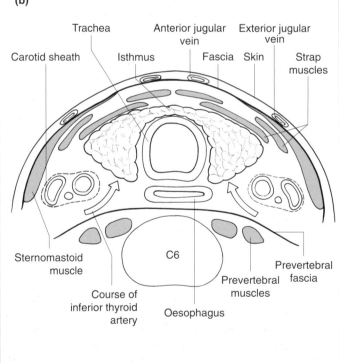

Three pairs of veins arise from a venous plexus on the surface of the gland. The *superior and middle thyroid veins* drain into the internal jugular vein. The *inferior thyroid veins* (often multiple) end in the left brachiocephalic vein.

Lymph drainage is directly into the thoracic duct and the right lymphatic duct.

Ectopic thyroid tissue

The thyroid gland develops from an outpouching of the pharynx, and descends into the neck, passing anterior to the hyoid bone and trachea.

Maldevelopment may cause thyroid tissue to be found anywhere along a line from the base of the tongue to its normal position. Less commonly, thyroid tissue may migrate inferiorly to the mediastinum or even to the pericardium or myocardium. The *thyroglossal duct* may persist as a midline structure extending superiorly from the isthmus of the gland and a *thyroglossal cyst* may be found at any site related to this. More commonly, part of the duct persists as the *pyramidal lobe* of the gland, extending superiorly from the isthmus or medial part of either lobe.

RADIOLOGY OF THE THYROID GLAND (Fig. 1.37)

Plain films

The normal thyroid is not seen on plain radiographs. If enlarged, it may be seen to displace the trachea or barium-filled oesophagus.

Ultrasound

Ultrasound of the gland with a high-frequency transducer provides excellent detail. The normal thyroid gland has a homogeneous echotexture of medium echogenicity. The carotid vessels may be seen as anechoic structures on either side of the gland. The strap muscles are seen as structures of low echogenicity. Linear echogenic lines may be seen separating the muscles. The prevertebral muscles may be identified posteriorly. Numerous vascular structures may be seen surrounding the gland, and its extreme vascularity is readily appreciated with colour flow imaging.

Nuclear medicine studies

Isotope scanning provides functional rather than anatomical detail. It is useful for identifying ectopic thyroid tissue. Technetium-99m- or iodine-labelled agents are used.

Fig. 1.37 Ultrasound of the thyroid gland showing left lobe.

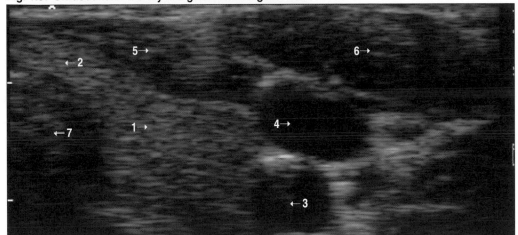

1. Left lobe of gland
2. Isthmus
3. Left common carotid artery
4. Left internal jugular vein
5. Strap muscle
6. Sternomastoid muscle
7. Trachea

Computed tomography

CT may be used to assess the gland in the axial plane. It shows as soft-tissue areas of high attenuation because of the iodine content. The surrounding structures of the neck may also be imaged. Imaging with short scan times during dynamic infusion of contrast gives the best images and definition of the gland and surrounding structures.

Magnetic resonance imaging

MRI can image the gland in any plane along with the surrounding structures. The gland is of higher signal intensity than surrounding muscles on T2-weighted images. The use of surface coils improves detail.

THE PARATHYROID GLANDS

These endocrine glands are small lentiform structures measuring approximately 6 mm in length, 3–4 mm in transverse diameter and 1–2 mm in AP diameter. They usually number four — two superior and two inferior glands — but any number from two to six is possible. The glands lie posterior to the thyroid gland within its fascial sheath in 90% of cases. The superior glands lie on the posterior border of the middle third of the thyroid, and the inferior glands lie near the lower pole of the thyroid.

The superior gland develops from the fourth pharyngeal pouch and does not migrate. The inferior parathyroid gland develops from the third pharyngeal pouch with the thymus and migrates inferiorly. Maldescent may cause the inferior parathyroid gland to be found in ectopic sites and this may be of clinical importance in the search for a parathyroid adenoma. The most common ectopic site is just below the inferior pole of the thyroid. Occasionally the gland descends into the superior mediastinum with the thymus. Less commonly it does not descend at all and remains above the superior parathyroid, or it may be found behind the oesophagus or in the posterior mediastinum.

RADIOLOGY OF THE PARATHYROID GLANDS

Cross-sectional imaging

The normal parathyroids are not seen radiologically. They may be imaged when enlarged. On ultrasound they are seen as hypoechoic structures lying posterior to the thyroid gland.

Nuclear medicine studies

The parathyroids may be imaged using a subtraction technique. Both the thyroid and parathyroid glands take up thallium-201 chloride. The thyroid (but not the parathyroids) takes up technetium-99m pertechnetate. By computerized subtraction of the technetium image from the thallium image, the parathyroids may be demonstrated.

Computed tomography

On CT the parathyroids appear as structures of lower attenuation than thyroid tissue. CT is of value in locating the abnormal ectopic gland.

THE NECK VESSELS

THE CAROTID ARTERIES IN THE NECK (Figs 1.38–1.40)

The left common carotid artery arises from the aortic arch in front of the trachea. It passes across this to lie on its left side in the root of the neck. The right common carotid arises from the brachiocephalic trunk behind the right sternoclavicular joint. The vessels have a similar course from this point. The common carotid artery passes upwards and slightly laterally. It is accompanied by the internal jugular vein on its lateral aspect, with the vagus nerve lying posteriorly between the two. All three structures are invested in the carotid sheath. The common carotid artery bifurcates into internal and external branches at the level of C4. The external carotid artery passes anteriorly and curves slightly posteriorly as it ascends to enter the substance of the parotid gland, where it terminates by dividing into maxillary and superficial temporal arteries. The internal carotid artery continues superiorly from its origin to the base of the skull, maintaining the relationship of the common carotid artery with the internal jugular vein and vagus nerve in the carotid sheath. It has a localized dilatation at its origin called the carotid sinus. It has no branches in the neck.

Fig. 1.38 Ultrasound of the carotid artery: longitudinal section.

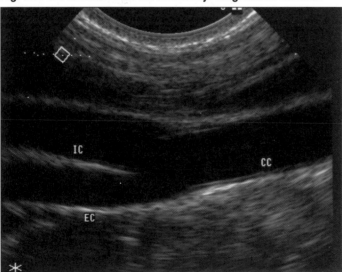

CC.	Common carotid artery
IC.	Internal carotid artery
EC.	External carotid artery

Anatomical relations of the common carotid artery within the carotid sheath

The anatomical relations are as follows:

- Posteriorly is the sympathetic trunk. It is separated from the transverse processes of C4 to C6 by the prevertebral muscles;
- Medially are the trachea and oesophagus with the phrenic nerve between them at first. At a higher level the the larynx, pharynx and phrenic nerve are medial, with the thyroid gland lying anteromedially; and
- Anterolaterally the artery is covered by sternomastoid and the strap muscles at first. Above the level of the cricoid cartilage, it is covered only by skin and fascia.

Anatomical relations of the internal carotid artery within the carotid sheath

These are as follows:

- Posteriorly is the sympathetic trunk, prevertebral muscles and transverse processes of C1–C3;
- Medially is the lateral wall of the pharynx; and
- Anterolaterally it is covered throughout its length by sternomastoid muscle. The styloid process and muscles separate it from the external carotid artery in its upper part.

The artery becomes anterior to the internal jugular vein at the base of the skull and enters the carotid canal. The internal jugular vein and vagus nerve pass through the jugular foramen.

Anatomical relations of the external carotid artery

At its origin, the internal carotid artery is lateral. As the external carotid artery ascends in the neck, it comes to lie in a more lateral plane than the internal carotid artery.

- Medially is the lateral wall of the pharynx at first. At a higher level it is separated from the internal carotid artery by the styloid process and its muscles; and
- Anterolaterally is the anterior part of sternomastoid at first. It then passes deep to the posterior belly of digastric and the stylohyoid muscles before entering the substance of the parotid gland.

Branches of the external carotid artery (Figs 1.39 and 1.40)

The branches of the external carotid artery anastomose freely with each other and with their partners on the opposite side. There are also several points of anastomosis with the internal carotid circulation and with branches of the subclavian artery.

Superior thyroid artery

This branch arises anteriorly close to the origin, and passes inferiorly to supply the thyroid gland, anastomosing with the inferior thyroid artery.

Ascending pharyngeal artery

This is a small branch that ascends deep to the external carotid on the lateral wall of the pharynx. It supplies the larynx and also gives rise to meningeal vessels, which pass through the foramen lacerum.

Lingual artery

This branch arises anteriorly and runs upwards and medially before curving downward and forwards towards the hyoid bone in a characteristic loop. It then runs under muscles arising from that bone to supply the tongue and floor of the mouth.

Facial artery

This vessel arises from the anterior surface of the external carotid artery above the level of the hyoid bone. It passes upward deep to the ramus of the mandible grooving the posterior part of the submandibular gland. It then curves downward under the ramus of the mandible and hooks around it to supply the muscles and tissues of the face. Its terminal branch anastomoses with a branch of the ophthalmic artery. It also supplies the submandibular gland, soft palate and tonsil.

Occipital artery

This arises posteriorly opposite the origin of the facial artery. It runs to the posterior part of the scalp, crossing the internal carotid and jugular vessels and terminates in tortuous occipital branches supplying the scalp. It gives off muscular branches in the neck. The stylomastoid artery arises from the vessel in two-thirds of people, passing superiorly through the stylomastoid foramen to supply the middle and inner ear. Meningeal branches enter the skull through the jugular foramen and condylar canal and supply the dura of the posterior cranial fossa.

Posterior auricular artery

This vessel arises posteriorly and ascends between the styloid process and parotid gland. It has muscular branches in the neck, and supplies the parotid, pinna and scalp, anastomosing with branches of the occipital artery. In one-third of people it gives rise to the stylomastoid artery.

Superficial temporal artery

This is the smaller of the two terminal branches. It arises within the parotid gland behind the neck of the mandible. It ascends over the posterior root of the zygomatic arch, dividing into tortuous anterior and posterior branches 5 cm above that point and supplies the scalp

and pericranium. It also gives branches to the parotid, temporomandibular joint, facial structures and outer ear. One of its branches anastomoses with the lacrimal and palpebral branches of the ophthalmic artery in yet another communication between internal and external systems.

Maxillary artery

This is the larger of the two terminal branches. It arises within the parotid gland behind the neck of the mandible. It supplies the upper and lower jaws, muscles of mastication, palate, nose and cranial dura mater. Its first (mandibular) part passes deep to the neck of the mandible. Its second (pterygoid) part runs forwards and upwards between temporalis and the lower head of lateral

Fig. 1.39 Carotid artery in the neck. (Courtesy of Prof. JB Coakley.)

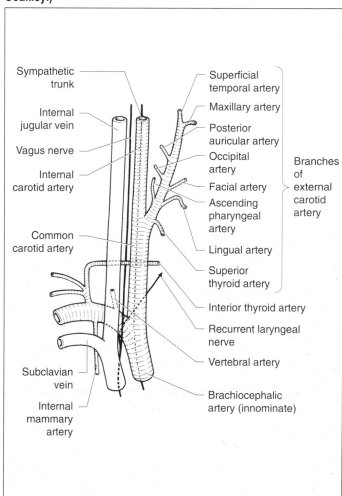

pterygoid. Its third (pterygopalatine) part passes between the upper and lower heads of lateral pterygoid through the pterygomaxillary fissure to enter the pterygopalatine fossa.

The maxillary artery has several important branches. The branches of the first part are:

- The middle meningeal artery enters the skull through the foramen spinosum and supplies the dura mater and bone of the cranium;
- The accessory meningeal artery may arise from this part or from the middle meningeal artery. It passes through the foramen ovale to supply dura mater and bone; and
- The inferior dental artery descends to supply the structures of the lower jaw.

The branches of the second part are the branches to temporalis, pterygoid and masseter muscles.

The branches of the third part are:

- The superior dental artery arises just as the artery enters the pterygopalatine fossa and supplies the structures of the upper jaw;
- The infraorbital artery enters the orbital cavity through the infraorbital fissure, running along the infraorbital groove to supply the contents of the orbit;
- The greater palatine artery descends from the pterygo-palatine fossa through the palatine canal and through the greater palatine foramen of the hard palate. It supplies the tonsil, palate, gums and mucous membrane of the roof of the mouth; and
- The sphenopalatine artery is the terminal part of the maxillary artery. It passes from the fossa through the sphenopalatine foramen into the cavity of the nose, branching to supply the nasal structures and the sinuses.

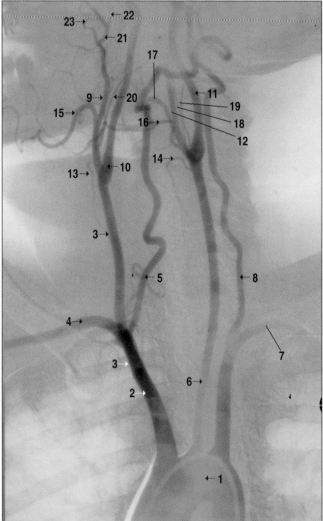

Fig. 1.40 Arch aortogram: subtraction film. The catheter is in the aortic arch. All branches of the external carotid are shown except the occipital artery. The facial artery is not filling on the right.

1. Arch of aorta
2. Brachiocephalic trunk
3. Right common carotid artery (superimposed upon the subclavian artery)
4. Right subclavian artery
5. Right vertebral artery
6. Left common carotid artery
7. Left subclavian artery
8. Left vertebral artery
9. Right external carotid artery
10. Sinus of right internal carotid artery
11. Left internal carotid artery
12. Left external carotid artery
13. Right superior thyroid artery (arising from the external carotid artery)
14. Left superior thyroid artery (arising from common carotid artery)
15. Right lingual artery
16. Left lingual artery
17. Left facial artery
18. Left ascending pharyngeal artery
19. Left posterior auricular artery
20. Right posterior auricular artery
21. Left maxillary artery
22. Middle meningeal artery (branch of left maxillary artery)
23. Left superficial temporal artery

RADIOLOGY OF THE CAROTID VESSELS (see **Figs 1.38** and **1.40**)

Ultrasound

The common carotid artery and its bifurcation may be imaged using a high-frequency probe (7.5 or 10 MHz). The external carotid artery may be distinguished from the internal carotid artery by identifying the superior thyroid branch. The carotid sinus is seen as a localized dilation of the common carotid artery at its bifurcation. Ultrasound is most useful for assessment of the inner walls of the vessels, which should appear smooth in the normal patient.

Angiography

This may be performed in the conventional manner, or using a digital system to 'subtract' overlying bone. It provides a visual map of the vessels injected. The carotid vessels may be demonstrated by injection of contrast through a catheter in the aortic arch, or by selective injection of the common carotid artery or of either carotid vessel. Selective injection of the common carotid artery is usually performed to assess this vessel and the cervical part of the internal carotid artery, which should be smooth and of even calibre. Selective injection of the external carotid is rarely performed. It may be necessary when demonstration of supply to vascular tumours or arteriovascular malformations is required. Both intracranial and extracranial pathology may cause pathological enlargement of external branches, owing to the numerous pathways of possible anastomosis. Selective injection of the internal carotid artery is performed to assess intracranial pathology.

Variations in the anatomy of the vessels may be seen. The left common carotid artery may arise with the brachiocephalic artery. The right common carotid artery may arise from the arch of the aorta. Occasionally, the common carotid arteries arise from a single trunk. Congenital absence of the internal or external carotid artery may occur rarely. The right subclavian artery may arise as the last branch of the arch in approximately 0.5% of people. In this situation it ascends to the right, passing behind the oesophagus and causes an oblique posterior indentation, which can be seen on a barium-swallow examination.

Computed tomography and magnetic resonance imaging

The carotid vessels may be identified by both modalities. Pathology in the neck may displace or involve the vessels, and symmetry between the two sides should be evident in normal cases. MRI has the advantage of being able to image the vessels in any plane. The vessels may be imaged at the thoracic inlet without any degradation from bony artefact, and coronal imaging allows assessment of their origin from the aortic arch.

VENOUS DRAINAGE OF THE HEAD AND NECK (**Fig. 1.41**)

The *facial vein* drains the anterior part of the scalp and facial structures. It forms at the angle of the eye and runs posteroinferiorly to the angle of the mandible.

The *superficial temporal vein* (which also drains the scalp) joins with the *maxillary vein* (which drains the infratemporal area) to form the retromandibular vein behind the angle of the mandible.

The *retromandibular vein* descends through the parotid gland deep to the facial nerve and superficial to the external carotid artery. Below this, it divides in two. The anterior branch joins with the facial vein to form the *internal jugular vein.* The posterior branch joins with the *posterior auricular vein* (which drains the posterior scalp) to form the *external jugular vein.*

The internal jugular vein is formed at the jugular foramen where it is a continuation of the sigmoid sinus. It descends in the carotid sheath lateral to its artery, then passes inferiorly to behind the medial end of the clavicle, where it is joined by the subclavian vein to become the *brachiocephalic vein.* It drains the petrosal sinus from within the cranium, as well as the facial vein. In addition, it receives the superior and middle thyroid veins as well as pharyngeal and lingual veins. The left internal jugular vein receives the thoracic duct. The right lymph duct usually drains into the right internal jugular vein.

The external jugular vein descends superficial to the sternomastoid muscle and pierces the cervical fascia above the midpoint of the clavicle to enter the subclavian vein.

The *anterior jugular vein* arises at the level of the hyoid bone near the midline. It passes downward and laterally, passing deep to sternomastoid to enter the external jugular vein behind the clavicle.

The *jugular arch* is a U-shaped communication between the two anterior jugular veins above the manubrium sterni.

The *vertebral vein* exits from the transverse foramen of C6 and runs down and forward to drain into the posterior aspect of the brachiocephalic vein.

Fig. 1.41 Veins of the face and neck. (Courtesy of Prof. JB Coakley.)

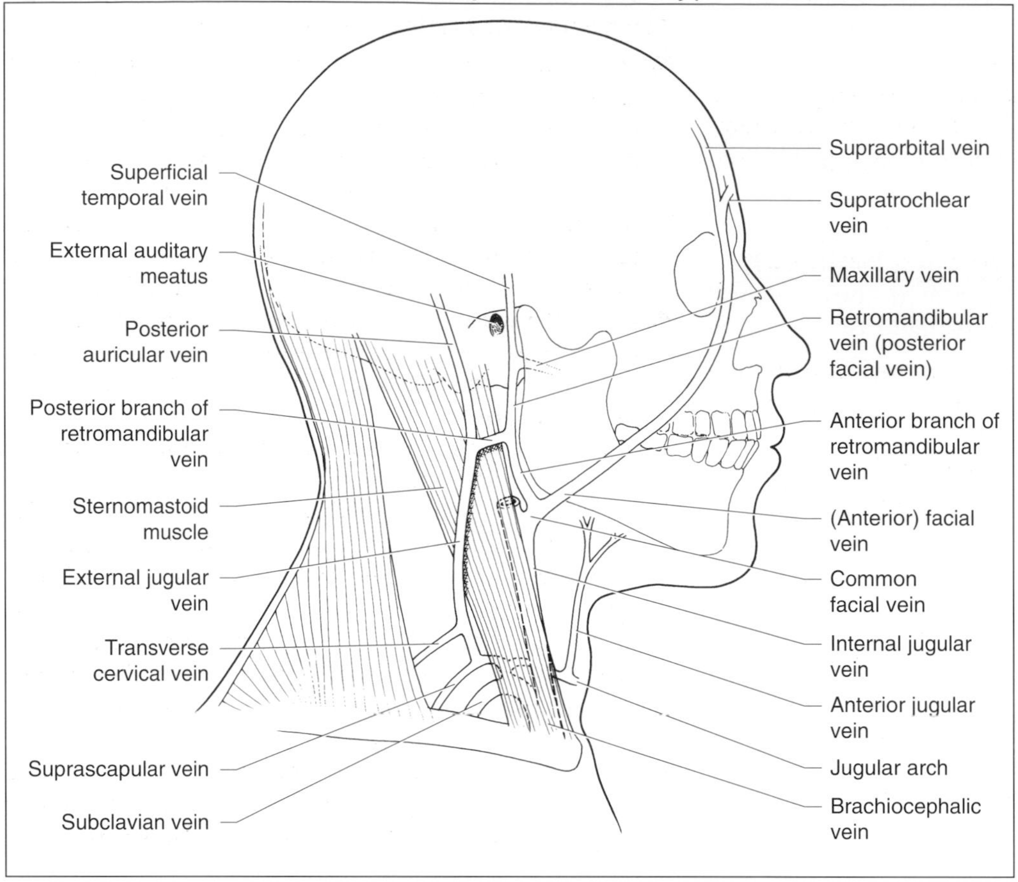

Superficial temporal vein

External auditary meatus

Posterior auricular vein

Posterior branch of retromandibular vein

Sternomastoid muscle

External jugular vein

Transverse cervical vein

Suprascapular vein

Subclavian vein

Supraorbital vein

Supratrochlear vein

Maxillary vein

Retromandibular vein (posterior facial vein)

Anterior branch of retromandibular vein

(Anterior) facial vein

Common facial vein

Internal jugular vein

Anterior jugular vein

Jugular arch

Brachiocephalic vein

Fig. 1.42 Subclavian angiogram.

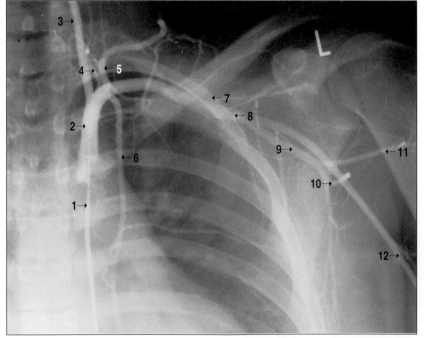

1. Angiographic catheter
2. Subclavian artery
3. Vertebral artery
4. Thyrocervical trunk
5. Costocervical trunk
6. Internal thoracic (mammary) artery
7. First rib
8. Axillary artery
9. Subscapular artery
10. Circumflex scapular artery
11. Circumflex humeral artery
12. Brachial artery

RADIOLOGY OF THE VEINS OF THE HEAD AND NECK

The veins of the face and scalp are not usually imaged specifically. The neck veins are identified on cross-sectional imaging techniques such as ultrasound, CT (see **Fig. 1.35**) and MRI.

THE SUBCLAVIAN ARTERIES IN THE NECK (**Figs 1.42 and 1.43**)

The right subclavian artery arises from the bifurcation of the brachiocephalic trunk behind the right sternoclavicular joint. The left subclavian artery arises from the arch of the aorta in front of the trachea at the level of the C3/C4 disc space. It ascends on the right of the trachea to behind the left sternoclavicular joint. From this point, both arteries have a similar course. The scalenus anterior muscle (which passes from the transverse processes of the upper cervical vertebrae to the inner border of the first rib) divides the artery into three parts. The first part arches over the apex of the lung and lies deeply in the neck. The second part passes laterally behind scalenus anterior muscle, which separates it from the subclavian vein. The third part passes to the lateral border of the first rib where it becomes the axillary artery.

Branches of the subclavian artery in the neck

The branches of the first part are as follows:

■ Vertebral artery. This crosses the dome of the pleura to enter the transverse foramen of C6. It passes through the transverse foramina of C6 to C1 then arches medially, passing behind the lateral masses of C1 before entering the cranial cavity through the foramen magnum. In the neck it supplies the vertebral muscles and the spinal cord. Within the vertebral transverse foramina, it is accompanied by the vertebral vein;

■ Internal mammary (thoracic) artery. This arises from the inferior aspect of the subclavian and descends behind the costal cartilages of the ribs about 2 cm from the lateral border of the sternum. It supplies the anterior mediastinum, the anterior pericardium, the sternum and anterior chest wall;

■ Thyrocervical trunk. This arises close to the medial border of scalenus and trifurcates almost immediately. Its branches are the inferior thyroid artery, which runs upwards and medially to enter the lower pole of the thyroid gland, and the suprascapular and transverse cervical arteries, which run laterally over the scalenus muscles to join in the scapular anastomosis and supply the muscles of the shoulder region; and

■ The costocervical artery, on the left. This usually arises from the second part on the right. It divides into superior intercostal and deep cervical branches.

Fig. 1.43 Arteries in the root of the neck.

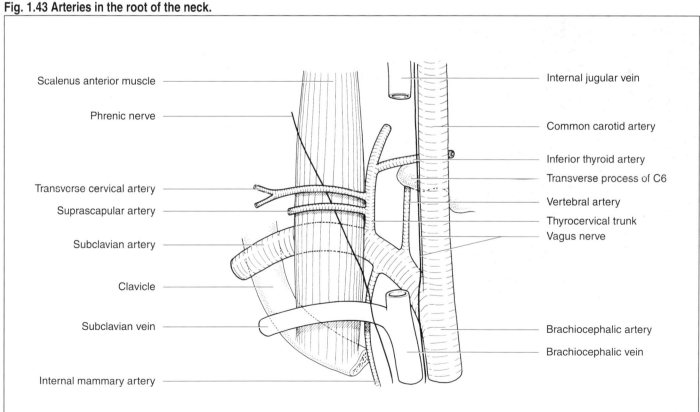

Scalenus anterior muscle

Phrenic nerve

Transverse cervical artery

Suprascapular artery

Subclavian artery

Clavicle

Subclavian vein

Internal mammary artery

Internal jugular vein

Common carotid artery

Inferior thyroid artery

Transverse process of C6

Vertebral artery

Thyrocervical trunk

Vagus nerve

Brachiocephalic artery

Brachiocephalic vein

The branch of the second part is the costocervical artery on the right side.

The branch of the third part is the dorsal scapular artery.

THE SUBCLAVIAN VEINS IN THE NECK (Fig. 1.44)

These are the continuation of the axillary veins from the outer border of the first rib to where they join with the internal jugular to form the brachiocephalic veins. As the vessel crosses the first rib, it grooves its superior surface. Anterior to the vein is the clavicle and posteriorly it is separated from the subclavian artery by the scalenus anterior muscle. It receives the external jugular vein on both sides. On the left it receives the thoracic duct (which drains lymph from the body except the right arm and the right side of the head and neck) just at its union with the internal jugular vein to form the left brachiocephalic vein. On the right, the right lymphatic duct (often several small ducts) drain into it as it unites with the internal jugular to form the right brachiocephalic vein.

RADIOLOGY OF THE SUBCLAVIAN VESSELS

Angiography

The subclavian arteries are best demonstrated by angiography (see **Fig. 1.42**).

The subclavian veins are best demonstrated by venography, with an injection into one of the veins in the arm.

Ultrasound

The subclavian vessels may be imaged at least in part by ultrasound. This is technically difficult, however, due to overlying bone and adjacent lung, neither of which transmit sound.

Computed tomography and magnetic resonance imaging

The subclavian vessels may be imaged by both modalities. Intravenous contrast improves visualization on CT. It is difficult to demonstrate more than a short segment on any single CT image and MRI is superior in this regard as the vessels can be imaged along their axis, demonstrating a greater length.

Fig. 1.44 Veins in the root of the neck.

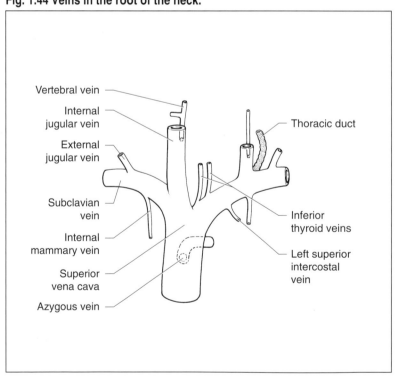

CHAPTER 2 *THE CENTRAL NERVOUS SYSTEM*

Cerebral hemispheres

Cerebral cortex

White matter

Thalamus, hypothalamus and pineal gland

Pituitary gland

Limbic lobe

Brainstem

Cerebellum

Ventricles, cisterns, CSF production and flow

Meninges

Arterial supply

Veins

Cross-sectional anatomy

CEREBRAL HEMISPHERES

The cerebral hemispheres fill the cranial vault above the tentorium cerebelli. Right and left hemispheres are connected by the corpus callosum and otherwise partly separated by the median longitudinal fissure. The hemispheres consist of cortical grey matter, white matter, basal ganglia, thalamus, hypothalamus, pituitary gland and the limbic lobe. The lateral ventricles form a cavity within each ventricle.

CEREBRAL CORTEX (Figs 2.1 and 2.2)

The superolateral surface of each cerebral hemisphere has two deep sulci, these are:

- The *lateral sulcus,* also known as the Sylvian fissure, which separates the frontal and temporal lobes;
- The *central sulcus* (of Rolando), which passes upwards from the lateral sulcus to the superior border of the hemisphere. This separates the frontal and parietal lobes.

The *parieto-occipital sulcus* on the medial surface of hemisphere separates the parietal and occipital lobes.

FRONTAL LOBE

The frontal lobe includes all the cortex anterior to the central sulcus and superior to the lateral sulcus. The motor cortex, premotor cortex and prefrontal area are associated with known functions.

Motor cortex

The motor cortex is the cortex on the gyrus anterior to the central sulcus, the precentral gyrus. It controls voluntary movement.

Premotor cortex

The premotor cortex is the anterior part of precentral gyrus and adjoining gyri. This too is associated with the control of voluntary movements. The posteroinferior part of the premotor area on the dominant hemisphere deals with the motor aspects of speech and is called *Broca's speech area.*

Prefrontal area

Anterior to the motor and premotor cortex, the frontal lobes are involved with intellectual, emotional and autonomic activity.

Fig. 2.1 Superolateral surface of the cerebral hemisphere.

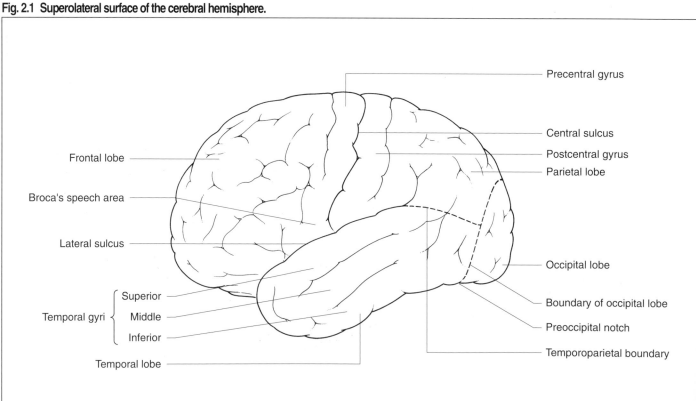

On the medial surface of the frontal lobe, above and parallel to the corpus callosum, is the callosal sulcus. Above this, the cingulate gyrus extends posteriorly from the frontal lobe into the parietal lobe. This, in turn, is separated superiorly from the remainder of the medial surface by the cingulate sulcus.

PARIETAL LOBE

This includes all the cortex from the central sulcus to a line from the parieto-occipital boundary to the posterior end of the lateral sulcus. Areas with known function include the sensory cortex and the parietal association cortex.

Sensory cortex

This is found on the gyrus posterior to the central sulcus and is known as the postcentral gyrus. This controls somatic sensations.

Parietal association cortex

This is posterior to the sensory cortex. This area is involved with recognition and integration of sensory stimuli.

TEMPORAL LOBE

The temporal lobe lies inferior to the lateral sulcus and is separated from the occipital lobe by an arbitrary line drawn from the preoccipital notch to the parieto-occipital sulcus (see **Fig. 2.1**). Two horizontal gyri separate the superolateral surface into superior, middle and inferior temporal gyri. Areas associated with known function include the auditory cortex and the temporal association cortex.

Auditory cortex

Found on the superior temporal gyrus, its function is the reception of auditory stimuli.

Temporal association cortex

Situated around the auditory cortex, this area is involved with the recognition and integration of auditory stimuli.

OCCIPITAL LOBE

The occipital lobe lies posterior to the parietal and temporal lobes. There is no anatomical separation of these lobes on the superolateral surface of the hemisphere.

Fig. 2.2 Medial surface of the cerebral hemisphere.

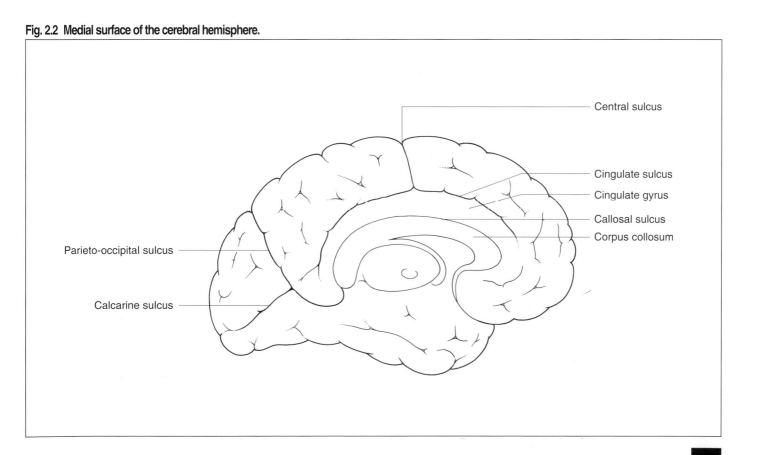

Fig. 2.3 CT scan of brain: (a) level of the pons; (b) level of midbrain; (c) level of the lateral ventricles.

1. Frontal sinus
2. Falx cerebri
3. Greater wing of sphenoid bone
4. Clivus
5. Petrous part of temporal bone
6. Left frontal lobe
7. Left temporal lobe
8. Temporal horn of right lateral ventricle
9. Pons

10. Prepontine cistern
11. Basilar artery
12. Right internal carotid artery
13. Fourth ventricle
14. Cerebellar peduncle
15. Right cerebellar hemisphere
16. Enhancement of the edge of the tentorium cerebelli
17. Transverse sinus
18. Temporalis muscle
19. Pinna of ear

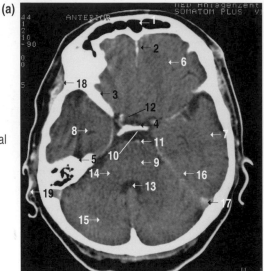

1. Frontal sinus
2. Falx cerebri
3. Interhemispheric fissure
4. Internal carotid artery
5. Anterior cerebral artery
6. Middle cerebral artery
7. Posterior cerebral artery
8. Interpeduncular cistern
9. Sylvian fissure (containing branches of the middle cerebral artery)
10. Midbrain

11. Cerebral peduncle
12. Aqueduct of Sylvius
13. Superior colliculus and quadrigeminal plate (tectum) of midbrain
14. Quadrigeminal cistern
15. Ambient cistern links 14 to 8)
16. Cerebellar vermis
17. Straight sinus
18. Superior sagittal sinus

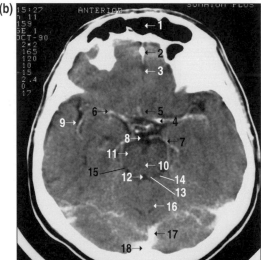

1. Frontal sinus
2. Falx cerebri
3. Sylvian fissure
4. Middle cerebral vessels in Sylvian fissure
5. Cavum septum pellucidum
6. Frontal horn of right lateral ventricle
7. Foramen of Munro
8. Third ventricle
9. Calcified habenular commissure
10. Calcified pineal gland
11. Calcification in choroid plexus in trigone of right lateral ventricle
12. Cisterna vena magna (part of quadrigeminal cistern)

13. Ambient wing cistern
14. Straight sinus
15. Superior sagittal sinus
16. Head of caudate nucleus
17. Right thalamic nucleus
18. Anterior limb of right internal capsule
19. Posterior limb of right internal capsule
20. Left globus pallidus (part of the left lentiform nucleus)
21. Left putamen (part of the left lentiform nucleus)
22. Claustrum
23. Insula
24. Deep white matter of frontal lobe
25. Grey matter of frontal lobe

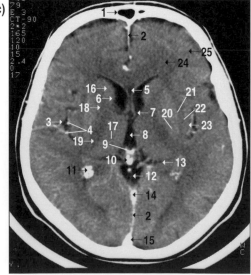

However, on the medial surface, the occipital lobe is separated from the parietal lobe by the parieto-occipital sulcus. A further deep sulcus of this surface, the calcarine sulcus, runs anteriorly from the occipital pole (see **Fig. 2.2**). Areas with known function include the visual cortex and the occipital association cortex.

Visual cortex

This surrounds the calcarine sulcus and receives visual stimuli from the opposite half field of sight.

Occipital association cortex

This lies anterior to the visual cortex and is involved with the recognition and integration of visual stimuli.

INSULA (OF REIL)

This is the cortex buried in the floor of the lateral sulcus and is crossed by branches of the middle cerebral artery. Its function is unknown, although the area closest to the sensory cortex is probably related to taste. The parts of the frontal, parietal and temporal lobes that overlie the insula are called the operculum.

RADIOLOGICAL FEATURES OF THE CEREBRAL CORTEX

Computed tomography

identification of lobes on CT slices depends on identification of their boundaries. The Sylvian cistern and fissure separating the frontal and temporal lobes are easily identified on axial CT slices (**Fig. 2.3**). The central sulcus that forms a boundary between the frontal and parietal lobes is less well seen, however. This lies at a transverse level just posterior to the anterior limit of the lateral ventricles.

The parieto-occipital sulcus on the medial surface of the hemisphere can be seen on CT at the level of the lateral ventricles (see **Fig. 2.3c**). The parieto-occipital junction on the lateral surface has no anatomical landmark but lies at approximately the same transverse level as the sulcus.

WHITE MATTER OF THE HEMISPHERES

There are three types of fibres within the cerebral hemispheres:

- Commissural fibres, which connect corresponding areas of the two hemispheres;
- Association (arcuate) fibres, which connect different parts of the cortex of the same hemisphere; and
- Projection fibres, which join the cortex to lower centres.

COMMISSURAL FIBRES

The corpus callosum (Figs 2.4 and 2.5)

The corpus callosum is a large midline mass of commissural fibres, each fibre of which connects corresponding areas of both hemispheres. It is approximately 10 cm long and becomes progressively thicker towards its posterior end. Named parts include the:

- *Rostrum* — this is the first part, which extends anteriorly from the anterior commissure (vide infra).
- *Genu* — this is the most anterior part where it bends sharply backwards;
- *Trunk (body)* — this is the main mass of fibres extending from the genu anteriorly to the splenium posteriorly. It lies below the lower free edge of the falx cerebri. The anterior cerebral vessels run on its superior surface; and
- *Splenium* — this is the thickened posterior end.

In cross-section, fibres from the genu that arch forward to the frontal cortex on each side are called *forceps minor*, and fibres from the splenium passing posteriorly to each occipital cortex are called *forceps major*. Fibres extending laterally from the body of the corpus callosum are called the **tapetum.** These form part of the roof and lateral wall of the lateral ventricle.

Habenular commissure

This small commissure is situated above and anterior to pineal body. It unites the habenular striae, which are

Fig. 2.4 Corpus callosum and other commissures.

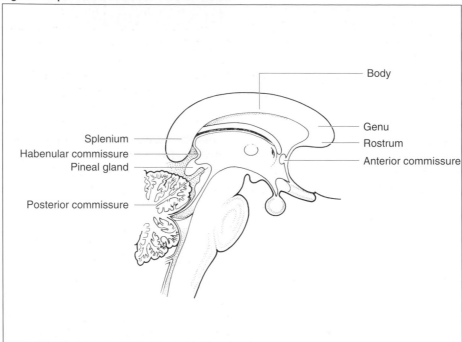

Fig. 2.5 MRI scan of brain: midline sagittal image.

1. Frontal lobe
2. Parietal lobe
3. Occipital lobe
4. Rostrum of corpus callosum
5. Genu of corpus callosum
6. Body of corpus callosum
7. Splenium of corpus callosum
8. Septum pellucidum of lateral ventricle
9. Foramen of Monro
10. Fornix
11. Massa intermedia of thalami
12. Third ventricle
13. Supraoptic recess of third ventricle
14. Suprapineal recess of third ventricle
15. Pineal gland
16. Optic chiasm
17. Midbrain (red nucleus)
18. Interpeduncular cistern

19. Aqueduct of Sylvius
20. Quadrigeminal plate (superior and inferior colliculi)
21. Quadrigeminal plate cistern
22. Fourth ventricle
23. Vermis of cerebellum
24. Pons
25. Anterior commisure
26. Prepontine cistern
27. Medulla oblongata
28. Tonsil of cerebellum
29. Cisterna magna
30. Clivus
31. Pituitary
32. Suprasellar cistern
33. Tentorium cerebelli
34. Spinal cord
35. Nasopharynx
36. Soft palate
37. Tongue

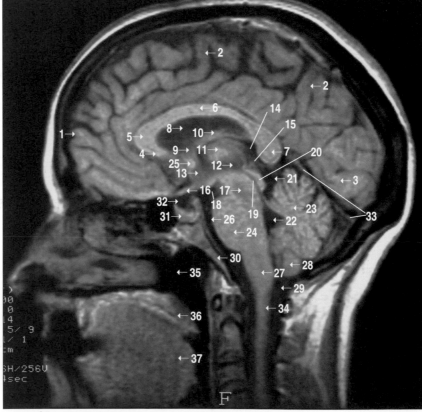

fibres from the olfactory centre that pass posteriorly along upper surface of each thalamus and unite in a 'U' configuration in this commissure.

Posterior commissure

This is situated anterior and inferior to the pineal body. It connects the superior colliculi, which are concerned with light reflexes (see brainstem).

PROJECTION FIBRES

These fibres join the cerebral cortex to lower centres. Some are afferent and some efferent. They are called the internal capsule where they lie lateral to the thalamus and the corona radiata as they fan out between the internal capsule and the cerebral cortex.

Internal capsule (see Fig. 2.3c)

This contains sensory fibres from the thalamus to the sensory cortex and motor fibres from the motor cortex to the pyramidal tracts of the spinal cord. In cross-section, the internal capsule has an anterior limb between the caudate and lentiform nuclei and a posterior limb between

Fig. 2.6 MRI scan of brain: coronal image through the third ventricle.

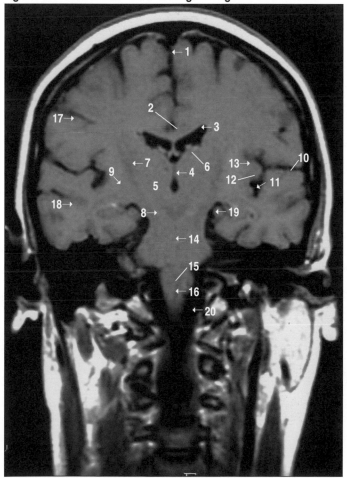

the lentiform nucleus and the thalamus. Both limbs meet at a right angle called the genu.

The anterior limb is composed mainly of frontopontine fibres. The genu and the anterior two-thirds of the posterior limb contain motor fibres. The most anterior fibres at the genu are those of the head. Fibres to the arm, hand, trunk, leg and perineum lie progressively more posteriorly. Haemorrhage or thrombosis of thalamostriate arteries supplying this area leads to paralysis of these muscles.

Behind these fibres on the posterior limb and on the retrolentiform part of the internal capsule are the sensory fibres. More posteriorly are the visual fibres that extend towards the occipital pole as the optic radiation. Most posterior of all are the auditory fibres.

RADIOLOGICAL FEATURES OF THE PROJECTION FIBRES

Plain films of the skull

Calcification of the habenular commissure is a common finding on skull radiographs. It is found anterior and superior to the pineal gland if this is also calcified. Typically the calcification is 'C'-shaped with the open part of the letter facing backwards. Some authors suggest that this calcification is in the choroid plexus of the third ventricles — the taenia habenulare — rather than in the commissure.

Computed tomography

The corpus callosum can be seen between the lateral ventricles on CT slices at a high ventricular level. The internal capsule is seen as a 'V'-shaped low-attenuation structure (see **Fig. 2.3c**) between the caudate and lentiform nuclei anteriorly and the lentiform and thalamus posteriorly.

Magnetic resonance imaging

The rostrum, genu, body and splenium can be seen on sagittal MRI (**Fig. 2.5**). The body of the corpus callosum can be seen in the roof of the third ventricle in coronal MRI scans through the third ventricle (**Fig. 2.6**).

1. Interhemispheric fissure
2. Body of corpus callosum
3. Body of lateral ventricle
4. Third ventricle
5. Thalamus
6. Body of caudate nucleus
7. Internal capsule
8. Cerebral peduncle
9. Lentiform nucleus (globus pallidus and putamen)
10. Lateral sulcus
11. Sylvian fissure
12. Insula
13. Claustrum
14. Pons
15. Medulla
16. Spinal cord
17. Parietal lobe
18. Temporal lobe
19. Ambient cistern
20. Cisterna magna

Fig. 2.7 Ultrasound of infant brain: coronal image through the frontal horns of the lateral ventricles.

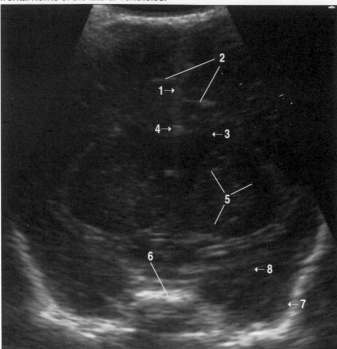

Ultrasound examination of the neonatal head

The corpus callosum is seen below the interhemispheric fissure on coronal scans where both its upper and lower surfaces are perpendicular to the beam (**Fig. 2.7**). It can be seen to extend laterally as the roof of the lateral ventricles. On midline sagittal scans, it is seen as a thin band of tissue between the pericallosal artery in the pericallosal sulcus, superiorly, and the fluid of the cavum septum pellucidum inferiorly.

1. Interhemispheric fissure
2. Sulci
3. Frontal horn of lateral ventricle
4. Corpus callosum
5. Putamen above, lentiform nucleus below, separated by internal capsule. (These three are not distinguished separately)
6. Nonaerated sphenoid sinus
7. Floor of middle cranial fossa
8. Temporal lobe

BASAL GANGLIA (Fig. 2.8)

This subcortical grey matter includes:

■ The corpus striatum — the caudate and lentiform nuclei;
■ The amygdaloid body; and
■ The claustrum.

CAUDATE NUCLEUS

This nucleus is described as having a head, body and tail. Its long, thin tail ends in the amygdaloid nucleus. The caudate nucleus is highly curved and lies within the concavity of the lateral ventricle. Thus its head projects into the floor of the anterior horn and its body into the floor of the body of the lateral ventricle. Its tail indents the roof of the inferior horn of this ventricle.

LENTIFORM NUCLEUS

This is shaped like a biconcave lens. It is made up of a larger lateral putamen and a smaller medial globus pallidus. Medially, it is separated from the head of the caudate nucleus anteriorly, and from the thalamus posteriorly by the internal capsule. A thin layer of white matter on its lateral surface is called the external capsule.

Strands of grey matter connect the head of the caudate nucleus with the putamen of the lentiform nucleus across the anterior limb of the internal capsule. The resulting striated appearance gives rise to the term '*corpus striatum*'.

The function of the corpus striatum is not well understood. It is part of the extrapyramidal system and influences voluntary motor activity. Cortical afferents enter the putamen and caudate nucleus, which send efferents to the globus pallidus. This in turn sends efferents to the hypothalamus, brainstem and the spinal cord.

CLAUSTRUM

This thin sheet of grey matter lies between the putamen and the insula. It is separated medially from the putamen by the external capsule and bounded laterally by a thin sheet of white matter (the extreme capsule) just deep to the insula. The claustrum is cortical in origin but its function is unknown.

RADIOLOGICAL FEATURES OF THE BASAL GANGLIA

Computed tomography

On axial CT the head of the *caudate nucleus* can be seen projecting into the anterior horn of the lateral ventricle on slices taken at ventricular level (see **Fig. 2.3c**). The head of the caudate nucleus is usually more radiodense than the lentiform nucleus or the thalamus, especially in older subjects. The tail of the caudate nucleus is seen as a thin, dense stripe on the superolateral margin of the lateral ventricle on higher cuts.

Bilateral calcification of the *globus pallidus* is occasionally seen on CT as a normal variant in older subjects.

The *claustrum* can be seen on CT (see **Fig. 2.3c**) as a high-attenuation stripe, separated from the putamen by the external capsule and from the insula by the extreme capsule.

Magnetic resonance imaging

MRI is sensitive to paramagnetic substances such as iron, which may be deposited in the globus pallidus, giving this a lower signal than the surrounding brain on T2-weighted images (see **Fig. 2.6**).

Ultrasound examination of the neonatal brain

Parasagittal scans (**Fig. 2.9**) show the caudate nucleus within the curve of the lateral ventricle. A caudothalamic groove, the site of the thalamostriate vein, can be identified.

1. Frontal horn of lateral ventricle
2. Body of lateral ventricle
3. Trigone/occipital horn of lateral ventricle
4. Temporal horn of lateral ventricle
5. Choroid plexus (echogenic)
6. Thalamus
7. Caudate nucleus
8. Cerebellum
9. Floor of anterior cranial fossa
10. Floor of middle cranial fossa
11. Floor of posterior cranial fossa

Fig. 2.8 Basal ganglia.

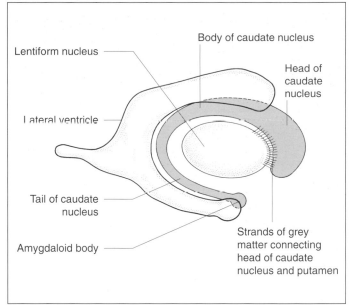

Fig. 2.9 Parasagittal ultrasound of the infant brain: 15° view. This section shows most of the lateral ventricle. The thalamus lies in its concavity with the caudate nucleus anterosuperior to it. The caudothalamic notch or groove is between these two and is a common site for haemorrhage.

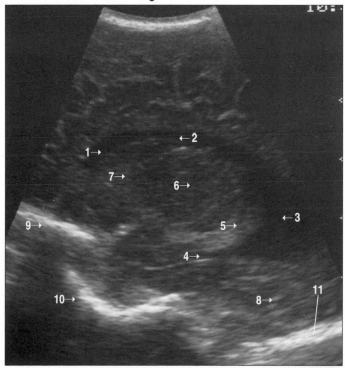

THALAMUS, HYPOTHALAMUS AND PINEAL GLAND

The structures around the third ventricle include the thalamus, hypothalamus and the pineal gland.

THALAMUS

These paired, ovoid bodies of grey matter lie in the lateral walls of the third ventricle, from the interventricular foramen anteriorly to the brainstem posteriorly. Each has its apex anteriorly and a more rounded posterior end called the pulvinar. The thalamus is related laterally to the internal capsule and, beyond that, to the lentiform nucleus. The body and tail of the caudate nucleus are in contact with the lateral margin of the thalamus. The superior part of the thalamus forms part of the floor of the lateral ventricle.

The thalamus is attached in approximately 60% of cases to the thalamus of the other side by the interthalamic adhesion or massa intermedia. This is not a neural connection.

Most thalamic nuclei are relay nuclei of the main sensory pathways. Medial and lateral swellings on the posteroinferior aspect of thalamus, called the medial and lateral geniculate bodies, are attached to the inferior and superior colliculi and are involved in the relay of auditory and visual impulses.

The thalamus receives its blood supply from thalamo-striate branches of the posterior cerebral artery.

HYPOTHALAMUS (Fig. 2.10)

The hypothalamus forms the floor of the third ventricle. It includes the following, starting anteriorly:

- Optic chiasm;
- Tuber cinereum — a sheet of grey matter between the optic chiasm and the mammillary bodies;
- Infundibular stalk — leading down to the posterior lobe of the pituitary gland;
- Mammillary bodies — small round masses in front of the posterior perforated substance in which the columns of the fornix (vide infra) end; and
- Posterior perforated substance — the interval between the diverging crura cerebri, which is pierced by central branches of the posterior cerebral artery.

Fig. 2.10 Anterior surface of brainstem.

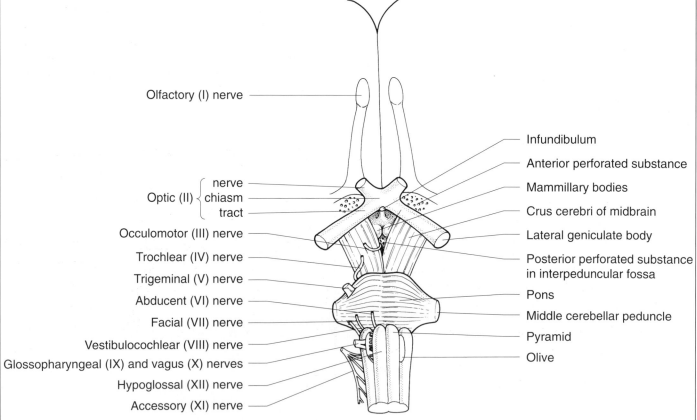

Olfactory (I) nerve

Optic (II) { nerve, chiasm, tract }

Occulomotor (III) nerve

Trochlear (IV) nerve

Trigeminal (V) nerve

Abducent (VI) nerve

Facial (VII) nerve

Vestibulocochlear (VIII) nerve

Glossopharyngeal (IX) and vagus (X) nerves

Hypoglossal (XII) nerve

Accessory (XI) nerve

Infundibulum

Anterior perforated substance

Mammillary bodies

Crus cerebri of midbrain

Lateral geniculate body

Posterior perforated substance in interpeduncular fossa

Pons

Middle cerebellar peduncle

Pyramid

Olive

The nuclei of the hypothalamus are connected by white matter, the medial forebrain bundle, to each other, to the frontal lobe anteriorly and to the midbrain posteriorly.

The function of the hypothalamus is control of autonomic activity. It has sympathetic and parasympathetic areas and plays a role in the regulation of temperature, appetite and sleep patterns.

The hypothalamus is supplied by branches of the anterior and posterior cerebral and posterior communicating arteries and is drained by the thalamostriate veins.

PINEAL GLAND (see **Figs 2.4** and **2.5**)

The pineal gland lies between the posterior ends of the thalami and between the splenium above and the superior colliculi below. It is separated from the splenium by the cerebral veins.

The pineal stalk has superior and inferior laminae. The superior lamina is formed by the habenular commissure and the inferior lamina contains the posterior commissure. Between these laminae is the posterior recess of the third ventricle.

RADIOLOGICAL FEATURES OF THE THALAMUS, HYPOTHALAMUS AND THE PINEAL GLAND

Skull radiographs
Pineal calcification is visible in some normal skull radiographs but in a greater percentage of CT scans (see the section on the skull, p. 9).

Computed tomography
The thalami can be seen on CT on each side of the third ventricle (see **Fig. 2.3c**). Their relationship to the posterior limb of the internal capsule and to the lentiform nucleus can be appreciated on this slice.

Magnetic resonance imaging
The structures forming the hypothalamus can be appreciated best on midline sagittal MRI (see **Fig. 2.5**). The optic chiasm, the tuber cinereum, the infundibular stalk and the interpeduncular cistern (containing the mammillary bodies and in the base of which lies the posterior perforated substance) can be identified.

Ultrasound examination of the neonatal brain
In the parasagittal plane (see **Fig. 2.9**), the echogenic thalamus can be seen within the 'C'-shaped curve of the lateral ventricle posterior to the caudate nucleus.

PITUITARY GLAND (Fig. 2.11)

The pituitary gland (hypophysis cerebri) lies in the pituitary fossa and measures 12 mm in its transverse diameter and 8 mm in its anteroposterior diameter.

The pituitary gland has a hollow stalk, the infundibulum, which arises from the tuber cinereum in the floor of the third ventricle. This stalk is composed of nerve fibres whose cell bodies are in the third ventricle. It is directed anteroinferiorly and surrounded by an upward extension of the anterior lobe, the tuberal part.

The anterior lobe is five times larger than the posterior lobe. It is developed from Rathke's pouch in the roof of the primitive mouth. (A tumour from remnants of the epithelium of this pouch is called a craniopharyngioma.) The anterior lobe produces hormones in response to release factors carried from the hypothalamus by hypophyseal portal veins.

The posterior lobe is made up of nerve fibres whose cell bodies lie in the hypothalamus and release hormones in response to impulses from these nerves.

The anterior lobe is adherent to the posterior lobe by a narrow zone called the pars intermedia. This is, in fact, developmentally and functionally part of the anterior lobe.

The *relations of the pituitary gland* are as follows:

- Above: the diaphragma sella (dura mater) and the optic chiasm anteriorly (8 mm above dura);
- Below: the body of sphenoid and the sphenoid sinus; and
- Laterally: the dura and the cavernous sinus and its contents, the internal carotid artery and abducens nerve with occulomotor, ophthalmic and trochlear nerves in its walls.

Fig. 2.11 Pituitary gland and cavernous sinus: coronal section.

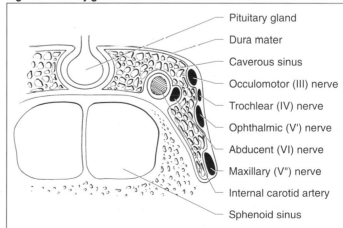

- Pituitary gland
- Dura mater
- Caverous sinus
- Occulomotor (III) nerve
- Trochlear (IV) nerve
- Ophthalmic (V') nerve
- Abducent (VI) nerve
- Maxillary (V") nerve
- Internal carotid artery
- Sphenoid sinus

Fig. 2.12 CT scan of scan of pituitary gland: coronal image.

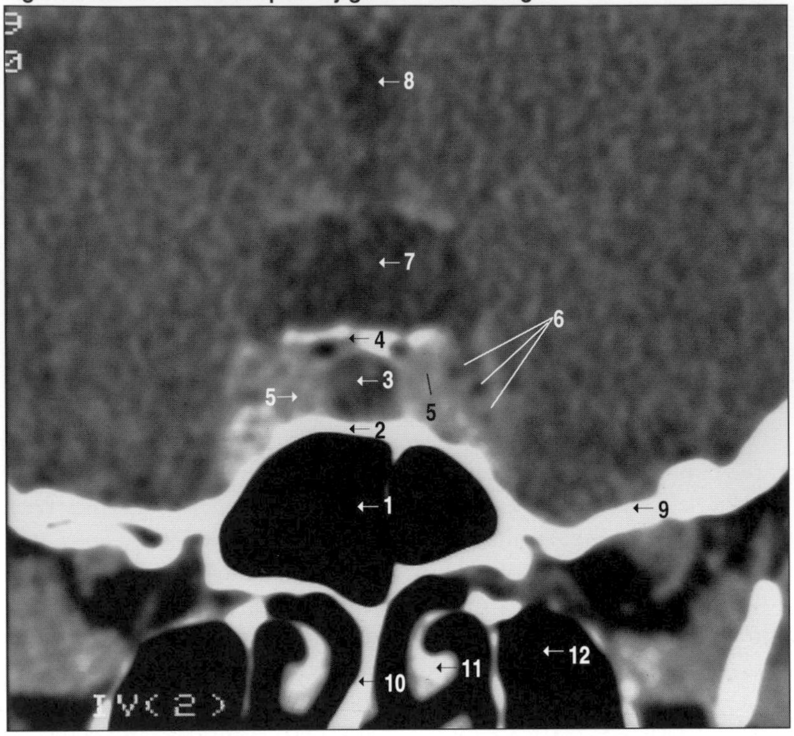

1. Sphenoid sinus
2. Floor of pituitary fossa
3. Pituitary gland
4. Pneumatized dorsum sellae
5. Cavernous sinus
6. Cranial nerves
7. Suprasellar cistern
8. Third ventricle
9. Floor of middle cranial fossa
10. Nasal septum
11. Superior nasal concha
12. Superior part of maxillary sinus

The cavernous sinuses are united by intercavernous sinuses, which surround the pituitary gland anteriorly, posteriorly and inferiorly.

BLOOD SUPPLY

Superior hypophyseal arteries, which arise from each internal carotid artery immediately after it pierces the dura, supply the hypothalamus and the infundibulum. A capillary bed in the infundibulum gives rise to portal vessels to the anterior lobe. The posterior lobe is supplied by inferior hypophyseal arteries from the internal carotid arteries in the cavernous sinus.

Venous drainage is to the cavernous and inter cavernous sinuses.

RADIOLOGICAL FEATURES OF THE PITUITARY GLAND

Skull radiographs

The appearance of the pituitary fossa is affected by disease processes in the gland. This is dealt with in the section on the skull.

Computed tomography (Fig. 2.12)

The pituitary gland is visible on axial scans, with the surrounding cavernous sinuses best seen in contrast-enhanced views. Coronal reconstruction is useful. The relation of the pituitary gland to suprasellar structures can be seen.

Magnetic resonance imaging (see Fig. 2.5)

Sagittal and coronal images are most useful. The normal pituitary has a heterogenous signal intensity and enhances with gadolinium contrast. Anterior and posterior components can be distinguished. High signal intensity in the posteroinferior part of the sella may be due to a normal fat pad. The sella itself is delineated by signal void of the bony cortex and by high-intensity signal of marrow in the clivus. The optic nerves and chiasm and the intracranial carotid vessels above, and the sphenoid sinus below, are seen clearly on sagittal sections.

LIMBIC LOBE (Fig. 2.13)

This is not an anatomical lobe as such but is functionally related to structures (including the hippocampus and the fornix) that surround the corpus callosum on the medial surface of the cerebral hemisphere.

It includes the cingulate gyrus, which curves around the genu and body of the corpus callosum and continues around the splenium as the splenial gyrus. This, in turn, is continuous with the dentate gyrus, which lies along the hippocampus so far as its anterior pole.

Also included in the limbic lobe are grey matter on the corpus callosum — called the induseum griseum — and white fibres that run along its length — the medial and lateral longitudinal striae.

HIPPOCAMPUS

This is a curved elevation in the floor of the inferior horn of the lateral ventricle. Its enlarged, ridged anterior end has the appearance of a paw — the pes hippocampi. The hippocampus consists of grey matter, with a fine covering of white matter called the alveus. Its function is concerned with behaviour patterns, emotion and recent memory.

FORNIX (see **Fig. 2.13**)

This is an efferent pathway from the hippocampus to the mammillary bodies. Fibres of the alveus converge on the medial border of the hippocampus as a band of fibres called the fimbria of the hippocampus. This becomes free of the hippocampus as the crus of the fornix (the posterior pillar of the fornix).

Each crus extends posteriorly to below the splenium of the corpus callosum, where it connects with that of the other side as the commissure of the fornix. Together the two crura form the body of the fornix. The body of the fornix extends anteriorly around the upper surface of the thalami. It is attached posteriorly to the undersurface of the corpus callosum and anteriorly to the inferior border of the septum pellucidum.

Above the interventricular foramen the body divides into two columns, which pass inferiorly between the foramen and the anterior commissure and form the anterior border of the interventricular foramen. The columns then pass to the hypothalamus and the mammillary bodies in which they terminate. Some fibres from the columns of the fornix, the habenular fibres, turn back over the thalamus to join posteriorly in the habenular commissure.

RADIOLOGICAL FEATURES OF THE LIMBIC LOBE

Magnetic resonance imaging
The body of the fornix is seen in midline sagittal MRI (see **Fig. 2.5**), extending from the undersurface of the corpus callosum posteriorly to the interventricular foramen anteriorly along the undersurface of the septum pellucidum.

Ultrasound examination of the neonatal brain
In the coronal plane at the level of the third ventricle (see **Fig. 2.7**) the curved 'C'-shaped echoes of the parahippocampal gyrus are used as a far-field landmark.

Fig. 2.13 Components of the limbic lobe.

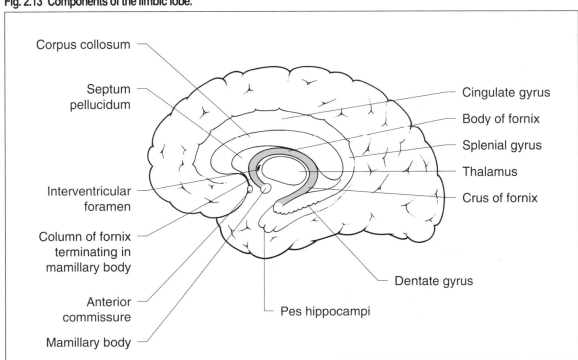

Corpus collosum

Septum pellucidum

Interventricular foramen

Column of fornix terminating in mamillary body

Anterior commissure

Mamillary body

Pes hippocampi

Cingulate gyrus

Body of fornix

Splenial gyrus

Thalamus

Crus of fornix

Dentate gyrus

THE BRAINSTEM (see Fig. 2.10)

The brainstem connects the cerebral hemispheres with the spinal cord and extends from just above the tentorial hiatus to just below the foramen magnum. It is bounded anteriorly by the clivus — basisphenoid above and the basiocciput below. The pons, the widest part of the brainstem, also grooves the apex of the petrous temporal bone on each side. This bony anterior boundary can cause an artefact in CT scanning of the brainstem, although it does not interfere with MRI studies.

The brainstem has three parts — from superior to inferior: the midbrain, the pons and the medulla.

MIDBRAIN

External features

Anteriorly two cerebral peduncles are seen separated by the interpeduncular fossa. These peduncles (crura cerebri) carry fibres from the internal capsule to the pons. The floor of the interpeduncular fossa is the posterior perforated substance.

The posterior surface of the midbrain presents four rounded prominences — the corpora quadrigemini or the superior and inferior colliculi. Each superior colliculus is joined by a superior brachium to the lateral geniculate body of the optic tract. Each inferior colliculus is joined by an inferior brachium to the medial geniculate body of the auditory system.

Below the colliculi, the superior cerebellar peduncles converge to form the superior boundary of the fourth ventricle. A thin sheet of white matter between these is the superior medullary velum.

Internal features

Cerebral peduncles have a ventral part, the crus cerebri (descending fibres), and a dorsal part, the tegmentum (ascending fibres), which are separated by the substantia nigra. Dorsal to the substantia nigra at the level of the superior colliculi, are paired red nuclei, which lie close to the median plane. These are part of the extrapyramidal pathway. That part of the midbrain posterior to the aqueduct is called the tectum or quadrigeminal plate.

Cranial nerves

The third (III) cranial nerve emerges from between the cerebral peduncles, while the fourth (IV) emerges from the dorsal surface of the midbrain and winds around its lateral aspect.

Blood supply

The basilar artery divides at the lower border of the midbrain into posterior cerebral and superior cerebellar arteries on each side. These sweep around the cerebral peduncles with the third and fourth nerves between them.

Posterior mesencephalic veins curve around each side of the midbrain towards the great cerebral vein.

RADIOLOGICAL FEATURES OF THE MIDBRAIN

Computed tomography

The midbrain is seen on CT at the level of the circle of Willis (see **Fig. 2.3b**). The crura can be identified anteriorly and the colliculi posteriorly. It is not always possible to identify the cerebral aqueduct.

On contrast-enhanced CT, the posterior cerebral arteries or the posterior mesencephalic veins may be seen passing around the midbrain.

Magnetic resonance imaging

Ferritin deposition in the substantia nigra and red nuclei may lead to a lower signal intensity here than in the remainder of the crus cerebri on T2-weighted MRI.

PONS

External features

Anteriorly, cerebellopontine fibres are seen to be continuous on each side with the middle cerebellar peduncle. A shallow groove is seen in the midline. The basilar artery may lie in this groove but often lies lateral to it.

The posterior surface of the pons forms the upper part of the floor of the fourth ventricle.

Cranial nerves

The fifth (V) cranial nerve emerges from the anterolateral surface of the pons.

The sixth (VI) cranial nerve emerges at the junction with the medulla close to the midline anteriorly.

The seventh and eighth (VII and VIII) cranial nerves emerge at the junction with the medulla laterally, that is, at the cerebellopontine angle.

Blood supply

The pons is supplied by pontine branches of the basilar artery.

Blood from the pons drains to the anterior ponto-mesencephalic vein and the inferior petrosal sinus.

RADIOLOGICAL FEATURES OF THE PONS

Computed tomography (see Fig. 2.3a)

The bony anterior relations of the pons — the clivus centrally and the petrous temporal bones laterally — may cause considerable artefact on CT scanning of this area, thus MRI may be superior for this reason.

On CT scans, the cerebellopontine fibres of the middle cerebellar peduncle can be seen as an area of low attenuation extending from the pons into each cerebellar hemisphere.

With contrast enhancement, the basilar artery may be seen anterior to the pons. A position to the right or left of the midline is not abnormal. Asymmetry of the cerebellopontine cisterns, however, is usually associated with pathology.

Magnetic resonance imaging

The anatomy already described can be seen. In particular even the trigeminal nerves can be seen entering its anterior surface and the seventh and eighth cranial nerves can be seen exiting at the cerebellopontine angle.

MEDULLA OBLONGATA

External features

Anteriorly, the ventral median fissure is deep in its superior part. A ridge on each side of this fissure is formed by pyramidal fibres and is called the pyramid. These fibres decussate in the lower medulla, obliterating the median fissure here. Lateral to the pyramid in the upper medulla is an oval bulge called the olive. Lateral to the olive lies the inferior cerebellar peduncle — known as the restiform body — joining the medulla to the cerebellum.

Posteriorly, the upper part of the medulla is open as the floor of the fourth ventricle, while its lower part is closed around the central canal. Dorsal median and lateral sulci define four columns below the ventricle — gracile columns medially and cuneate columns laterally.

A correspondingly named tubercle is found at the upper end of each column.

Cranial nerves

The ninth and tenth (IX and X) cranial nerves emerge posterior to the olive.

The eleventh (XI) cranial nerve has medullary rootlets that arise inferior to those of X, and cervical rootlets that arise form the upper spinal cord and enter the foramen magnum to unite with the medullary roots.

The twelfth (XII) cranial nerve arises from several rootlets posterior to the olive.

Blood supply

The vertebral and basilar arteries supply the anterior part of the medulla, while the posterior inferior cerebellar artery supplies its posterior part.

Venous drainage is to the occipital sinus posteriorly and the inferior petrosal sinus anteriorly. Inferior medullary veins communicate with spinal veins.

RADIOLOGICAL FEATURES OF THE MEDULLA OBLONGATA

Computed tomography

Sections through the lower medulla are difficult to distinguish from those through the upper cervical cord unless the atlas or foramen magnum can be identified. The upper medulla can be identified easily by the presence of the fourth ventricle and cerebellum posteriorly.

Magnetic resonance imaging

Magnetic resonance imaging of the medulla gives superior images because of the lack of bony artefact (see **Fig. 2.5**). The ventral sulcus can be seen anteriorly on axial sections with the pre- and postolivary sulci laterally. The olives give a square configuration to the medulla on this section. The fourth ventricle is seen posteriorly, especially on sagittal sections, with its midline foramen leading to the vallecula. The most inferior part of the fourth ventricle is called the obex. This may be sealed during surgery of the cervical cord syrinx.

Cervical myelography

Contrast medium may extend into the cranium and outline the medulla anterior to the cisterna magna. The expanded upper medulla with its nerve rootlets can be seen.

CEREBELLUM (Fig. 2.14)

The cerebellum lies in the posterior fossa. It is separated from the occipital lobe by the tentorium and from the pons and midbrain by the fourth ventricle. It is connected to the brainstem by three pairs of cerebellar peduncles:

■ Superior cerebellar peduncles (brachium conjunctivum) to the midbrain;
■ Middle cerebellar peduncles (brachium pontis) to the pons; and
■ Inferior cerebellar peduncles (restiform body) to the medulla.

The cerebellum lies on the occipital bone posteriorly and close to the mastoid anteriorly. It is related to the dural sinuses, especially the sigmoid sinuses.

The superior surface of the cerebellum slopes upwards from posterior to anterior. A CT slice of upper cerebellum, therefore, contains cerebellum anteriorly and occipital lobes posterolaterally.

The surface of the cerebellum has numerous shallow sulci that separate tiny parallel folia. Deep fissures separate the hemispheres into lobules.

There are two hemispheres with the midline vermis between.

HEMISPHERES

The two hemispheres extend laterally and posteriorly. These are separated by a shallow median groove superiorly and by a deep groove inferiorly. A midline posterior cerebellar notch lodges the falx cerebelli.

The hemispheres are divided into lobules by fissures, the deepest of which is the horizontal fissure, which extends from the convex posterior border into the depth of the hemispheres. The primary fissure (fissura prima) divides the superior surface.

On each side below the middle cerebellar peduncle is the *flocculus*. This is a small ventral portion of the hemisphere that is almost completely separate from the remainder. It extends laterally from the midline as a slender band with an expanded end. It lies close to the lateral recess and choroid plexus of the fourth ventricle.

The *tonsils* are the most anterior inferior part of the hemispheres and lie close to the midline.

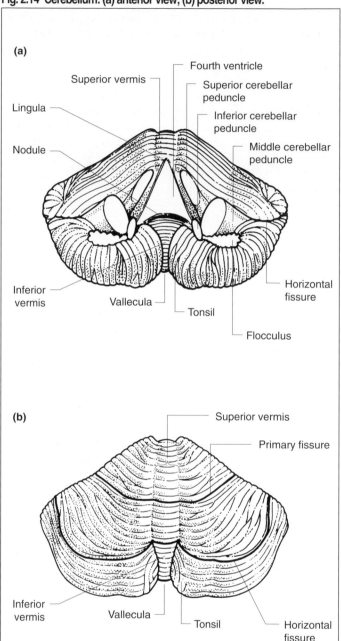

Fig. 2.14 Cerebellum: (a) anterior view; (b) posterior view.

The cerebellum, like the cerebrum, has a cortex of grey matter and deeper white matter. There are deep nuclei within the hemispheres, the largest of which is the dentate nucleus.

VERMIS

The vermis is the narrow midline portion of the cerebellum. Superiorly this is merely a low median elevation not clearly separated from the hemispheres; however, inferiorly the vermis is quite separate and lies in a deep cleft called the vallecula. The vermis is separated into named parts by fissures, each part except the lingula corresponding to an adjoining lobule of the cerebellar hemispheres. The most anterior part of the superior vermis is the lingula, which lies on the superior medullary velum (a thin sheet of white matter between the superior cerebellar peduncles). The most anterior part of the inferior vermis is the nodule.

THE FUNCTION OF THE CEREBELLUM

The cerebellum is important in muscle co-ordination and in the regulation of muscle tone and of posture. Unilateral lesions of the cerebellum affect the ipsilateral side of the body.

ARTERIAL SUPPLY

Three pairs of arteries supply the cerebellum, namely the:

- Posterior inferior cerebellar arteries (PICA) from the vertebral arteries supply the inferior vermis and the inferior part of the hemispheres;
- Anterior inferior cerebellar arteries (AICA) from the basilar artery supply the anterolateral aspect of the undersurface of the hemisphere; and
- Superior cerebellar arteries also from the basilar artery supply the superior aspect of the cerebellum.

VENOUS DRAINAGE

(See section on veins of the posterior fossa, p. 80.)

The precentral cerebellar vein and the superior vermian vein drain to the great cerebral vein. The remainder of the cerebellar veins drain to the nearby dural sinuses as follows:

- The superior and posterior parts to the straight and transverse sinuses; and
- The inferior aspect to the inferior petrosal, sigmoid and occipital sinuses.

RADIOLOGICAL FEATURES OF THE CEREBELLUM

Computed tomography

On CT sections taken through the pons (see **Fig. 2.3a**), the cerebellum is seen separated from the pons by the fourth ventricle and connected to the pons on each side of this by the middle cerebellar peduncles. At this level the cerebellum is bounded anteriorly by the petrous temporal bones.

On higher slices (see **Fig. 2.3b**) the cerebellum is separated from the temporal and occipital lobes antero-laterally by the tentorial margins. Close to its bony attachment, the tentorium can be easily seen on contrast-enhanced CT due to the contained superior petrosal sinus.

The superior vermis can be seen between the occipital lobes on CT sections through the thalamus.

VENTRICLES, CISTERNS, CSF PRODUCTION AND FLOW

VENTRICLES (Figs 2.15 and 2.16)

These are fluid-filled spaces within the brain related to the development of the nervous system as a tubular structure with a central canal.

Two lateral ventricles represent expansion of the most anterior part of the ventricular system into each cerebral hemisphere. The third ventricle, the aqueduct and the fourth ventricle are midline in position and are continuous with the central canal of the cord. The ventricular system is also continuous with the subarachnoid space around the brain via foramina in the fourth ventricle.

The ventricles are lined with ependyma, which is invaginated by plexuses of blood vessels called the choroid plexus. These vessels produce cerebrospinal fluid (CSF).

THE LATERAL VENTRICLES (see Fig. 2.15)

There is a lateral ventricle within each cerebral hemisphere. Each is 'C'-shaped, with the limbs of the 'C' facing anteriorly and a variably developed posterior extension from its midpoint. Each is described as having an anterior (frontal) horn, a body (atrium), an inferior (temporal) horn and a posterior (occipital) horn. An interventricular foramen at the junction of the anterior horn and the body connects each lateral ventricle with the third ventricle.

Anterior horn

This extends into the frontal lobe. Its roof and anterior extremity is formed by the corpus callosum, its rostrum and genu, and fibres radiating from these, are formed by the tapetum. The head of the caudate nucleus makes a prominent impression in the floor and lateral wall of the anterior horn. The medial wall is formed by the septum pellucidum. There is no choroid plexus in the anterior horn.

Body

This is within the parietal lobe. As with the anterior horn, the roof and lateral wall of the body of the ventricle are formed by the corpus callosum and its fibres — the tapetum — and the medial wall is formed by the septum pellucidum. The thalamus lies in the floor medially, with the body of the caudate nucleus laterally and the thalamostriate groove and thalamostriate vein between. The body of the fornix lies above the thalamus and the choroid plexus is invaginated into the cavity of the ventricle between these.

Inferior horn

This extends anteriorly into the temporal lobe. It curves down and laterally from the body of the ventricle as it extends anteriorly and then curves somewhat medially towards the temporal pole. Its lateral wall is formed by the fibres of the tapetum. The caudate nucleus lies in the floor of the anterior horn, and the body curves around in the concavity of the ventricle so that its tail lies in the roof of the inferior horn with the amygdaloid nucleus at its anterior end. The hippocampus forms the floor of the inferior horn with the pes hippocampi anteriorly and the crus of the fornix arising from this (cf. the fornix).

The choroid plexus of the body of the lateral ventricle is continuous with that of the inferior horn.

Occipital horn

This is the posterior extension of the lateral ventricle that extends into the occipital lobe. The posterior convexity of the body from which it arises is called the trigone of the lateral ventricle. The occipital horn may be absent or poorly developed or may extend the full depth of the lobe. The posterior horns of the two lateral ventricles are often asymmetrical and are bilaterally well developed in only 12% of subjects. If the posterior horn is present on one side only it is usually the left side.

The lateral wall of the occipital horn is formed by tapetal fibres and the optic radiation. Its floor is formed by grey matter in the depth of the collateral sulcus and its medial wall by grey matter in the depth of the calcarine sulcus. There is no choroid plexus in the occipital horn.

THE CHOROID PLEXUS OF THE LATERAL VENTRICLE

The choroid plexus of the lateral ventricle is responsible for the production of most of the CSF. It extends from the inferior horn through the body to the interventricular foramen where it is continuous with that of the third ventricle.

The vessels supplying this are the anterior and posterior choroidal arteries. The anterior choroidal artery, a branch of the internal carotid artery, enters the choroidal plexus in the anterior part of the inferior horn. The posterior choroidal arteries are branches of the posterior cerebral artery; these are variable in number and pass into the body of lateral ventricle behind and above the thalamus and into the posterior part of the inferior horn below the thalamus.

The veins draining the plexus unite to form the choroidal vein, which begins in the inferior horn and passes anteriorly to the interventricular foramen, where it joins the thalamostriate vein to form the internal cerebral vein on each side.

Fig. 2.15 The ventricular system.

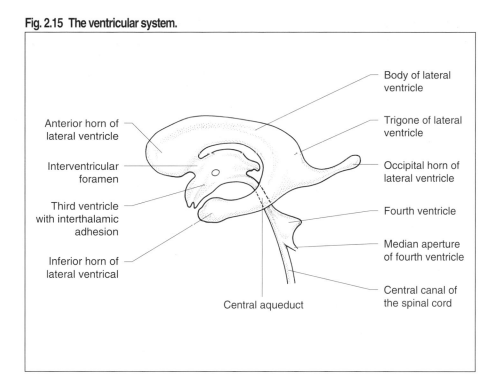

Labels (clockwise from left):
- Anterior horn of lateral ventricle
- Interventricular foramen
- Third ventricle with interthalamic adhesion
- Inferior horn of lateral ventrical
- Central aqueduct
- Body of lateral ventricle
- Trigone of lateral ventricle
- Occipital horn of lateral ventricle
- Fourth ventricle
- Median aperture of fourth ventricle
- Central canal of the spinal cord

THE THIRD VENTRICLE
(see **Figs 2.15** and **2.16**)

This is a slit-like space between the thalami. Its width is between 2 and 10 mm and increases with age. Its lateral walls are formed by the thalami and are limited inferiorly by the subthalamic (hypothalamic) groove. The thin anterior wall of the third ventricle between the anterior commissure above to the optic chiasm below is called the lamina terminalis. The extension of the cavity above the optic chiasm is called the supraoptic recess. The floor of the third ventricle is formed by the structures of the hypothalamus, including the pituitary gland whose hollow stalk is the infundibular recess of the ventricle. Posteriorly, the ventricle extends as a small pineal recess into the pineal stalk and above this into a recess whose size varies from 1 mm–3 cm — known as the suprapineal recess. The roof of the third ventricle is formed anteriorly by the anterior commissure, the column of the fornix and the interventricular foramen. Behind this the roof is formed by the body of the fornix, with the choroid plexus invaginating below it into the upper part of the ventricle.

The thalami are connected across the ventricle in 60% of subjects by a non-neural connection, the massa intermedia or interthalamic adhesion.

THE CEREBRAL AQUEDUCT
(see **Figs 2.15** and **2.16**)

This is a narrow channel connecting the posterior end of the third ventricle with the superior end of the fourth ventricle. Measuring 1.5 cm in length and 1–2 mm in diameter, it passes through the brainstem with the tectum (the quadrigeminal plate) posterior to it and the tegmentum and cerebral peduncles anteriorly. The nuclei of the third, fourth and fifth cranial nerves surround the aqueduct and are called the periaqueductal grey matter.

THE FOURTH VENTRICLE
(see **Figs 2.15** and **2.16**)

Posterior to the pons and the medulla, the aqueduct widens as the fourth ventricle and narrows again in the inferior part of the medulla as the central canal of the medulla and of the spinal cord.

The floor of the fourth of the fourth ventricle is diamond-shaped (the rhomboid fossa) and is formed by the posterior surface of the pons and of the upper part of the medulla. The roof is formed superiorly by the superior cerebellar peduncles, with the superior medullary velum between,

Fig. 2.16 Third and fourth ventricles and related midline sagittal structures.

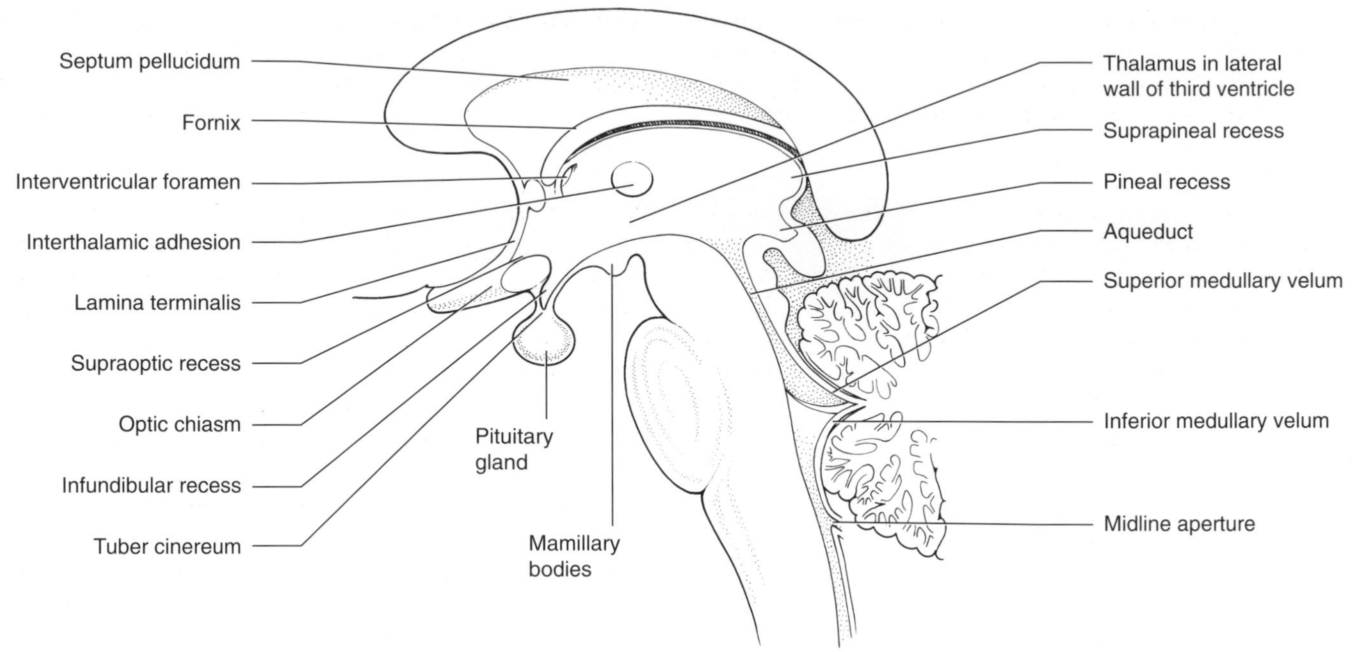

Septum pellucidum
Fornix
Interventricular foramen
Interthalamic adhesion
Lamina terminalis
Supraoptic recess
Optic chiasm
Infundibular recess
Tuber cinereum
Pituitary gland
Mamillary bodies
Thalamus in lateral wall of third ventricle
Suprapineal recess
Pineal recess
Aqueduct
Superior medullary velum
Inferior medullary velum
Midline aperture

and inferiorly by the inferior cerebellar peduncles and the inferior medullary velum. Over these lies the cerebellum.

In the lower part of the roof of the fourth ventricle there are three openings, one median and two lateral. The median aperture (of Magendie) is a large opening in the inferior medullary velum beneath the cerebellum, which communicates with the cisterna magna. The cavity of the fourth ventricle is prolonged laterally under the inferior cerebellar peduncle on each side as the lateral recesses of the ventricle. The lateral apertures (of Luschka) are at the apex of these recesses and open anteriorly just behind the eighth cranial nerve into the pontine cistern.

The fourth ventricle tends to be symmetrical in its anatomy (as do the third ventricle and the aqueduct) and minor asymmetry may be a sign of pathology.

The choroid plexus of the fourth ventricle invaginates the lower part of its roof and is supplied by a branch of the inferior cerebellar artery.

RADIOLOGICAL FEATURES OF THE VENTRICULAR SYSTEM

Skull radiographs

The ventricular system cannot be seen by plain skull radiography but the position of the lateral ventricles is often indicated in adults by calcification of its choroid plexus. This is seen on a lateral view in the parietal area about 2.5 cm above the pineal. On OF or FO views it is seen to be nearly always symmetrical and bilateral.

The normal position of the fourth ventricle is indicated by Twining's Line, which runs from the tuberculum sellae to the internal occipital protuberance. The midpoint of this line lies within the fourth ventricle near its floor.

Computed tomography

The ventricular system can be visualized on axial CT scans. Starting on the lowest cuts (see **Fig. 2.3a**), the fourth ventricle can be seen as a slit-like CSF-filled structure between the brainstem and the cerebellum. Sections taken through the midbrain (see **Fig. 2.3b**) may show the aqueduct with high-attenuation periaqueductal grey matter. The third ventricle becomes visible on higher cuts (see **Fig. 2.3c**) as a slit-like space between the thalami. At this level, the anterior horns of the lateral ventricles can be seen separated by the septum pellucidum with the head of the caudate nucleus indenting their lateral wall.

The posterior horns are visible also on this section and calcified choroid plexus is commonly seen in the trigone of the lateral ventricles. The temporal horns are not usually visible unless they are dilated. Higher cuts show the bodies of the lateral ventricles separated by the septum pellucidum or by the corpus callosum. The body and tail of the caudate nucleus can be seen as a high-attenuation structure in its lateral wall.

Magnetic resonance imaging (see Figs 2.5 and 2.6)

In the axial plane, anatomical features similar to CT images are seen; however, posterior fossa views are superior to CT because of the lack of bone artefact. Sagittal MRI images show the third ventricle, aqueduct and fourth ventricle in continuity with each other and with the central canal of the medulla and of the spinal cord. The communication of the fourth ventricle with the cisterna magna at the foramen of Magendie can also be seen. The recesses of the third ventricle can be seen particularly well on this view.

Ultrasound scanning of the neonatal brain

The anterior fontanelle is used as an acoustic window, and angled coronal and sagittal views of the ventricular system are obtained. In anterior coronal views (see **Fig. 2.7**), the frontal horns are seen as triangular in cross-section, with the medial wall indented by the head of the caudate nucle-

us. The echogenic roof is formed by the corpus callosum.

More posteriorly, the third ventricle may be seen as a slit-like space between the thalami. If not enlarged this space may not be visible in the normal scan. Superolateral communications with the lateral ventricles at the foramina of Monro can be identified. The bodies of the lateral ventricles are also approximately triangular in cross-section, indented inferiolaterally by the thalamus medially and the body of the caudate nucleus laterally. Between these is the thalamostriate groove, which contains echogenic choroid plexus posteriorly and the thalamostriate vein anteriorly. The mean width of the lateral ventricles is measured at the level of the body and is 9 mm in a 30-week premature infant and 12 mm in the full-term infant.

The *cava septi pellucidi and vergae* lie between the frontal horns and bodies of the two lateral ventricles. These are, in fact, a single structure with that part posterior to the foramen of Monro being named the cavum vergae. They are not normally connected with the remainder of the ventricular system and the term 'fifth ventricle', which is sometimes used, is therefore misleading. The cavum vergae begins to close from posterior to anterior in the sixth gestational month and progresses to complete obliteration of both spaces by 2 months of age in 85% of infants. Scans through the posterior part of the body of the lateral ventricle show echogenic divergent bands of the glomus of the choroid plexus. The fluid-filled ventricle around the choroid plexus is not always seen.

Midline sagittal scanning identifies the cavum septi pellucidi above and anterior to the third ventricle. The echogenic choroid plexus of the third ventricle can be seen with the interthalamic adhesion inferior to this. The aqueduct is seldom visible in the normal scan but the echogenic cerebellar vermis helps identify the roof and cavity of the fourth ventricle.

Parasagittal scans (see **Fig. 2.9**) show the full sweep of the lateral ventricle, with the choroid plexus in the floor of the body and in the roof of the inferior horn. The head of the caudate nucleus can be identified anteriorly, the thalamus posterior to this and the thalamocaudate notch between.

Pneumoencephalography and air or contrast ventriculography

These have been replaced by the imaging modalities of CT, MRI and ultrasound scanning for visualization of the ventricles.

THE SUBARACHNOID CISTERNS (Fig. 2.17)

Since the brain and the skull show marked differences in shape, the subarachnoid space is deep in several places, particularly around the base of the brain. These deep spaces are called cisterns and are named according to nearby brain structures. They contain more CSF than the ventricles.

CISTERNA MAGNA (CEREBELLO-MEDULLARY CISTERN)

This lies behind the medulla and below the cerebellar hemispheres and receives CSF from the median aperture of the fourth ventricle. It is continuous through the foramen magnum with the spinal subarachnoid space, and continues superiorly for a variable distance behind the cerebellum. On each side, its lateral part contains the vertebral artery and its posterior inferior cerebellar branch.

PONTINE CISTERN

This lies between the pons and the clivus and is continuous below with the cisterna magna and above with the interpeduncular cistern. It receives CSF from the lateral apertures of the fourth ventricle. The pontine cistern contains the basilar artery and its pontine and labyrinthine branches.

INTERPEDUNCULAR CISTERNS

This cistern lies between the cerebral peduncles of the midbrain and the dorsum sellae. It is continuous below with the pontine cistern, laterally with the ambient cisterns and superiorly with the suprasellar cisterns. It contains the posterior part of the arterial circle of the base of the brain.

QUADRIGEMINAL CISTERN

This cistern lies posterior to the quadrigeminal plate of the midbrain. It lies between the splenium above and the vermis below and is limited posteriorly by the tentorium and falx. Also called the cistern of the great vein, it contains the venous confluence of the straight and inferior sagittal sinuses to form the great vein (of Galen), which in turn is joined by the internal cerebral and the basal vein on each side.

AMBIENT CISTERNS

These extend around both sides of the midbrain between the interpeduncular cistern anteriorly and the quadrigeminal cistern posteriorly. Lateral extensions of the superior part of the ambient cisterns around the posterior part of the thalamus are called the ambient wing

Fig. 2.17 The subarachnoid cisterns.

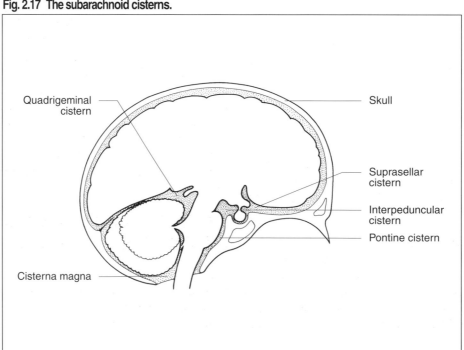

cisterns. The posterior cerebral artery and the basal vein lie in the anterior part of each ambient cistern.

SUPRASELLAR CISTERNS

This cistern is above and to the side of the pituitary fossa; it lies between the anterior part of the floor of the third ventricle above and diaphragma sellae below. It is continuous posteriorly with the interpeduncular cistern and extends laterally into the Sylvian cistern at the lower end of the Sylvian fissure. The optic nerves pass to the chiasm in the anterior part of the suprasellar cistern and the part of the cistern anterior to this is sometimes referred to as the chiasmatic cistern. The anterior part of the circle of Willis lies in the supersellar cistern.

PERICALLOSAL CISTERN

The suprasellar and chiasmatic cisterns continue superiorly as the cistern of the lamina terminalis and around the superior surface of the corpus callosum as the pericallosal cistern. This is in turn continuous posteriorly with the quadrigeminal cistern below the splenium. The pericallosal cistern contains branches of the anterior cerebral artery.

RADIOLOGICAL FEATURES OF THE SUBARACHNOID CISTERNS

Pneumoencephalography
The brain is imaged by viewing air in the cisterns. This is now replaced by CT scanning.

Computed tomography
The cisterns are visible on axial CT scanning as CSF-filled spaces between parts of the brain and the skull. On slices through the midbrain (see **Fig. 2.3b**) the interpeduncular, ambient and quadrigeminal cisterns are seen around the midbrain. Anterior to the interpeduncular cistern is the suprasellar cistern and posterior to the quadrigeminal cistern is the superior vermian cistern. On cuts at the level of the superior part of the lateral ventricles, the pericallosal cistern can be seen between the falx and the genu of the corpus callosum anteriorly, and between the splenium and the falx posteriorly.

Magnetic resonance imaging
The marked difference in relaxation constants between water and brain tissue results in particularly good demonstration of small structures in cisterns where they are surrounded by CSF. Thus the optic nerve and chiasm in the suprasellar cistern and the acoustic nerve in the pontine cistern and vessels in all cisterns are seen well on MRI.

Cervical myelography
Cisternal puncture may be used to introduce contrast media into the cisterna magna and the spinal subarachnoid space. A needle is introduced above level C2 and directed upwards. At a depth of about 3 cm the needle is felt to penetrate the atlanto-occipital membrane and to enter the cisterna magna. Structures at risk of injury by this procedure include the spinal cord and the medulla oblongata anterior to the cistern, and the posterior inferior cerebellar artery and its branches within the cistern.

CEREBROSPINAL FLUID PRODUCTION AND FLOW

The total volume of CSF is about 150 ml, 25 ml of which is within and around the spinal cord. It is produced at 0.4 ml per minute independent of CSF pressure. CSF is produced by the choroid plexuses of all ventricles but principally by that of the lateral ventricles. It flows through the interventricular foramina into the third ventricle, through the cerebral aqueduct to the fourth ventricle and from the ventricular system via the midline aperture into the cisterna magna and via the lateral apertures into the pontine cisterns. Some diffusion occurs with fluid from the spinal canal.

From the basal cisterns, some fluid flows down and bathes the spinal cord; the remainder passes upward through the tentorial hiatus and diffuses over the surface of the cerebral hemispheres. Pulsation of arteries within the cisterns may play a role in the directional flow of CSF.

CSF is absorbed through the arachnoid villi. These are herniations of arachnoid through holes in the dura into the venous sinuses. These are most numerous in the superior sagittal sinus and in its laterally projecting blood lakes. In the child, these villi are discrete; with age they aggregate into visible clumps called arachnoid granulations (Pacchionian granulations). These indent the inner table of the skull beside the dural venous sinuses.

About one-third of the CSF is either absorbed along similar spinal villi or escapes along nerve sheaths into the perineural lymphatics. This absorption is passive and dependant on hydrostatic pressure differences.

RADIOLOGICAL FEATURES OF CSF PRODUCTION AND FLOW

Knowledge of the circulatory pathway of CSF is important in diagnosis since ventricular dilation proximal to the point of obstruction of its flow indicates the site of the lesion. Thus a lesion obstructing the cerebral aqueduct causes dilatation of the lateral and third ventricles but not the fourth. Arachnoiditis blocking the exit foramina of the fourth ventricle causes dilatation of all four ventricles.

Skull radiographs

Arachnoid (Pacchionian) granulations are seen as relative translucencies or small bony defects. Tangential views show that they are indentations of the inner table only. They are most frequently found along the superior sagittal sinus but are also seen around the torcula (*cf.* venous sinuses). Calcium deposition can occur at the arachnoid granulations and may cause calcification, which is visible on plain films at these sites.

Radionuclide cisternography

The radionuclide is injected into the CSF via the lumbar route. After 1–3 hours the isotope can be seen in the basal cisterns — the cisterna magna, the pontine and interpeduncular cisterns and the quadrigeminal cistern. After 3–6 hours the radionuclide is seen in the Sylvian and interhemispheric fissures. By 24 hours activity surrounds the brain. In children, the CSF flow is more rapid, with the basal cisterns reached at 15-30 minutes and isotope surrounding the brain at 12 hours. At no time is activity normally seen within the ventricles.

Magnetic resonance imaging

MRI can be used to study flow phenomena of CSF, for example an abnormal degree of signal loss is seen in the aqueduct in normal pressure hydrocephalus.

MENINGES

Three layers of meninges cover the brain and spinal cord (*cf.* spinal meninges). These are, from without inwards — the dura mater, the arachnoid mater and the pia mater.

DURA MATER

This is a tough membrane described as having two layers. The outer layer is, in fact, the periosteum of the inner aspect of the skull and is continuous through all the foramina and sutures of the skull with the periosteum on the outside of the skull. The inner layer is the dura mater proper. This is, however, densely adherent to the outer layer, in all places except where the layers separate around the dural venous sinuses and where the inner layer projects inwardly as the falx cerebri and cerebelli, and as the tentorium cerebelli and the diaphragma sellae.

The *falx cerebri* is a sickle-shaped dural septum in the median sagittal plane attached to the crista galli in the midline of the floor of the anterior cranial fossa and along the midline of the inner aspect of the vault of the skull to the margins of the superior sagittal sinus. Posteriorly it is wider; here it is attached to the upper surface of the tentorium cerebelli enclosing the straight sinus. It projects into the interhemispheric fissure and its inferior free edge lies close to the corpus callosum. The inferior sagittal sinus is within this free edge.

The *diaphragma sellae* is a horizontal fold of dura that almost completely covers the pituitary fossa with a small opening for the pituitary stalk.

The *tentorium cerebelli* is a horizontal septum of dura mater that separates the occipital lobes from the superior surface of the cerebellum. Its posterior concave border is attached to each posterior clinoid process and along the upper border of the petrous bones, enclosing the superior petrosal sinus on each side. It is attached to the occipital bone along the margins of the transverse sinuses to the internal occipital protuberence. The anterior free edge of the tentorium, called the tentorial notch, is attached to the anterior clinoid processes and surrounds the midbrain. There is no venous sinus in this free edge. The tentorium is sloped upwards from its attached edge to its free edge and has a midline ridge where the falx cerebri is attached to its superior surface.

The *falx cerebelli* is a low elevation of dura that projects a small distance into the cerebellar interhemispheric fissure. It is attached from the internal occipital protuberence along the internal occipital crest to the posterior margin of the foramen magnum. The small occipital venous sinus lies in its attached edge.

ARACHNOID MATER

This layer of meninges is a delicate membrane, which is impermeable to CSF. It lines the dura mater, separated from it only by a thin layer of lymph in the subdural (potential) space. It is separated from the pia mater by the subarachnoid space, which contains the CSF. The arachnoid mater projects into the interhemispheric fissure and into the root of the Sylvian fissure but otherwise does not dip into the sulci. It surrounds the cranial and spinal nerves in a loose sheath so far as their exit from the skull and vertebral canal.

Arachnoid mater herniates through holes in the dura into the venous sinuses and venous lakes as arachnoid villi (*cf.* CSF absorption) and only in these villi is the arachnoid pervious to CSF.

PIA MATER

This meningeal layer is closely adherent to the brain surface and dips into all the sulci. It continues along all the cranial and spinal nerves and fuses with their epineurium. It is also invaginated into the surface of the brain by the entering cerebral arteries. It invaginates with the choroid vessels into the ventricles, and the layer of pia mater and ependyma together thus formed over these vessels is called the tela choroidea of the ventricles.

ARTERIAL SUPPLY OF THE MENINGES

The arterial supply is found mostly between the periosteal and inner layers of the dura mater. Most of the supratentorial dura is supplied by the middle meningeal artery with additional supply in:

- The anterior cranial fossa from meningeal branches of the ophthalmic and anterior and posterior ethmoid arteries; and
- Over the cavernous sinus by meningeal branches of the carotid artery and by the accessory meningeal artery from the maxillary artery, which passes through the foramen ovale.

The posterior fossa meninges are supplied by meningeal branches of the vertebral artery, with some additional supply from meningeal branches of the occipital artery through the mastoid and jugular foramina and from meningeal branches of the ascending pharyngeal artery through the jugular foramen and the hypoglossal canal.

THE NERVE SUPPLY OF THE MENINGES

The meninges are supplied supratentorially, mostly by the ophthalmic division of the trigeminal nerve with some supply in the middle cranial fossa by the maxillary and mandibular divisions of this nerve. In the posterior fossa, the meninges are supplied by meningeal branches of the ninth and tenth cranial nerves, with the dura around the foramen magnum being innervated by the C1–C3 nerves.

RADIOLOGICAL FEATURES OF THE MENINGES

Extradural haematoma

This occurs when a vessel in the extradural (potential) space between dura and bone is torn by trauma. In the majority of cases the middle meningeal artery is affected, and the resulting haematoma strips the dura mater from the skull in the area of the parietal bone.

Subdural haematoma

This is also due to traumatic bleed into a potential space, in this case the space between the dura mater and the arachnoid mater. Bleeding into this space occurs when a bridging vein is torn and, because the dura and arachnoid are not very adherent, blood can easily pass between them over a large area and tends to do so in a thin layer. The subdural space and therefore subdural haematoma can extend into the interhemispheric fissure and the root of the Sylvian fissure but not into the other sulci.

Subarachnoid haemorrhage

This occurs into the subarachnoid space between the arachnoid and pia mater from spontaneous or traumatic rupture of one of the vessels, usually an artery, in this space. Subarachnoid blood can then be seen in the cisterns and extending into the sulci and fissures on the brain surface close to the site of bleeding.

Skull radiographs

Dural calcification on skull radiographs is common in older subjects. This can occur anywhere over the vault but is difficult to see if close to the skull, unless tangential views are obtained. Calcification of the falx cerebri or of the tentorium can be seen on OF or FO views.

Computed tomography

Above the level of the petrous temporal bones (see **Fig. 2.3a**) the cerebral hemispheres are separated from the cerebellum by the tentorium. This is best seen on contrast-enhanced scans because of its contained venous sinuses. The tentorium is seen as a high-attenuation linear structure extending laterally from the midbrain to the inner table of the skull. Since the tentorium slopes upwards towards the tentorial notch, higher slices (see **Fig. 2.3b**) show the margins of the tentorium much closer to the midline. Only a small portion of the upper cerebellum and vermis and the superior vermian cistern are visible between these margins. The occipital lobes may meet the falx in the midline posterior to the tentorium on these slices giving a 'Y'-shaped configuration to the dural folds here.

The falx cerebri is seen on higher cuts (see **Fig. 2.3c**) anteriorly and posteriorly extending into the interhemispheric fissure almost to the corpus callosum.

ARTERIAL SUPPLY OF THE CNS (Figs 2.18–2.20)

The arterial supply of the CNS is derived from the internal carotid and vertebral arteries. Anastomoses exist between the internal and external carotid arteries but little or no supply to the normal brain is derived from the latter artery.

All arteries entering the surface of the brain are end arteries, that is, they have no precapillary anastomosis with other arteries and obstruction of these arteries causes infarct of the supplied territory (see **Fig. 2.18**).

Fig. 2.18 Distribution of the cerebral arteries: (a) superolateral surface of the cerebral hemisphere; (b) medial surface of the cerebral hemisphere.

Anterior cerebral artery

Middle cerebral artery

Posterior cerebral artery

(a)

Posterior cerebral artery

Anterior cerebral artery

(b)

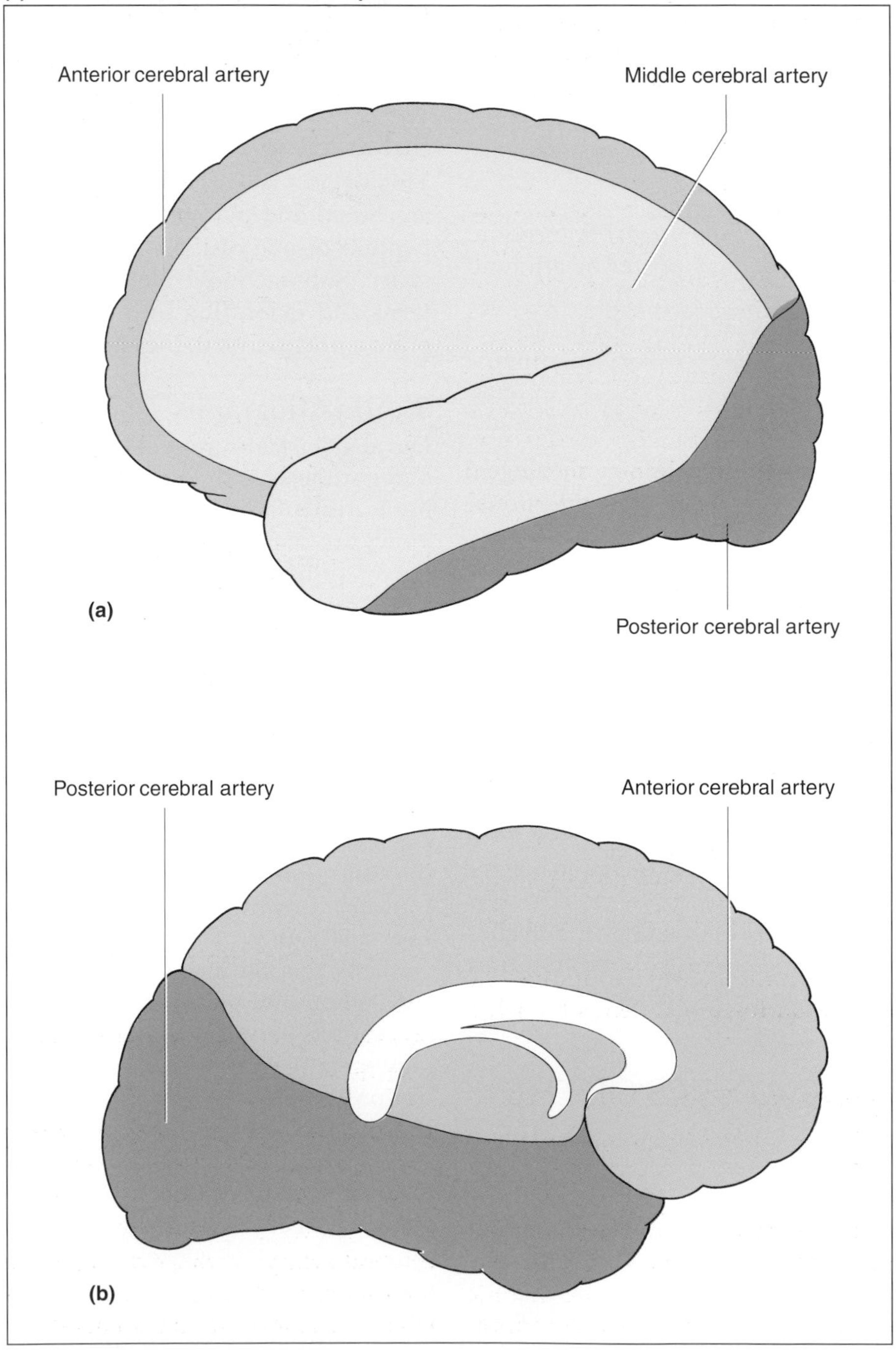

INTERNAL CAROTID ARTERY
(see **Figs 2.19** and **2.20**)

(See also the section on the carotid artery in neck.)

Once the carotid artery enters the carotid canal it has a very tortuous course — six bends in all before its terminal division. The reason for this tortuosity is unknown but it may have a role in reducing the pulsating force of the blood supply to the brain.

The artery passes forwards and medially in the petrous bone where it is separated from the middle and inner ear by only a thin plate of bone. It then passes upwards in the foramen lacerum in the middle cranial fossa into the cavernous sinus. The artery travels anteriorly in the cavernous sinus with the third, fourth, sixth and the ophthalmic division of the fifth cranial nerves on its lateral side (see **Fig. 2.11**). The sympathetic nerves around this part of the artery are called the cavernous plexus and these supply branches to the eye. Anteriorly, in the cavernous sinus, the artery curves upwards again and pierces the dura and arachnoid mater to enter the subarachnoid space medial to the anterior clinoid process. The artery then turns posteriorly and finally curves upwards and divides into the anterior and middle cerebral arteries at the anterior perforated substance. The cavernous and supraclinoid portions of the internal carotid artery are referred to as the carotid siphon.

BRANCHES OF THE INTERNAL CAROTID ARTERY

The cervical portion has no branches. Two small branches each arise from the petrous and cavernous parts of the internal carotid artery. These are seldom visible on angiography. These are:

- The caroticotympanic artery to the ear drum;
- The pterygoid artery to the pterygoid canal and plate;
- The cavernous artery to the walls of the cavernous sinus; and
- The meningohypophyseal artery, which supplies the dura of the anterior cranial fossa and sends branches to the pituitary.

Ophthalmic artery (see Fig. 2.20)
This is the first large (visible on angiography) branch of the internal carotid artery and is its first branch after emerging from the cavernous sinus. It passes anteriorly and enters the optic foramen inferior and lateral to the optic nerve. It then crosses the optic nerve superiorly and passes to the medial wall of the orbit. The ophthalmic artery supplies the orbital contents and also has supra-

Fig. 2.19 The arterial circle of Willis and arteries of the brainstem.

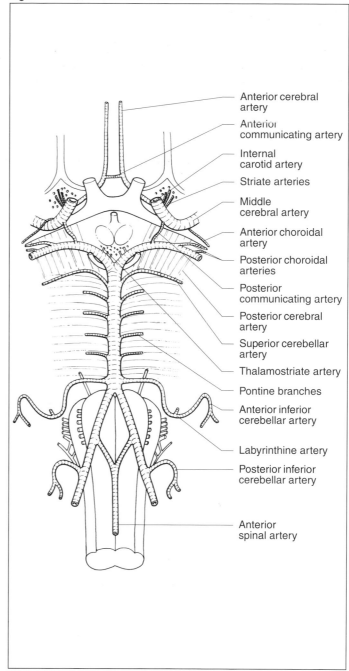

- Anterior cerebral artery
- Anterior communicating artery
- Internal carotid artery
- Striate arteries
- Middle cerebral artery
- Anterior choroidal artery
- Posterior choroidal arteries
- Posterior communicating artery
- Posterior cerebral artery
- Superior cerebellar artery
- Thalamostriate artery
- Pontine branches
- Anterior inferior cerebellar artery
- Labyrinthine artery
- Posterior inferior cerebellar artery
- Anterior spinal artery

trochlear and supraorbital branches to supply the skin over the eyebrow.

Posterior communicating artery
This runs posteriorly to anastomose with the posterior cerebral artery. Although usually small, this artery is occasionally so large on one side that the posterior cerebral artery on this side can be said to arise from the internal carotid artery. Such an artery is referred to as a fetal posterior communicating artery.

Fig. 2.20 Internal carotid angiogram: (a) AP view; (b) lateral view. The posterior communicating artery does not fill in this case.

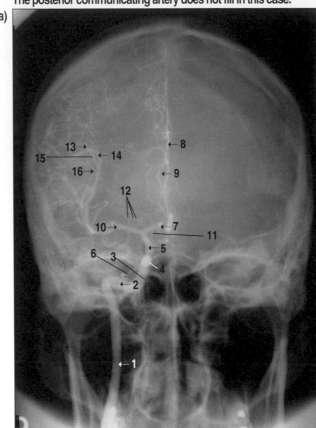

(a)

1. Internal carotid artery in the neck
2. Petrous part of the internal carotid artery (carotid canal)
3. Cavernous part of the internal carotid artery
4. Carotid siphon
5. Intracranial part of the internal carotid artery
6. Ophthalmic artery
7. A1 segment of the anterior cerebral artery
8. Pericallosal artery
9. Callosomarginal artery
10. Middle cerebral artery
11. Anterior choroidal artery
12. Lenticulostriate arteries: medial and lateral
13. Sylvian point
14. Posterior parietal artery
15. Angular artery
16. Posterior temporal artery

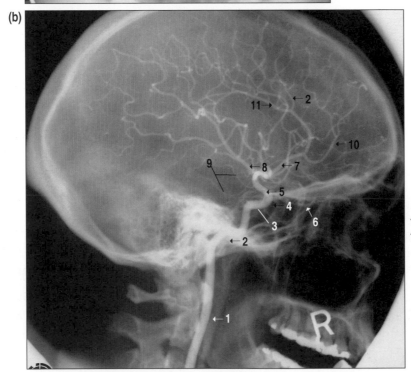

(b)

1. Internal carotid artery in the neck
2. Internal carotid artery in the petrous bone
3. Internal carotid artery in the cavernous sinus
4. Carotid siphon
5. Intracranial part of the internal carotid artery
6. Ophthalmic artery
7. Anterior cerebral artery
8. Middle cerebral artery
9. Anterior choroidal branches
10. Callosomarginal artery
11. Pericallosal artery

Anterior choroidal artery

This vessel is small but is readily identifiable on angiograms. It passes posteriorly giving branches to the crus cerebri and to the lateral geniculate body before entering the lateral ventricle at the anterior tip of its inferior horn to supply the choroid plexus of this ventricle (along with the posterior choroidal arteries of the posterior cerebral artery). It supplies branches also to the basal ganglia and to the hippocampus.

Striate arteries

These are perforating arteries to the lentiform and caudate nuclei and the internal capsule.

The terminal division of the internal carotid artery is into the anterior cerebral and middle cerebral arteries.

Anterior cerebral artery

This arises from the internal carotid artery at the anterior perforated substance and passes anteriorly, superior to the optic chiasm. It winds around the genu of the corpus callosum and passes posteriorly on its superior surface to supply the medial and superolateral aspect of the cerebral hemisphere posteriorly so far as the parieto-occipital surface (see **Fig. 2.18**).

The branches are as follows:

■ *Recurrent artery (of Heubner)* — the only branch of the precommunicating segment, this artery passes posteriorly and gives branches to the lentiform nucleus;
■ *Anterior communicating artery* — this joins it to the anterior cerebral of the other side;
■ *Frontopolar artery* — this arises before the vessel curves over the superior surface of the corpus callosum. It passes anterosuperiorly towards the anterior pole of the frontal lobe;
■ *Callosomarginal artery* — this arises near the genu and passes up to the superior border of the hemisphere at the frontoparietal region;
■ *Pericallosal artery* — this is the continuation of the anterior cerebral artery on the superior surface of the corpus callosum; and
■ *Central branches* — these travel to the corpus callosum, the septum pellucidum, the anterior part of the lentiform nucleus and to the head of the caudate nucleus.

Middle cerebral artery

This is the largest and most direct of the branches of the internal carotid artery and is, therefore, the most prone to embolism. It passes laterally and ends as branches on the insula, the overlying opercula and most of the lateral surface of the cerebral hemisphere.

The branches of the middle cerebral artery are:

■ *Medial and lateral striate (or lenticulostriate) arteries* — these arise at the anterior perforated substance and are seen on AP angiograms arising from the upper surface of the middle cerebral artery trunk. They have a tortuous course superiorly, running at first medially for a short distance then laterally and finally medially again. On lateral angiograms they are usually hidden by overlying branches of the middle cerebral vessels. One of these branches tends to be larger than the others and is called the artery of cerebral haemorrhage as it is the artery of the brain most frequently ruptured. The striate arteries supply the basal ganglia and the anterior part of the internal capsule.
■ *Cortical branches* — these arise in the insula and pass superiorly and inferiorly to supply its surface before turning at a sharp angle to supply the inner surface of the overlying opercula and then exiting from the lateral fissure. They then turn again to emerge as branches that supply most of the lateral surface of the hemisphere as follows:
— Frontal branches;
— Parietal branches;
— Angular branches; and
— Superior temporal branches.

VERTEBROBASILAR SYSTEM (Fig. 2.21; see Fig. 2.19)

The vertebral artery arises from the posterosuperior aspect of the first part of the subclavian artery. The artery enters the foramen tranversarium of the sixth cervical vertebra (occasionally the seventh, fifth or fourth) and ascends through the foramina of the upper six (or seven, five or four) cervical vertebrae. Within the foramen, the artery passes anterior to the ventral ramus of the spinal nerve and is accompanied by sympathetic nerves from the inferior cervical ganglion and a plexus of veins that unite inferiorly to form the vertebral vein. Having exited from its foramen, the vertebral artery passes posterior to the lateral mass of the atlas and enters the skull through the foramen magnum. It pierces the dura and arachnoid mater and passes anterior to the medulla until it unites with its fellow at the lower border of the pons.

Fig. 2.21 Vertebral angiogram: (a) AP view; (b) lateral view.

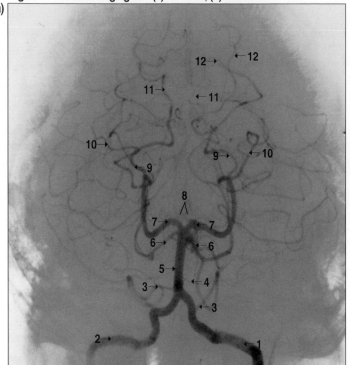

1. Left vertebral artery
2. Right vertebral artery (reflux of contrast)
3. Posterior inferior cerebellar artery
4. Anterior inferior cerebellar artery
5. Basilar artery
6. Superior cerebellar artery
7. Posterior cerebral artery
8. Thalamoperforate branches
9. Internal occipital artery
10. Posterior temporal artery
11. Calcarine branch of the internal occipital artery
12. Parieto-occipital branch of the internal occipital artery

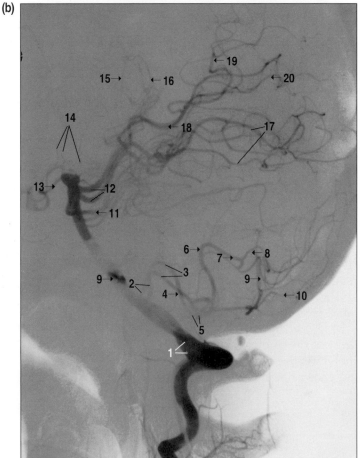

1. Vertebral artery
2. Posterior inferior cerebellar artery (PICA) — anterior medullary segment
3. Lateral medullary segment of PICA
4. Posterior medullary segment of PICA
5. Inferior tonsillar loop of PICA
6. Supratonsillar loop of PICA
7. Retrotonsillar segment of PICA
8. Vermis branch of PICA
9. Tonsillohemispheric branch of PICA
10. Hemispheric branch
11. Superior cerebellar artery
12. Posterior cerebral artery
13. Posterior communicating artery
14. Thalamoperforate branches of posterior cerebral artery
15. Medial posterior choroidal branches
16. Lateral posterior choroidal branches (arise distal to **15**)
17. Superior vermian branches of **11**
18. Internal occipital branch of **12**
19. Parieto-occipital artery
20. Calcarine artery

In the neck the branches (small branches rarely seen on angiograms) are as follows:

■ *Spinal branches* to the vertebrae and passing into the intervertebral foramina help to supply the spinal cord; and
■ *Muscular branches* to the deep muscles of the neck. These anastomose with the branches of the occipital and ascending pharyngeal arteries.

Within the skull the branches are as follows:
■ *Meningeal branch* to the cerebellar fossa and falx;
■ *Posterior spinal artery* (more frequently arises from PICA), descends as two branches anterior and posterior to the dorsal roots;
■ *Anterior spinal artery* unites with its fellow anterior to the medulla and descends as a single anterior spinal artery;
■ *Small branches to the medulla oblongata;*
■ *Posterior inferior cerebellar artery (PICA)* — the largest branch of the vertebral artery. It is occasionally absent. This artery has a tortuous course passing posteriorly and ascending at first to the lower border of the pons. It then courses inferolaterally around the fourth ventricle to reach the inferior surface of the cerebellum in the midline. It supplies branches to the lateral part of the medulla and to the choroid plexus of the fourth ventricle. PICA terminates as:
■ The *medial branch (inferior vermian artery)* to the inferior vermis and adjacent inferior surface of the cerebellar hemispheres; and
■ The *lateral branch* to the lateral aspect of the inferior surface of the cerebellum.

BASILAR ARTERY

Formed by the union of the two vertebral arteries at the lower border of the pons, the basilar artery lies close to (but seldom exactly in) the midline, anterior to the pons in the pontine cistern. When it deviates away from the midline it does so to the side away from that of a dominant vertebral artery.

The branches of the basilar artery are as follows:

■ *Pontine artery* — these are several small branches to the adjacent pons;
■ *Labyrinthine (internal auditory) artery,* which is a small branch (not visible on angiography) to the IAM with the seventh and eight cranial nerves;
■ *Anterior inferior cerebellar artery (AICA),* which runs laterally and posteriorly. It supplies the anterior and lateral aspect of the undersurface of the cerebellum and may form a loop into and out of the IAM with the labyrinthine artery arising from the summit of the loop;
■ *Superior cerebellar artery,* which arises very close to the terminal division of the basilar artery and runs laterally around the cerebral peduncle of the midbrain to the superior surface of the cerebellum, which it supplies. This artery also sends branches to the pons and to the pineal gland; and
■ *Right and left posterior cerebral arteries* — the basilar artery terminates by dividing into these.

POSTERIOR CEREBRAL ARTERIES

The posterior cerebral artery receives the posterior communicating artery of the internal carotid artery to complete the circle of Willis. It runs laterally and posteriorly around the cerebral peduncle parallel and superior to the superior cerebellar artery, and separated from this artery laterally by the tentorium. It reaches the inferior surface of the occipital lobe and supplies this and the inferior part of the temporal lobe.

The branches of the posterior cerebral artery are as follows:

■ *Small branches* to cerebral peduncle, the posterior thalamus, the medial geniculate body and the quadrigeminal plate.
■ *Thalamostriate arteries* — branches that enter the posterior perforated substance to supply the thalamus and the lentiform nucleus.
■ *Medial and lateral posterior choroidal arteries* — one medial and one or two lateral arteries on each side. These pass around the lateral geniculate body supplying branches to this, to reach the posterior part of the inferior horn of the lateral ventricle to supply (with the anterior choroidal artery) the choroid plexus of this ventricle.

Cortical branches are as follows:

■ The *posterior temporal branch*, which supplies the inferior aspect of the posterior part of the temporal lobe; and

■ The *internal occipital branch*, which passes to the medial aspect of the occipital lobe and divides terminally into *calcarine and parieto-occipital arteries*.

THE ARTERIAL CIRCLE OF WILLIS (Fig. 2.22; see Fig. 2.19)

This anastomosis between right and left internal carotid arteries, their branches and the posterior cerebral arteries forms a circle that encloses the optic chiasm and the pituitary stalk in the suprasellar and interpeduncular cisterns. The arteries taking part can be identified in **Fig. 2.19**.

The circle of Willis is subject to many variations, most commonly involving the posterior communicating artery. This vessel may be hypoplastic (22%) or may be large and associated with reduction in size of the proximal part of the ipsilateral posterior cerebral artery so that the posterior cerebral artery effectively receives its supply from the middle cerebral artery (15%). Such an artery is called a 'fetal' posterior communicating artery. Other variants include a hypoplastic anterior communicating artery (3%) or hypoplastic proximal segment of the anterior cerebral artery on one side, with both anterior cerebral vessels supplied from that of the other side (2%).

RADIOLOGICAL FEATURES OF THE ARTERIAL SUPPLY OF THE CNS

Plain radiographs

The arteries are not visible unless calcified. This occurs most commonly in the carotid siphon near the pituitary fossa.

Angiography of the carotid and vertebral system (see Figs 2.20 and 2.21)

This can be achieved via the aortic arch by a single femoral artery injection. The internal (or common) carotid arteries are catheterized in turn and views of both vertebral arteries are usually possible via contrast injection into one vertebral artery, with retrograde filling of the other from the basilar artery. The left vertebral artery is catheterized first since the vertebral arteries are often unequal in size and the right vertebral artery is bigger in only 20% of cases. Variation also occurs in the origin of

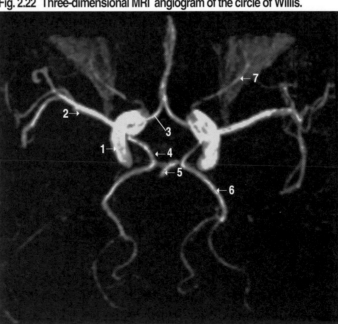

Fig. 2.22 Three-dimensional MRI angiogram of the circle of Willis.

1. Internal carotid artery
2. Middle cerebral artery
3. Anterior cerebral artery
4. Posterior communicating artery
5. Basilar artery
6. Posterior cerebral artery
7. Ophthalmic artery

the vertebral artery with the left vertebral artery arising directly from the arch of the aorta, between the origins of the left common carotid and left subclavian arteries in 5% of cases (see also aortic arch).

On the lateral view of the internal carotid angiogram (see **Fig. 2.20b**) the sharp angulation of the branches of the middle cerebral artery at the upper and lower borders of the insula approximately form a triangle, which is called the *Sylvian triangle.*

The uppermost point of these vessels as seen on AP views (see **Fig. 2.20a**) is called the *Sylvian point.* The Sylvian vessels and the Sylvian points should appear symmetrical on both sides.

The *arterial supply of the right and left side of the brain* are connected at the anterior communicating artery and at the union of the vertebral arteries as the basilar artery. Competence of these communications is demonstrated angiographically by selectively injecting contrast into one carotid artery while maintaining steady pressure on that of the other side.

Computed tomography

Contrast enhancement aids visualization of vessels on CT scanning. On scans at the level of the pons (see **Fig. 2.3a**) the basilar artery is visible in the pontine cistern between the clivus and the pons. It may deviate from the midline towards the side of the dominant vertebral artery.

At the level of the suprasellar cistern (see **Fig. 2.3b**) some of the vessels of the circle of Willis, particularly the posterior cerebral arteries as these wind around the midbrain, may be seen.

The anterior cerebral arteries and its branches may be seen in the interhemispheric fissure (see **Fig. 2.3b**). Branches of the middle cerebral artery may be identified in the Sylvian fissure.

Magnetic resonance imaging

This is good for visualization of vessels. Vessels in cisterns are particularly well seen because of the difference between the relaxation constants of CSF (water) and that of the vessel wall. MRangiography allows visualization of the Circle of Willis and its branches (see **Fig. 2.22**).

Ultrasound

On neonatal ultrasound of the brain, the collagen sheaths of the vessels give them echogenicity, and on real-time studies, pulsation of the middle cerebral vessels can be seen in the insula. The anterior cerebral artery can be seen in the interhemispheric fissure on coronal scanning and, on parasagittal scanning, the pericallosal and callosomarginal may be identifiable.

Radionuclide cerebral angiogram

During the arterial phase in the AP position a five-pointed star pattern is formed by the two carotid arteries, the two middle cerebral arteries and by the two anterior cerebral arteries, which are superimposed upon each other.

VENOUS DRAINAGE OF THE BRAIN

The veins draining the central nervous system do not follow the same course as the arteries that supply it. Generally, venous blood drains to the nearest venous sinus, except in the case of that draining from the deepest structures, which drain to deep veins. These drain, in turn, to the venous sinuses.

VENOUS SINUSES (Fig. 2.23)

These are large low-pressure veins within the folds of dura — between fibrous dura and endosteum except for the inferior sagittal and the straight sinuses which are between two layers of fibrous dura. They receive blood from the brain and the skull (diploic veins) and communicate with veins of the scalp and face (emissary veins).

The *superior sagittal sinus* starts anteriorly and runs posteriorly in the midline to the internal occipital protuberence. Veins enter the sinus obliquely against the flow of blood. Three or four venous lakes project laterally from the sinus between the dura and the endosteum. Into these the arachnoid (Pacchionian) granulations and villi project to return CSF to the blood. Posteriorly the sinus turns to one side, usually the right, to become the transverse sinus.

The *inferior sagittal sinus* runs in the lower free edge of the falx cerebi. Posteriorly it joins with the great cerebral vein to become the straight sinus.

The *straight sinus* runs in the tentorium where the falx is attached to it to the internal occipital protuberence — the confluence of the sinuses (torcula herophili). Here it turns to one side, usually the left, to become the transverse sinus.

The *transverse and sigmoid sinuses* — the transverse sinuses run right and left from the confluence of the sinuses to the mastoid bone where they turn inferiorly and become the sigmoid sinus (the transverse and sigmoid sinus are sometimes referred to together as the lateral sinus) which continues at the jugular foramen as the internal jugular vein. A focal dilatation of the vein within the foramen is called the jugular bulb.

The *cavernous sinus* (see **Fig. 2.11**) — this sinus is on either side of the pituitary gland and the body of the sphenoid bone connected across the midline by intercavernous sinuses. The carotid artery passes through this sinus as do the third, fourth and sixth cranial nerves and the ophthalmic and maxillary divisions of the fifth. After emerging from the sinus the carotid artery folds back on itself so that it comes to lie on the roof of the sinus. Above

Fig. 2.23 Superficial cerebral veins and venous sinuses.

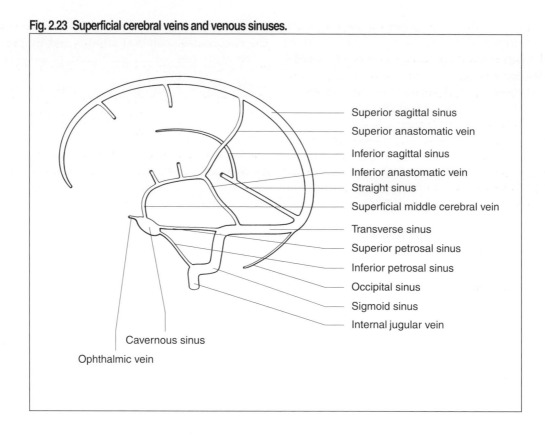

Superior sagittal sinus

Superior anastomatic vein

Inferior sagittal sinus

Inferior anastomatic vein

Straight sinus

Superficial middle cerebral vein

Transverse sinus

Superior petrosal sinus

Inferior petrosal sinus

Occipital sinus

Sigmoid sinus

Internal jugular vein

Cavernous sinus

Ophthalmic vein

the sinus lies the optic tract. The cavernous sinus receives the ophthalmic vein, the sphenoid sinus and the superficial middle cerebral vein and drains via the petrosal sinuses to the sigmoid sinus and the beginning of the internal jugular vein.

The *superior petrosal sinus* runs from the cavernous to the transverse sinus in the attached margin of the tentorium on the superior border of the petrous part of the temporal bone.

The *inferior petrosal sinus* runs from the cavernous sinus to the transverse sinus at the base of the petrous temporal bone.

SUPERFICIAL CEREBRAL VEINS (see **Fig. 2.23**)

These veins are very variable. They drain to the nearest dural sinus — thus the superolateral surface of the hemisphere drains to the superior sagittal sinus while the posteroinferior aspect drains to the transverse sinus. These named veins are variably seen:

- *The superior anastomostic vein (of Trolard)*, which runs from the posterior end of the lateral sulcus posterosuperiorly to the superior sagittal sinus in the parietal region;
- *The inferior anastomotic vein (of Labbé)*, which runs posteroinferiorly from the posterior end of the lateral sulcus to the transverse sinus; and
- *The superficial middle cerebral vein*, which runs anteriorly along the lateral sulcus to drain via the sphenoid sinus to the cavernous sinus.

DEEP CEREBRAL VEINS (**Fig. 2.24**)

Three veins unite just behind the interventricular foramen (of Monro) to form the internal cerebral vein. These are:

- *The choroid vein*, which runs from the choroid plexus of the lateral ventricle;
- *The septal vein*, which runs from the region of the septum pellucidum in the anterior horn of the lateral ventricle; and
- *The thalamostriate vein,* which runs anteriorly in the floor of the lateral ventricle in the thalamostriate groove between the thalamus and the lentiform nucleus.

The point of union of these veins is called the venous angle.

The *internal cerebral veins* of each side run posteriorly in the roof of the third ventricle and unite beneath the splenium of the corpus callosum to form the great cerebral vein.

The *great cerebral vein (of Galen)* is a short (1-2 cm long), thick vein that passes posterosuperiorly behind the splenium of the corpus callosum in the quadrigeminal cistern. It receives the basal veins and posterior fossa veins and drains to the anterior end of the straight sinus where this unites with the inferior sagittal sinus.

The *basal vein (of Rosenthal)* begins at the anterior perforated substance by the union of three veins:

■ The anterior cerebral vein, which accompanies the anterior cerebral artery;
■ The deep middle cerebral vein from the insula; and
■ The striate veins from the inferior part of the basal ganglia via the anterior perforated substance.

The basal vein of each side passes around the midbrain to join the great cerebral vein.

Fig. 2.24 Deep cerebral veins.

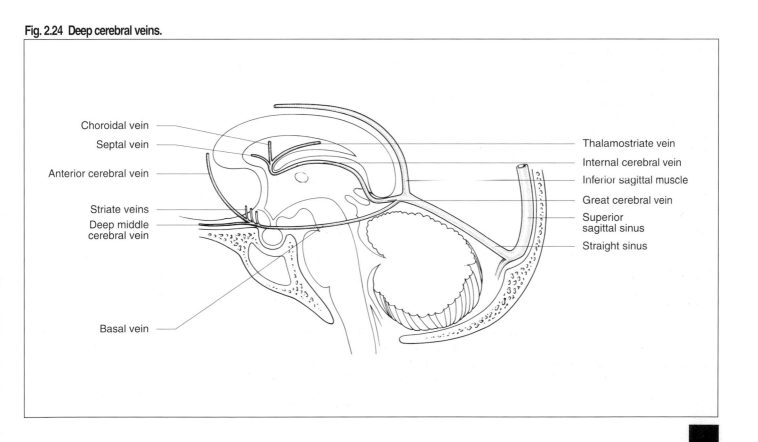

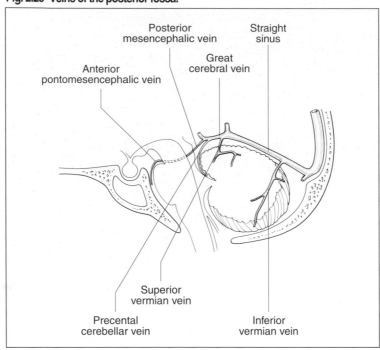

Fig. 2.25 Veins of the posterior fossa.

VEINS OF THE POSTERIOR FOSSA (Fig. 2.25)

The *anterior pontomesencephalic vein* runs on the anterior surface of the pons and midbrain in relation to the basilar artery. Inferiorly it drains via the petrosal veins to the superior petrosal sinuses. Superiorly this vein is connected to posterior mesencephalic vein.

The *posterior mesencephalic vein* runs around the upper midbrain to drain into the great cerebral vein.

The *precentral cerebellar vein* arises between the cerebellum and the posterior midbrain in the midline and passes superiorly to drain to the great cerebral vein.

The *superior vermian vein* drains also to the great vein while the *inferior vermian veins* (paired) drain to the straight sinus.

RADIOLOGICAL FEATURES OF THE CEREBRAL VEINS AND VENOUS SINUSES

Skull radiographs

The course of the venous sinuses can be seen where these groove the inner plate of bone. The arachnoid granulations may also indent the skull and show as lucencies on each side of the superior sagittal sinus on the skull radiograph (see section on the radiology of the skull, pp. 2–13).

Angiography during the venous phase (Fig. 2.26)

Superficial veins are seen to fill before deep veins and frontal veins before posterior veins. Of the superficial veins the superior or inferior anastomotic vein are often visualized but both are seldom seen on one angiogram. The deep veins are more constant than the superficial veins and were used to visualize the ventricular system before the widespread use of CT, with the thalamostriate vein indicating the size of the lateral ventricle, and the internal cerebral veins indicating the position of the roof of the third ventricle. Similarly, change in position of other deep veins may indicate the presence of a mass lesion nearby.

Contrast-enhanced computed tomography (see Fig. 2.3)

The tentorium and falx are seen as relatively hyperdense structures due to the venous sinuses that they enclose. Venous sinuses may also be seen at the internal occipital protuberence. On CT, at the level of the midbrain the posterior mesencephalic vein may be seen winding around

Fig. 2.26 Venous phase of internal carotid angiogram.

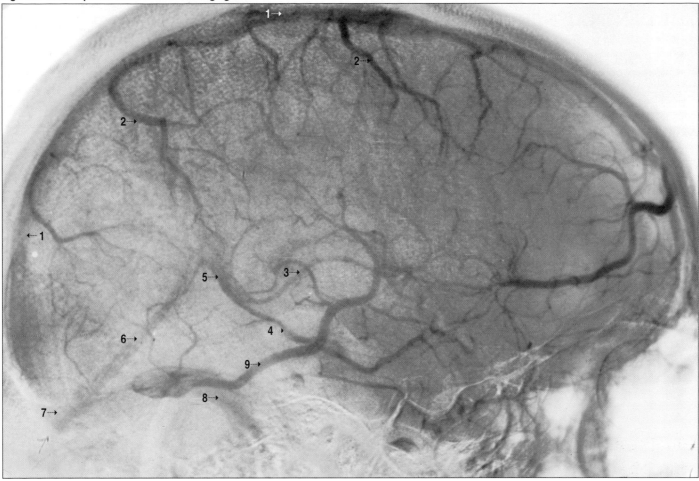

1. Sagittal sinus
2. Superficial cortical veins
3. Internal cerebral vein
4. Basal vein of Rosenthal
5. Great vein of Galen
6. Straight sinus
7. Torcula herophili (confluence of sinuses)
8. Transverse sinus
9. Inferior anastomotic vein of Labbé

the upper midbrain. In higher CT slices, the posterior end of the internal cerebral veins and the great cerebral vein may be seen in the quadrigeminal cistern.

Radionucleotide brain scans

Radionucleotide brain scans with diffusable tracers out-line vascular structures within the cranium. The venous sinuses are particularly well seen, especially the superior sagittal sinus and the transverse sinuses. That the right transverse sinus is usually bigger than the left is easily seen; however, enlargement of the left transverse sinus is seen in 30% of scans and is also normal.

CROSS-SECTIONAL ANATOMY OF THE CENTRAL NERVOUS SYSTEM

AXIAL SECTION THROUGH THE POSTERIOR FOSSA, PONS AND TEMPORAL LOBES (Fig. 2.27; see Fig. 2.3a)

At this level, the anterior cranial fossa is bounded by the frontal bone anteriorly and the frontal sinus can be seen within this. The middle cranial fossa is separated from the anterior fossa by the greater wing of the sphenoid bone on each side and is bounded laterally by the squamous part of the temporal bone. The occipital bone surrounds the posterior cranial fossa. The internal occipital protuberence, the site of the confluence of the venous sinuses, is seen in the midline posteriorly. The transverse sinus is usually visible in part near this. The petrous temporal bone extends anteromedially between the middle and posterior cranial fossae. The clivus forms the bony anterior boundary of the posterior cranial fossa in the midline.

A variable amount of frontal lobes separated by the interhemispheric fissure are seen in the anterior third of this scan if the level is above the orbital plate of the frontal bone. In the middle cranial fossa, the temporal lobes are seen and the temporal horns of the lateral ventricle may be distinguished within these. In the posterior fossa, the pons lies anteriorly in the midline. The prepontine cistern containing the basilar artery separates the pons from the clivus. The cerebellum occupies the remainder of the posterior fossa with the vermis in the midline and the hemispheres laterally. The pons is separated from the cerebellum in the midline by the fourth ventricle and connected to the cerebellum by the middle cerebellar peduncles on each side.

Fig. 2.27 Axial CT scan: level of the pons.

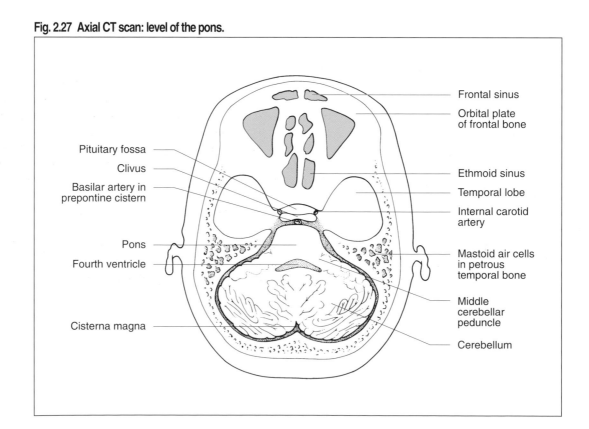

Fig. 2.28 Axial CT scan: level of the midbrain.

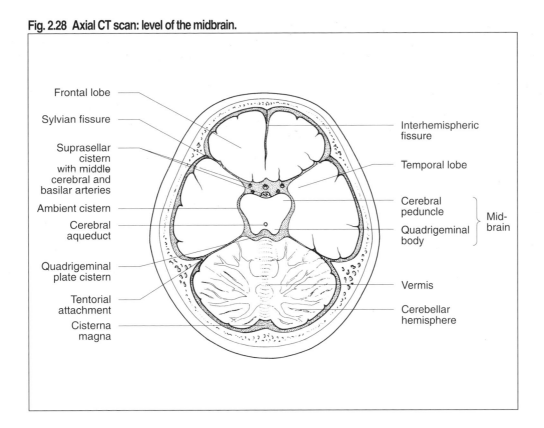

AXIAL SECTION AT THE LEVEL OF THE MIDBRAIN (**Fig. 2.28**; see **Fig. 2.3b**)

At this level, the brain is surrounded by the frontal bone anteriorly, the squamous temporal bones laterally and the occipital bone laterally.

The frontal lobes, separated by the interhemispheric fissure and the falx cerebri, occupy the anterior third of this cross-section. The temporal lobes lie in the middle third of the section and are separated from the frontal lobe by the Sylvian fissure. The middle cerebral artery and its branches can be seen within the Sylvian fissure. Posteriorly lies the cerebellum with its hemispheres and the midline vermis. The borders of the tentorium may be visible in contrast-enhanced scans, allowing distinction of the temporal and occipital lobes laterally from the cerebellum medially.

The midbrain is visible in the midline and the contours of the cerebral peduncles, separated by the interpeduncular cistern, can be seen on its anterior border. The ambient cistern surrounds the lateral aspects of the midbrain. The colliculi (quadrigeminal bodies) can be seen on the posterior aspect of the midbrain. The quadrigeminal plate cistern lies posterior to the colliculi. The great cerebral vein may be visible within this but is usually better seen on higher scans. In the posterior part of the midbrain the aqueduct may be visible.

Anterior to the midbrain is the hexagonally shaped suprasellar cistern. This contains the internal carotid artery and its branches, which form the circle of Willis.

Fig. 2.29 Axial CT scan: level of the third ventricle.

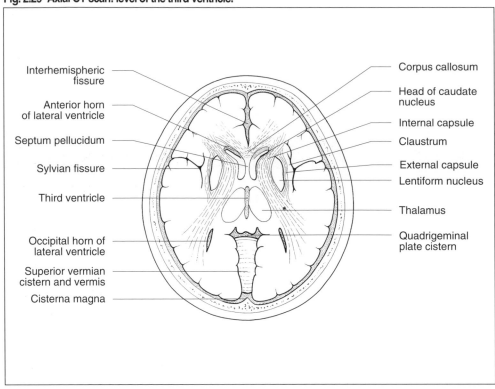

Labels (left side): Interhemispheric fissure; Anterior horn of lateral ventricle; Septum pellucidum; Sylvian fissure; Third ventricle; Occipital horn of lateral ventricle; Superior vermian cistern and vermis; Cisterna magna

Labels (right side): Corpus callosum; Head of caudate nucleus; Internal capsule; Claustrum; External capsule; Lentiform nucleus; Thalamus; Quadrigeminal plate cistern

AXIAL SECTION THROUGH THE THIRD VENTRICLE, THALAMI AND THE INTERNAL CAPSULES (Fig. 2.29; see Fig. 2.3c)

At this level, the brain is surrounded by the frontal bone anteriorly, the temporal and parietal bones laterally and the occipital bones posteriorly.

The ventricles and CSF cisterns are the most prominent features of this section. In the anterior part of the scan, the frontal horns of the lateral ventricle are seen close to the midline, separated by the thin septum pellucidum, the two walls of which may be separated to form the cavum septum pellucidum. The lateral wall of the frontal horn is concave where it is indented by the head of the caudate nucleus.

The trigones of the body of the lateral ventricles are seen posteriorly. The choroid plexus is prominent within this part of the ventricle and may be calcified.

The third ventricle is a narrow slit-like structure in the midline starting anteriorly just behind the frontal horns of the lateral ventricle. The interventricular foramina of Monro may be visible at this point.

The upper part of the quadrigeminal cistern, the cistern of the great veins can be seen with the posterior ends of the internal cerebral veins uniting here to form the great cerebral vein. The pineal gland lies within this cistern and the habenular commissure, if calcified, can be sometimes seen anterior to the pineal gland.

The anterior part of this section is occupied mostly by the frontal lobes, which are separated by the interhemispheric fissure and the falx cerebri. The middle third contains the basal ganglia, the thalamus and the internal capsule. The head of the caudate nuclei lie between the frontal horns of the lateral ventricles and the anterior limb of the internal capsule. The thalami lie on each side of the third ventricle and medial to the posterior limb of the internal capsule. The lentiform nucleus lies lateral to the internal capsule, with the globus pallidus situated medially and the putamen laterally. A thin sheet of grey matter, the claustrum, can be seen lateral to the putamen, separated from it by the external capsule and separated from the insula by the extreme capsule. The insula is the floor of the Sylvian fissure, and the part of the frontal, parietal and temporal lobes overlying this are called the opercula.

The posterior part of the temporal lobes and the occipital lobes occupy the posterior third of this cross-section. A small portion of the vermis and the superior vermian cistern can be seen in the midline between the leaves of the tentorium.

CHAPTER 3 *THE SPINAL COLUMN AND ITS CONTENTS*

Vertebral column

Joints of the vertebral column

Ligaments of the vertebral column

Intervertebral discs

Blood supply of the vertebral column

Spinal cord

Spinal meninges

Blood supply of the spinal cord

THE VERTEBRAL COLUMN

The vertebral column has 33 vertebrae — 7 cervical, 12 thoracic, 5 lumbar, 5 sacral (fused) and 4 coccygeal (fused) vertebrae.

The spine of the fetus is flexed in a smooth 'C' shape. This is referred to as the 'primary curvature' and is retained in the adult in the thoracic and sacrococcygeal areas. Secondary extension results in lordosis — known as the 'secondary curvature' — of the cervical and lumbar spine.

A TYPICAL VERTEBRA (**Fig. 3.1**; see **Figs 3.4** and **3.5**)

A typical vertebra has a vertebral body anteriorly and a neural arch posteriorly. The neural arch consists of pedicles laterally and of laminae posteriorly.

The pedicles are notched superiorly and inferiorly so that adjoining pedicles are separated by an intervertebral foramen, which transmits the segmental nerves. There are 31 segmental spinal nerves — 8 cervical, 12 thoracic, 5 lumbar, 5 sacral and 1 coccygeal. The first seven cervical nerves emerge above the correspondingly named vertebra; the others emerge below.

A transverse process arises at the junction of the pedicle and the lamina and extends laterally on each side. The laminae fuse posteriorly as the spinous process.

Articular processes project superiorly and inferiorly from each lamina. Articular facets on these processes face posteriorly on the superior facet and anteriorly on the inferior facet. The part of the lamina between the superior and inferior articular facets on each side is called the pars interarticularis.

THE CERVICAL VERTEBRAE

Typical cervical vertebra (Fig. 3.1)

The most distinctive feature is the presence of the foramen tranversarium in the transverse process. This transmits the vertebral artery (except C7) and its accompanying veins and sympathetic nerves.

Small lips are seen on either side of the superior surface of the vertebral body, with corresponding bevels on the inferior surface. Small synovial joints, called *neurocentral joints (of Luschka)*, are formed between adjacent cervical vertebral bodies at these sites.

The cervical vertebral canal is triangular in cross-section. The spinous processes are small and bifid, while the articular facets are relatively horizontal.

The atlas — C1 (Fig. 3.2)

The atlas has no body as it is fused with that of the axis to become the odontoid process. A lateral mass on each side has a superior articular facet for articulation, with the occipital condyles in the atlanto-occipital joint, also an inferior articular facet for articulation with the axis in the atlantoaxial joint.

The anterior arch of the atlas has a tubercle on its anterior surface and a facet posteriorly for articulation with the odontoid process.

Fig. 3.1 Cervical vertebra.

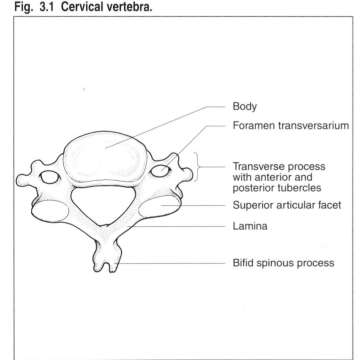

- Body
- Foramen transversarium
- Transverse process with anterior and posterior tubercles
- Superior articular facet
- Lamina
- Bifid spinous process

Fig. 3.2 The atlas: superior view.

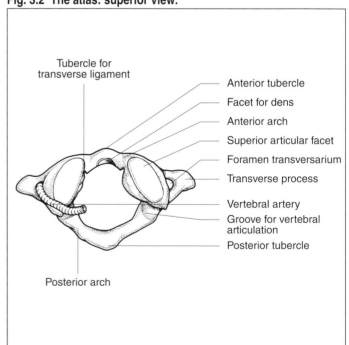

- Tubercle for transverse ligament
- Anterior tubercle
- Facet for dens
- Anterior arch
- Superior articular facet
- Foramen transversarium
- Transverse process
- Vertebral artery
- Groove for vertebral articulation
- Posterior tubercle
- Posterior arch

The posterior arch is grooved behind the lateral mass by the vertebral artery as it ascends into the foramen magnum.

The axis — C2 (Fig. 3.3)

The odontoid process, which represents the body of the atlas, bears no weight. Like the atlas, the axis has a large lateral mass on each side that transmits the weight of the skull to the vertebral bodies of the remainder of the spinal cord. Sloping articular facets on each side of the dens are for articulation in the atlantoaxial joint.

Vertebra prominens — C7

This name is derived from its long, easily felt, nonbifid spine. Its foramen tranversarium is small or absent and usually transmits only vertebral veins.

THE THORACIC VERTEBRAE (Fig. 3.4)

These have articular facets on the lateral aspect of the vertebral bodies for articulation with the ribs. A demifacet is found on the upper and lower aspect on each side

Fig. 3.3 The axis: (a) lateral view; (b) anterior view.

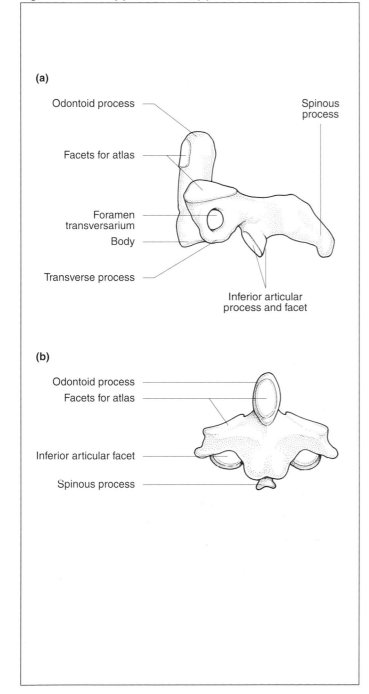

(a)

Odontoid process

Spinous process

Facets for atlas

Foramen transversarium

Body

Transverse process

Inferior articular process and facet

(b)

Odontoid process

Facets for atlas

Inferior articular facet

Spinous process

Fig. 3.4 Typical thoracic vertebra: (a) lateral view; (b) superior view.

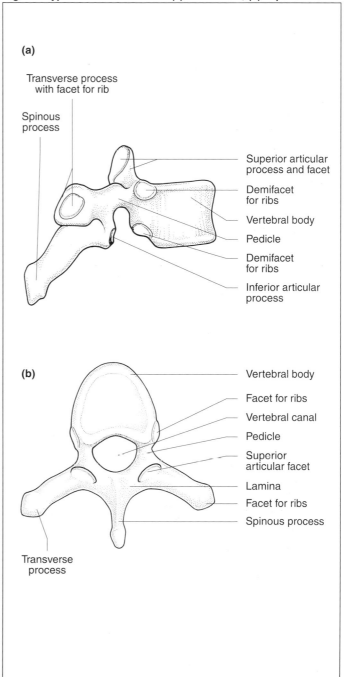

(a)

Transverse process with facet for rib

Spinous process

Superior articular process and facet

Demifacet for ribs

Vertebral body

Pedicle

Demifacet for ribs

Inferior articular process

(b)

Vertebral body

Facet for ribs

Vertebral canal

Pedicle

Superior articular facet

Lamina

Facet for ribs

Spinous process

Transverse process

Fig. 3.5 Typical lumbar vertebra: (a) lateral view; (b) superior view.

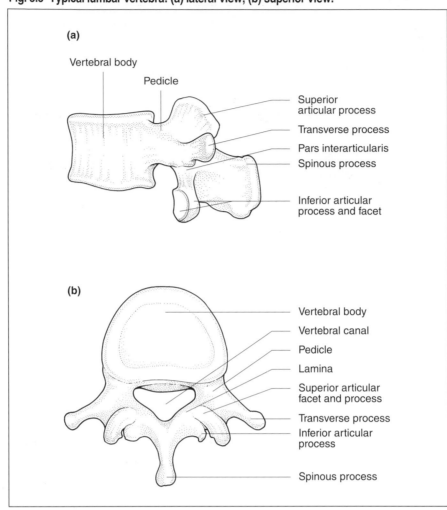

(a)

Vertebral body

Pedicle

Superior articular process

Transverse process

Pars interarticularis

Spinous process

Inferior articular process and facet

(b)

Vertebral body

Vertebral canal

Pedicle

Lamina

Superior articular facet and process

Transverse process

Inferior articular process

Spinous process

on T2–T10 vertebrae. T1 has a complete facet superiorly and a demi-facet inferiorly, while a single complete facet is seen at midlevel on T11 and T12. Articular facets are also found on the anterior surface of the transverse processes for the costotransverse articulations.

The spinous processes of the thoracic vertebrae are long and slope downward.

The facets on the articular processes are relatively vertical.

THE LUMBAR VERTEBRAE (Fig. 3.5)

These have bigger vertebral bodies and strong, square, horizontal spinous processes. The articular facets face each other in a sagittal plane.

The transverse processes of the upper four lumbar vertebrae are spatulate and increase in size from above downwards. The transverse process of the fifth lumbar vertebra is shorter but strong and pyramidal and, in contrast to those of the other vertebrae, does not arise from the junction of the pedicle and lamina but from the lateral aspect of the pedicle and the vertebral body itself.

THE SACRUM (Figs 3.6 and 3.7)

This is composed of five fused vertebrae. It is triangular in shape and concave anteriorly. A central mass is formed on the pelvic surface by the fused vertebral bodies. The superior border of the central mass is the most anterior

Fig. 3.6 The sacrum: (a) pelvic surface; (b) dorsal surface.

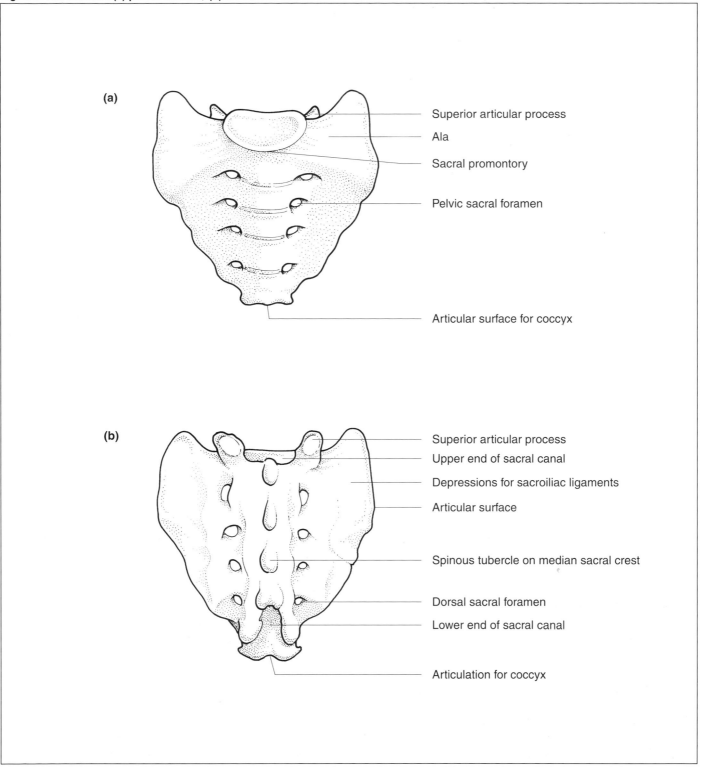

(a)

Superior articular process

Ala

Sacral promontory

Pelvic sacral foramen

Articular surface for coccyx

(b)

Superior articular process

Upper end of sacral canal

Depressions for sacroiliac ligaments

Articular surface

Spinous tubercle on median sacral crest

Dorsal sacral foramen

Lower end of sacral canal

Articulation for coccyx

part of the sacrum and is called the sacral promontory. Four anterior sacral foramina on each side transmit the sacral anterior primary rami. Lateral to these is the lateral mass of the sacrum, the upper anterior surface of which is called the ala of the sacrum.

On the posterior surface the laminae are also seen to be fused. The fusion of the spinous processes forms a median sacral crest. A sacral hiatus of variable extent inferiorly is caused by non-fusion of the laminae of S5 and often S4 in the midline. The transverse processes are rudimentary. Four posterior sacral foramina transmit the posterior primary rami. The sacral hiatus transmits the fifth sacral nerve.

Laterally there is a large articular facet, called the auricular surface, for articulation with the pelvis in the sacroiliac joint.

Differences between the male and female sacrum include:

- The width of the body of the first sacral vertebra is less than that of the ala in the female and wider in the male;
- The articular surface of the S1 joint occupies two vertebrae in the female and two-and-one-half vertebrae in the male; and
- The anterior surface of the female sacrum is flat superiorly and curves forward inferiorly, while that of the male is uniformly concave.

THE COCCYX

This comprises four vertebrae that are fused into a triangular bone that forms part of the floor of the pelvis.

Fig. 3.7 Lateral view of the sacrum showing the sacroiliac joint surface.

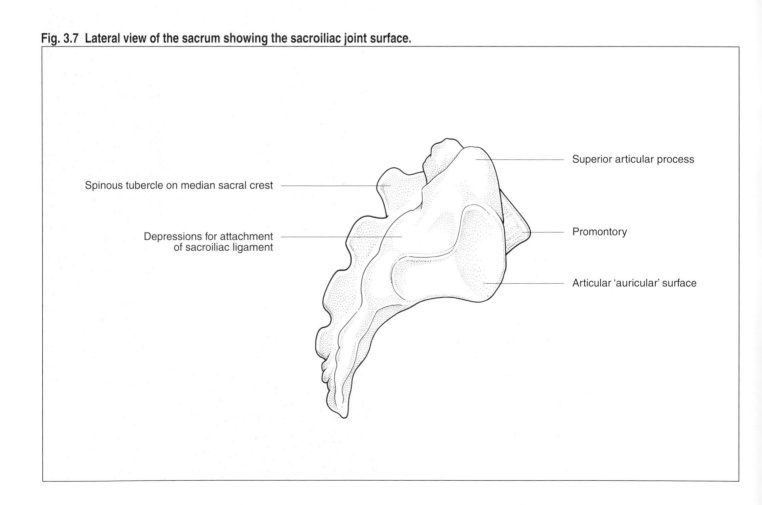

Spinous tubercle on median sacral crest

Depressions for attachment of sacroiliac ligament

Superior articular process

Promontory

Articular 'auricular' surface

RADIOLOGICAL FEATURES OF THE VERTEBRAE

Radiographs of the vertebral column (Figs 3.8 and 3.9)

The component parts of the vertebrae — the body, pedicles, laminae, and the transverse, articular and spinous processes — can be seen. Oblique views, particularly of the lumbar spine, are used for better visualization of the neural foramina and the pars interarticularis.

The point of exit of the basivertebral veins can be seen on lateral views as a defect in the cortex of the posterior surface of the vertebral body.

The anteroposterior (AP) *width of the spinal canal* is measured on a lateral film from the posterior cortex of the vertebral body to the base of the spinous process. The lower limit of normal is taken as 13 mm in the cervical spine at C5 level and 15 mm in the lumbar spine at L2.

The *interpedicular distance* is measured on AP views (and more easily on AP tomography) and reflects the

Fig. 3.8 AP radiograph of thoracic spine.

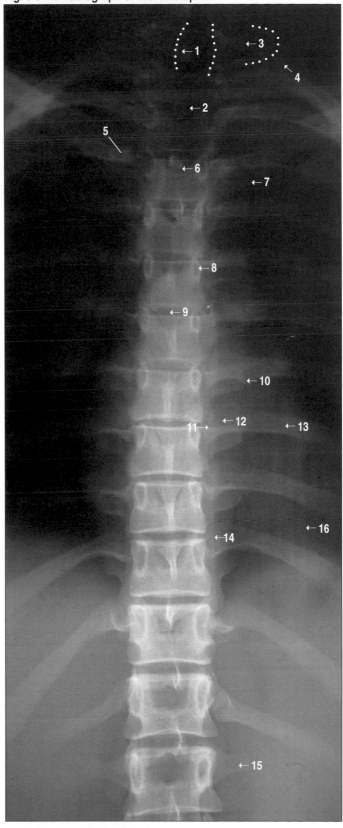

1. Trachea
2. Spinous process of C7
3. Left transverse process of C7
4. Tubercle of first rib, articulating with transverse process T1
5. Medial end of clavicle
6. Superior margin of manubrium sterni
7. Lateral margin of manubrium sterni
8. Left pedicle of T5
9. T5/T6 intervertebral disc space
10. Tubercle of seventh rib, articulating with transverse process of T7
11. Head of eighth rib
12. Neck of eighth rib
13. Shaft of eighth rib
14. Left paraspinal line
15. Left transverse process of L1
16. Dome of left hemidiaphragm

width of the spinal cord. It is maximum in the cervical spine at C5/C6 and in the thoracic spine at T12 since these are the sites of expansion of the cord for the limb plexuses.

Transitional vertebrae with features intermediate between the two types of typical vertebrae are developmental anomalies. These occur at the atlanto-occipital junction where the atlas may be assimilated into the occipital bone or where an extra bone may occur — known as the occipital vertebra. Transitional vertebrae may be found at the cervicothoracic junction at the level of C7; these may have long, pointed transverse processes with or without true rib (cervical rib) formation. Similarly, at the thoracolumbar junction, vestigial ribs may be seen on T12 or L1 vertebrae. At the lumbosacral junction, the last lumbar vertebra may be partly or completely fused with the sacrum — known as sacrilazation — or the first sacral segment may be separated from the remainder of the sacrum — known as lumbarization. In these cases it is important to avoid confusion in level identification, particularly prior to surgery.

Radiographs of the cervical spine

The alignment of the cervical spine with respect to the foramen magnum can be assessed radiographically. The following lines have been described:

- *Chamberlain's line* (on a lateral view): from the posterior tip of the hard palate to the posterior lip of the foramen magnum. Less than 2 mm of odontoid is normally above this;
- *McGregor's line* (on a lateral view): from the posterior tip of the hard palate to the base of the occiput (often easier to identify than the lip of the foramen magnum). Less than 5 mm of odontoid should lie above this; and
- *Digastric line* (on an OF view of the skull): the atlanto-occipital joints should be below a line between the digastric notches of both mastoid processes.

These relationships are abnormal in basilar invagination.

Radiographs of the thoracic spine (see Fig. 3.8)

In AP views of the thoracic spine, *paraspinal lines* are seen between the paravertebral soft-tissue shadows where these are covered with pleura and the air in the lungs. Only lymph nodes, intercostal vessels, sympathetic nerves and fat normally lie between the vertebrae and pleura so that displacement of the paraspinal lines on a radiograph is a marker of pathology in these structures or in the vertebrae (see also mediastinal lines).

Fig. 3.9 Oblique radiograph of lumbar spine.

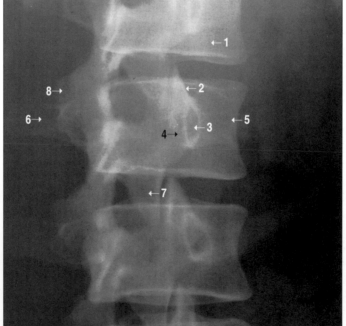

1. Vertebral body of L2
2. Superior articular process of L3
3. Pedicle of L3
4. Pars interarticularis
5. Transverse process of L3
6. Transverse process of L3
7. Inferior articular process of L3
8. Spinous process of L3

Radiographs of the lumbar spine

Anterior wedging of the L5 vertebra is a normal finding on lateral radiographs, as is narrowing of the L5/S1 disc space and should not be taken as a sign of disease.

Oblique views of the lumbar spine (see **Fig. 3.9**) are used to visualize the intervertebral foramina and the pars interarticularis.

Ossification of the vertebrae

Typical vertebrae have three primary ossification centres, the body and on each side of the neural arch. These appear in the eighth fetal week. Secondary centres appear for the upper and lower parts of the body, for each transverse process and for the spinous process at 16 years and fuse by the 25th year.

The atlas has only three primary ossification centres — one for the anterior arch and one each for each lateral mass. These unite at 6 years of age. Failure to fuse posteriorly results in a *posterior spina bifida.* Occasionally, there are two centres for the anterior arch that fuse at 8 years of age. Failure of fusion of these centres causes an *anterior spina bifida.*

The axis has two extra centres — those for the odontoid process. The odontoid process in adulthood may remain separated from the axis by a cartilaginous disc and simulate an ununited fracture.

The *seventh cervical vertebra* has also has two extra centres — for the attachment of costal processes on each side.

Lumbar vertebrae have extra primary centres for the mamillary processes on each side. In the lumbosacral spine, defects in ossification of the neural arch give rise to a *spina bifida defect* in 5–10% of the population. Other defects such as *persistent epiphysis in the transverse process* are also common and should not be mistaken for a fracture line.

Axial computed tomography (Figs 3.10 and 3.11)

The vertebral body anteriorly and the pedicles, laminae and spinous process posteriorly are seen as a bony ring around the spinal canal. Transverse processes are seen lateral to this and because they are not truly horizontal they appear separate from the remainder of the vertebra in several cuts.

Where the slice passes through the intervertebral foramen, it is seen as a gap between the body and the posterior vertebral elements. The intervertebral foramen being oval in shape appears narrower in cuts through its upper and lower ends.

The dimensions of the spinal canal can be measured directly. Lower limits of normal for the midsagittal distance is taken as 12–15 mm and 20 mm for the interpedicular distance. Other factors in spinal stenosis can also be determined, for example the soft-tissue elements such as the ligamenta flava, the thickness of the lamina (14 mm is the upper

Fig. 3.10 CT scan through L4 vertebral body.

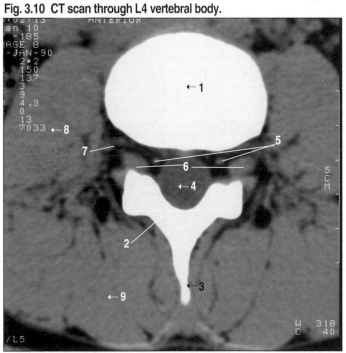

1. Body of L4
2. Right lamina of L4
3. Spinous process of L4
4. Thecal sac containing cauda equina
5. Epidural veins
6. Dorsal root ganglia of L4 nerve
7. Intervertebral foramen of L4/L5
8. Psoas muscles
9. Erector spinae muscles

Fig. 3.11 CT scan through L4/L5 intervertebral disc space.

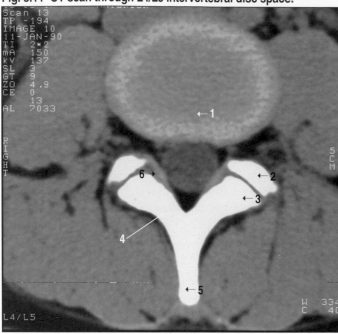

1. Disc of L4/L5
2. Inferior articular process of L4
3. Superior articular process of L5
4. Right lamina of L5
5. Spinous process of L5
6. Ligamentum flavum

limit of normal) and the development of bony spurs at the disc margins and at the facet joints.

Magnetic resonance imaging (Fig. 3.12)

MRI is widely used now to visualize the spinal column and its contents. T1-weighted spin-echo images give information on discs and vertebrae, the intervertebral foramina and facet joints and an outline of the spinal cord. The vertebrae have a low-signal outer rim surrounding the high-signal cancellous bone. The basivertebral veins are seen in the posterior midline of the vertebral body.

1. Pons
2. Medualla oblongata
3. Spinal cord
4. Cisterna magna
5. Prepontine cistem
6. Interpeduncular cistem
7. Cerebellum
8. Cerebellar tonsil
9. Occipital lobe
10. Arch of atlas
11. Odontoid process
12. Basivertebral vein of C3
13. C3/C4 disc space
14. Soft palate
15. Tongue
16. Epiglottis
17. Clivus
18. Sphenoid sinus

Fig. 3.12 MRI scan of the cervical spine: mid-sagittal section.

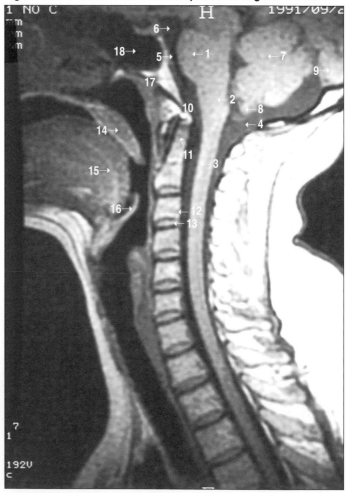

JOINTS OF THE VERTEBRAL COLUMN

Although the movement between individual vertebrae is small, the additive effect of this is great, allowing significant movement of the vertebral column. Maximum movement is at the atlanto-occipital and atlantoaxial joints and at the cervicothoracic and thoracolumbar junctions.

The joints between the vertebral bodies at the *inter vertebral discs* are secondary cartilaginous joints. The surface of the vertebral bodies in contact with the disc are coated with hyaline cartilage.

Small synovial joints between vertebral bodies called *neurocentral joints* occur in the cervical spine as already described.

Facet joints occur between the articular processes of the neural arches of the vertebrae. These are synovial joints with a simple capsule attached just beyond the margins of the articular surface. The capsules are looser in the cervical spine than in the thoracic or lumbar spine.

The *atlanto-occipital joint*, between the occipital condyle on each side of the foramen magnum and the superior articular surface of the atlas, is a synovial joint. A fibrous capsule surrounds the synovial membrane and is thickened posteriorly and laterally. In addition, the joint is strengthened by the anterior atlanto-occipital membrane (from the anterior margin of the foramen magnum to the anterior arch of the atlas) and by the posterior atlanto-occipital membrane (from the posterior margin of the foramen magnum to the posterior arch of the atlas). These joints act as a single joint and allow flexion and extension (nodding of the head) and some lateral motion.

Three joints make up the *atlantoaxial joint*:

- A small synovial joint between the anterior surface of the dens and the posterior aspect of the anterior arch of the atlas; and
- A synovial joint between each lateral mass of the atlas and of the axis.

These joints are strengthened by:

- The *membrana tectoria*, which is an upward continuation of the posterior longitudinal ligament from the axis to the anterior margin of the foramen magnum; and
- The *cruciform ligament*, which has a transverse band attached to the atlas and a vertical band anterior to the membrana tectoria from the posterior aspect of the body of the axis to the margin of the foramen magnum; and
- The *apical and alar ligaments* join the tip of the dens to the margin of the foramen magnum.

The atlantoaxial joint allows rotation about a vertical axis of the head and atlas on the axis.

The *sacroiliac joints* (see **Fig. 3.7**) between the auricular surfaces (so called because of their ear shape) of the sacrum and ilium on each side are true synovial joints with cartilage-covered articular surfaces and a synovial capsule. The articular surfaces have several elevations and depressions that fit into each other and contribute to the stability of the joint. The fibrous capsule is thickened posteriorly with the dense sacroiliac ligaments, which are the strongest ligaments in the body. Accessory ligaments include the iliolumbar ligament from the transverse process of the fifth lumbar vertebra to the iliac crest and the sacrotuberous and sacrospinous ligaments from the sacrum to the ischial tuberosity and ischial spine respectively. Only a small amount of rotatory movement is allowed at this joint, with some increase in the range of movement during pregnancy.

RADIOLOGICAL FEATURES OF THE JOINTS OF THE VERTEBRAL COLUMN

Plain radiographs

The distance from the anterior border of the odontoid process to posterior border of the anterior arch of the atlas — the *atlantoaxial distance* — is used as a measure of the integrity of the atlantoaxial joint. Normal measurements are up to 3 mm in the adult and 5 mm in the child — the latter reflects the presence of unossified cartilage in the young spine.

The *sacroiliac joints* lie obliquely at an angle of approximately 25° to the sagittal plane and are best radiographed by oblique views. Alternatively, by placing the patient in the prone position, the diverging beams passing at approximately 25° pass through both joints simultaneously.

The plane of the sacroiliac joints is perpendicular to the plane of the facet joint of the same side and thus these support each other structurally. As a result of this relationship, AP oblique views show best the facet joint nearest the film and the sacroiliac joint furthest from the film.

Facet (apophyseal joint) arthrography

This may be performed to visualize these joints or as a prelude to injection of anaesthetic or steroid or other agents, which are injected by a posterior oblique approach under fluoroscopic control. On AP views the joints are seen as smooth, oval, synovial cavities. On a lateral view, the joint cavity is 'S'-shaped. In spondylolysis, adjacent facet joints may be seen, on arthrography, to communicate via an abnormal tract.

Computed tomography

The facet joints are well seen on axial CT. The articular process anterior to the joint is that of the vertebra above, while that posterior to the joint is that of the vertebra below.

The sacroiliac joints and the dense sacroiliac ligament are also seen on axial views. Reconstruction in other planes is useful in addition to axial views of the atlanto-occipital and atlantoaxial joints.

Magnetic resonance imaging

Using MRI, the facet joints are seen on axial views, where the joint space is seen as a region of high signal intensity between the low-intensity cortical bone of the articular processes.

Disease processes

Some disease processes, for example rheumatoid arthritis, affect synovial rather than cartilaginous joints. In the spine this is manifest as involvement of the joints about the atlas and axis (this can lead to erosion of the dens, which is surrounded by synovial joints), the facet joints and the sacroiliac joints. Of the joints between the vertebral bodies, only the neurocentral joints of the cervical vertebrae are involved.

Fig. 3.13 Ligaments of the vertebral column.

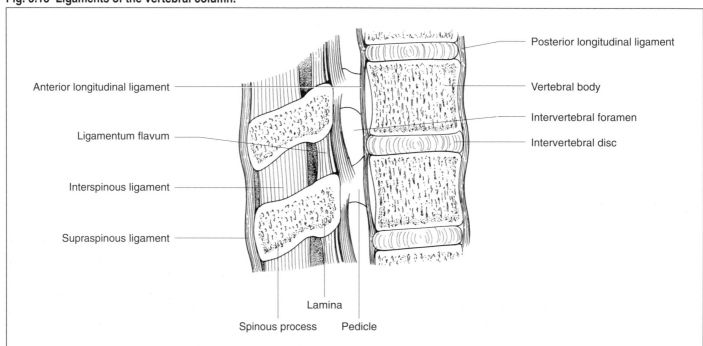

LIGAMENTS OF THE VERTEBRAL COLUMN (Fig. 3.13)

The *anterior longitudinal ligament* extends from the basilar part of the occipital bone along the anterior surface of the vertebral bodies and intervertebral discs so far as the upper sacrum. It is firmly attached to the discs and less firmly attached to the anterior surface of the vertebral bodies.

The *posterior longitudinal ligament* passes along the posterior surface of the vertebral bodies from the body of the axis to the sacrum. It is firmly attached to the intervertebral discs but is separated from the posterior surface of the vertebral bodies by the emerging basivertebral veins. The posterior longitudinal ligament continues superiorly as the membrana tectoria from the posterior aspect of the body of the axis to the anterior margin of the foramen magnum.

The *supraspinous ligament* is attached to the tips of the spinous processes from the seventh cervical vertebra to the sacrum. Above level C7 it is represented by the *ligamentum nuchae*, which is a fibrous septum lying in the midline saggital plane that extends from the spines of the cervical vertebrae to the external occipital protuberance and the external occipital crest.

Adjoining laminae are connected by *ligamenta flava*, which pass from the anterior surface of one lamina to the posterior surface of the lamina below. The yellow colour that gives them their name is due to their significant content of elastic tissue. They are the only markedly elastic ligament in man and can stretch on flexion without forming folds on extension that could impinge on dura.

Relatively weak ligaments connect adjacent transverse processes — the *intertransverse ligaments* — and adjacent spinous processes — the *interspinous ligaments*.

RADIOLOGICAL FEATURES OF THE LIGAMENTS OF THE VERTEBRAL COLUMN

Lumbar puncture for myelography

A needle is passed between and parallel to the spinous processes (i.e. with slight cranial angulation): (i) through the skin and subcutaneous tissues; (ii) through the supraspinous and interspinous ligaments; (iii) through the ligamenta flava if these join in the midline (a gap between these to admit midline vessels is variable in size); and (iv) through the dura to the subarachnoid space.

Myelogram

The *posterior longitudinal ligament* as it passes posterior to the disc may bulge slightly and impinge upon the thecal sac in myelography. This effect is more marked in extension and disappears in flexion.

Computed tomography and magnetic resonance imaging (see Figs 3.11 and 3.12)

The ligaments can be viewed directly on CT and MRI. The ligamentum flavum lies within the spinal canal arising from the lamina. Since the lamina slopes posteroinferiorly, the ligamentum flavum appears thicker in successively lower axial slices.

THE INTERVERTEBRAL DISCS

The vertebral bodies are joined by fibrocartilaginous discs, which are adherent to thin cartilaginous plates on the vertebral bodies above and below them. The discs are wedge-shaped in the cervical and lumbar regions and consequently contribute to lordosis in these regions; however, they are flat in the thoracic region. The intervertebral discs contribute one fifth of the total height of the vertebral column.

Each disc has a central nucleus pulposis, which is gelatinous in the young subject and becomes more fibrous with age. This is surrounded by an annulus fibrosis of tough fibrous tissue. The annulus is relatively thin posteriorly and this is the usual site of rupture in the degenerate disc.

RADIOLOGICAL FEATURES OF THE INTERVERTEBRAL DISCS

Plain radiographs

The disc space rather than the disc itself is visible. The disc space at L5/S1 level is narrow and this should not be taken as a sign of disease.

Discography

Discography is performed by injection of contrast medium through the annulus fibrosis into the nucleus pulposis of the intervertebral disc. It is usually performed in the lumbar region to establish if a disc above a proposed fusion is normal. Discography is also performed prior to chemonucleolysis. It can be performed by a posterior approach through the dura or by a posterolateral approach without going through the dura.

A normal disc is seen to have a smooth, central, unilocular or bilocular nucleus pulposis, and contrast medium remains within the confines of the annulus fibrosis.

Computed tomography (see Fig. 3.11)

On CT, the intervertebral discs are seen as low-attenuation structures between the vertebral bodies. It is not possible to distinguish between the nucleus pulposis, and the annulus fibrosis.

Magnetic resonance imaging

Multiple discs can be examined simultaneously by sagittal MRI (see **Fig. 3.12**). The annulus fibrosis has a lower water content than the nucleus pulposis and thus these can be distinguished from each other.

BLOOD SUPPLY OF THE VERTEBRAL COLUMN

The vertebral bodies and associated structures are supplied by the ascending cervical artery and intercostal and lumbar segmental arteries.

Venous drainage of the vertebral bodies is by a pair of basivertebral veins that emerge from the posterior surface of the body to drain to the internal vertebral venous plexus, which in turn drains to the segmental veins. These large valveless veins allow reflux of blood draining from other viscera into the vertebral bodies and are a potential route of spread of disease — particularly malignancy — into the vertebral bodies.

RADIOLOGICAL FEATURES OF THE BLOOD SUPPLY OF THE VERTEBRAL COLUMN

Spinal angiography

The blood supply to the vertebral bodies arises from the same arteries that supply the spinal cord. In spinal angiography, therefore, the relevant hemivertebra is opacified when the radicular arteries are opacified.

THE SPINAL CORD (Fig. 3.14; see Fig. 3.15)

The spinal cord extends from the medulla oblongata at the foramen magnum to the conus medullaris distally. It extends the entire length of the vertebral canal in a 3-month old fetus but, because of greater growth in length of the vertebral column than the spinal cord, the conus lies at the level of the L3 vertebra at birth and at the lower limit of L1 or upper limit of L2 at the age of 20 years. The conus may lie even higher in the flexed position that may be used during myelography.

Beyond the conus medullaris, a prolongation of pia mater extends as a thin cord — the filum terminale. This is attached to the posterior aspect of the first coccygeal segment.

From the spinal cord, 31 segmental nerves arise on each side — 8 cervical, 12 thoracic, 5 lumbar, 5 sacral and 1 coccygeal.

Although there is no trace of segmentation on the surface of the cord, the part of the spinal cord from which a pair of spinal nerves arises is called a spinal segment. Each spinal nerve arises from a series of rootlets, which fuse to form a dorsal root, with a dorsal root ganglion that carries sensory nerves and a ventral root with motor and autonomic nerves. The dorsal and ventral roots unite at the intervertebral foramen to form the spinal nerve.

Fig. 3.14 Cross-section of the thoracic spinal cord.

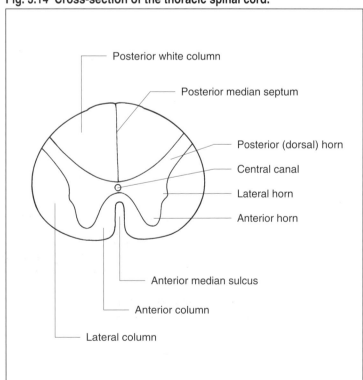

Posterior white column

Posterior median septum

Posterior (dorsal) horn

Central canal

Lateral horn

Anterior horn

Anterior median sulcus

Anterior column

Lateral column

Spinal nerves C1–C7 exit above the pedicle of the corresponding vertebra and all other spinal nerves exit below the pedicle of the corresponding vertebra. Thus the C8 nerve passes under the pedicle of C7 (there is no C8 vertebra) and the L5 nerve passes under the pedicle of the L5 vertebra. Having left the vertebral canal, the spinal nerves divide into dorsal and ventral rami, each of which carry motor and sensory nerves.

Owing to the difference in length of the spinal cord and the vertebral canal, the spinal segment from which a nerve arises is separated from the correspondingly named vertebra and the exit foramen. Thus cord segments in the lower cervical spine are one level above the exit foramina, those in the lower thorax two levels above and those in the lumbar spine three levels above their exit foramina.

Similarly, expansions in the diameter of the spinal cord due to the brachial plexus (C5–T1) and the lumbosacral plexus (L2–S3) cause expansion of vertebral interpedicular distances at higher levels — C4–T2, maximal at C6 for the brachial plexus, and T9–L1/2 (the conus) for the lumbar plexus.

Nerve roots take an increasingly greater downward course from cord to exit foramen in the cervical, thoracic and lumbar spinal cord. The lumbar, sacral and coccygeal roots that exit below the conus at L1/2 are contained within the dura so far as its lower limit at S2 and are called the cauda equina.

CROSS-SECTION OF THE SPINAL CORD (**Fig. 3.15**; see **Fig. 3.14**)

The spinal cord is somewhat elliptical in cross-section, with its greater diameter from side to side. It has a deep anterior median sulcus, which contains the anterior spinal artery. A smaller posterior sulcus is continued within the substance of the cord as a posterior median septum.

A small *central canal* transmits cerebrospinal fluid (CSF) and is continuous above with the fourth ventricle. It extends inferiorly for 5–6 mm into the filum terminale. While this canal is truly central in the upper lumbar cord, it lies anterior to the midline in the cervical and thoracic cord and is posteriorly placed in the conus. A fusiform dilation of the central canal in the conus about 10 mm long and triangular in cross-section is termed the *terminal ventricle.*

Around the central canal is an 'H'-shaped area of *grey matter*, the anterior horns of which have cell bodies of the motor neurones and the posterior horns have cells in the sensory pathways. In the thoracic and upper lumbar regions, lateral horns are found that have cell bodies for sympathetic neurones.

Outside the grey matter is the *white matter* of the cord, which has long ascending and descending tracts (see **Fig. 3.15**). The posterior (dorsal) columns, between the

Fig. 3.15 Cross-section of the spinal cord showing the main descending tracts (on right) and ascending tracts (on left).

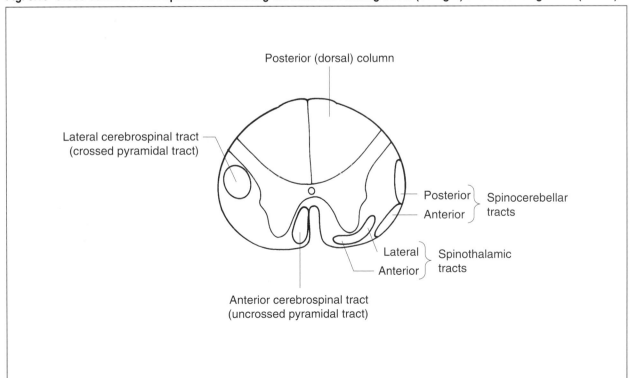

posterior horns, have tracts that convey sensations of pressure, vibration, position, movement and touch. Other sensations are carried in the lateral columns to the thalamus — the spinothalamic tracts — and to the cerebellum — the spinocerebellar tracts. Descending tracts from the motor cortex to the motor neurones of the anterior horns of the spinal cord — pyramidal tracts — also pass in the lateral white columns. Other pyramidal tracts are found in the anterior columns.

Fig. 3.16 Meninges of the spinal cord.

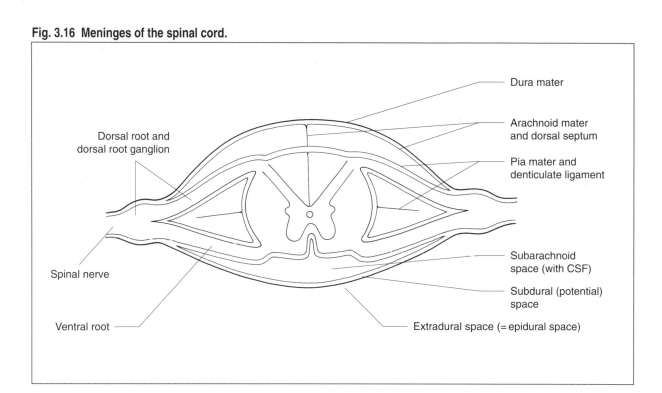

THE SPINAL MENINGES (Fig. 3.16)

Three layers of meninges — the pia, arachnoid and dura mater — cover the spinal cord as well as the brain. All three layers extend along the nerve roots to the intervertebral foramina.

The *pia mater* is applied closely to the surface of the spinal cord, entering its anterior and posterior sulci just as it does on the brain surface. The pia is thickened laterally between the nerve roots as the *denticulate ligament,* so called because of teeth-like projections that attach to the dura at intervals. Inferiorly the pia is thickened with some glial tissue as the filum terminale.

The *arachnoid mater* lines the dura and forms an incomplete posterior median septum. The subarachnoid space, which contains CSF, lies between the arachnoid and the pia mater. The subarachnoid space extends along the nerve roots to the intervertebral foramina, allowing visualization, in myelography, of the nerve roots in their sheaths to this point. The subdural space is a potential space between the arachnoid and the dura and contains only lubricating serous fluid.

The *dura mater* is a loose sheath around the spinal cord representing the inner layer of the cerebral dura. The outer periosteal layer is represented by the periosteum of the vertebral bodies with the extradural — or epidural — space between these layers. The extradural (epidural) space contains loose areolar tissue, fat and a plexus of veins. It extends laterally for a short distance beyond the intervertebral foramina along the spinal nerves.

The dural sac or thecal sac extends inferiorly so far as the S2 vertebral level. Below this the arachnoid and dura blend with the pia on the filum terminale.

THE BLOOD SUPPLY OF THE SPINAL CORD (Figs 3.17 and 3.18)

The spinal cord is supplied by two posterolateral spinal arteries that supply the posterior white columns and part of the grey matter of the dorsal horns, and a single midline anterior spinal artery that supplies the remainder (i.e. two thirds of the cross-sectional area) of the spinal cord. At the lower end of the cord (i.e. the conus) the anterior artery divides in two and anastomoses with each posterior spinal artery. A small 'twig' continues on the filum teminale.

The posterolateral spinal arteries arise by one or two branches on each side from the vertebral artery or, more commonly, its posterior inferior cerebellar branch. The anterior spinal artery also arises from the vertebral artery by union, in the midline, of a branch from each side. These arteries receive further supply at intervals along the length of the cord from branches of the deep cervical branch of the subclavian artery, the cervical part of the vertebral artery and by branches from the intercostal and first lumbar arteries.

These segmental branches pass into the intervertebral foramen and along the nerve roots towards the spinal cord. Branches along the anterior nerve root may arise with or separate from those to the posterior nerve root. The majority of these are *radicular arteries* (i.e. supply mainly the nerve root) but some are *radiculomedullary arteries* and give a significant supply to the cord. The level of origin and number of radiculomedullary arteries is variable but there are usually four to nine and they arise mainly in the lower cervical, lower thoracic and upper lumbar regions. One of these is often larger than the others and is called the *arteria radicularis magna* or the *artery of Adamkiewicz*. This arises at the lower thoracic level between T8 and T12 (on the left side in two-thirds of cases) and supplies the cord both above and below this level. Radicullomedullary arteries reinforce the supply of both the anterior and posterior spinal arteries and their supply to the cord is critical to its function.

VENOUS DRAINAGE OF THE SPINAL CORD

The spinal cord drains to a plexus of veins anterior and posterior to the cord, which in turn drains along the nerve roots to segmental veins. The plexus communicates with:

- The veins of the medulla at the foramen magnum;
- The vertebral veins in the neck;
- The azygous veins in the thorax; and
- The lumbar veins in the lumbar region.

Fig. 3.17 Arterial supply of the spinal cord.

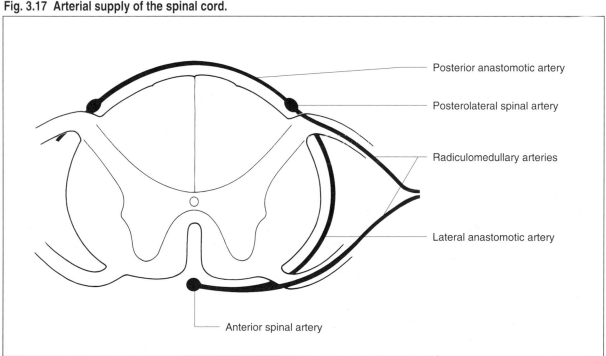

Posterior anastomotic artery

Posterolateral spinal artery

Radiculomedullary arteries

Lateral anastomotic artery

Anterior spinal artery

RADIOLOGICAL FEATURES OF THE SPINAL CORD, ITS MENINGES AND BLOOD SUPPLY

Myelographic technique

Lumbar puncture for myelography is performed at a level below the termination of the cord, that is below L1/2 and above the likely level of abnormality — often L5–S1. The highest point of the iliac crest is at L4 and this is used as a landmark to identify the interspaces above and below this. The anatomy of both cisternal and cervical puncture has already been described.

Nerve roots leave the cord anterolaterally; they are therefore foreshortened in AP views and are best seen in *oblique views*.

Inadvertant injection of contrast other than into the CSF in the subarachnoid space causes characteristic patterns due to the anatomy of the spinal meninges. *Extradural injection* between the dura and the vertebral bone causes collection of contrast around the dura and extension of contrast along the nerve roots to beyond the intervertebral foramina. *Subdural injection* between the dura and the arachnoid gives an angular collection of slow-moving contrast on AP views, which extends along the nerve roots only so far as the intervertebral foramen. In both subdural and extradural injection, contrast is dense because it is not mixed with CSF. Injection *into* an *epidural vein* is recognized by rapid disappearance of contrast with blood flow.

Myelographic appearance

Cervical

On the AP view, the cervical expansion, maximal at C6, can be seen. The cord occupies 50–75% of the interpedicular distance. Nerve roots and their sheaths can be seen leaving the cord almost horizontally. The odontoid peg and spinal vessels, vertebral arteries or posterior inferior cerebellar arteries (PICA) may cause normal filling defects. On lateral views, the transverse ligament of the atlas may cause a filling defect posterior to the odontoid peg.

Thoracic

On the AP view, a thin line of contrast on each side outlines the spinal cord, which fills most of the interpedicular distance. The path of the nerve roots is, as a result, short but somewhat more vertical than in the cervical region. On lateral views, the cord is seen to be more anterior in position than in the cervical region.

Fig. 3.18 Origin of the blood supply to the spinal cord.

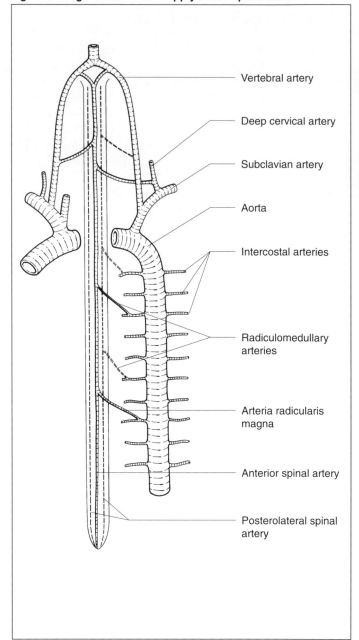

Vertebral artery

Deep cervical artery

Subclavian artery

Aorta

Intercostal arteries

Radiculomedullary arteries

Arteria radicularis magna

Anterior spinal artery

Posterolateral spinal artery

Lumbar (Fig. 3.19)

The spinal cord tapers sudddenly to end as the conus medullaris at L1/L2 level. The filum terminale can be seen as a long, thin, central, filling defect extending from the conus to the end of the thecal sac. It is surrounded by the nerve roots, the cauda equina, which lie laterally until they reach their exit points. The S1 nerve root can be identified passing to the first sacral foramen. The lumbar roots pass around beneath the pedicle of the correspondingly numbered vertebra. Roots are compressed by a protrusion of the disc above the exit level (e.g. L5 root is compressed by a disc at L4/5 level).

The level at which the thecal sac ends is variable and may lie at the L5/SI level or extend to the S2 level. The thecal sac fills 30–80% of the interpedicular distance and is also variable on the lateral view, usually lying close to the vertebral bodies and discs but occasionally a wide epidural space separates the thecal sac from the L5/S1 disc space and may hide a disc protrusion here.

In lumbar myelography in the *young subject,* the cord is seen to extend to a lower level than in the adult. The normal conus may have a bulbous appearance in the child.

1. Nerves of the cauda equina in the thecal sac, outlined by contrast
2. Body of L4
3. Left superior articular process of L4
4. Left pedicle of L4
5. Left L4 root
6. Left L5 nerve root
7. L4/L5 disc space

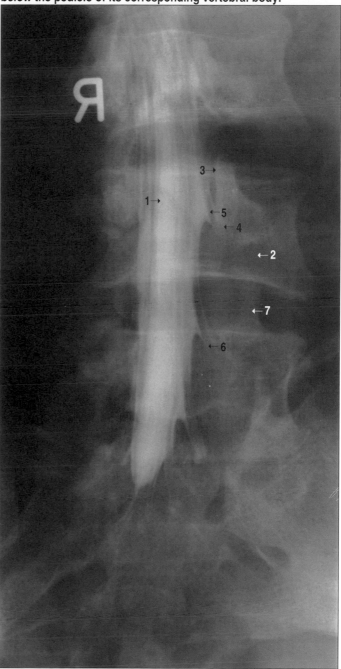

Fig. 3.19 Lumbar myelogram: left posterior oblique view to show nerve roots. Below the level of C7 each nerve root emerges *below* the pedicle of its corresponding vertebral body.

Computed tomography (see Figs 3.10 and 3.11)

CT of the spinal cord can be performed with or without intrathecal contrast. In noncontrast views, low-density epidural fat outlines the thecal sac. The CSF is of water density and the higher density cord is seen within it. The cord is elliptical in cross-section, with its wide axis lying transversely in the cervical region and in the centre of the subarachnoid space. In the thoracic region, the cord is circular in cross-section and lies more anteriorly. No cord is visible in cuts taken below the level of L2.

Without intrathecal contrast, nerve roots are difficult to see within the thecal sac; however, at the intervertebral foramen they can be seen, since here they are outlined by fat. For the same reason, the dorsal root ganglion may also be seen here. With contrast, the sheath of the nerve roots fill and the individual roots of the cauda equina may also be seen.

Spinal angiography

This is a lengthy procedure involving contrast injection into the vertebral arteries, the deep cervical arteries, several intercostal and lumbar arteries and the sacral branch of the internal iliac artery to identify the radiculo-medullary arteries, which are variable in number and level of origin. No single injection will opacify the entire anterior spinal artery. The main feeding vessel in spinal angiomas may arise distant from the lesion and may be missed if a thorough examination is not performed.

The arteria radicularis magna usually arises on the left side between T8 and T12. When opacified it is seen to turn cranially from its origin towards the midline of the spinal cord and to bifurcate into a small ascending and a large descending contribution to the anterior spinal artery. This angiographic feature is called the 'hairpin appearance'.

Angiographically directed *embolization* of angiomatous vessels is sometimes possible.

Bronchial angiography

In the catheterization of intercostal arteries and their branches, such as for bronchial angiography and in particular for bronchial embolization, there is a risk of damage to the blood supply of the cord by embolization to the radiculomedullary branches.

Magnetic resonance imaging (see Fig. 3.12)

MRI is useful for imaging the spinal cord — it is noninvasive and the entire cord can be seen in a few sagittal images. The spinal cord is well seen against the CSF in either T1- or T2-weighted images. The enlargements of the cord in the cervical and lower thoracic areas are visualized, and the cauda can be seen close to the posterior aspect of the subarachnoid space beyond the lower limit of the cord. Differentiation between grey and white matter within the cord is not always possible. A thin line of low-T1, high-T2 signal intensity seen down the centre of the normal cord on sagittal sections is not the central canal but represents a truncation artefact.

Nerve roots are visible especially where they are outlined by fat in the intervertebral foramen. Epidural fat is invariably present posteriorly and, to a lesser extent, anteriorly. The amount of epidural fat in the nerve roots increases from their cranial to their caudal ends. In contrast-enhanced MRI, bright epidural veins contrast with negligable signal from nerve roots. The spinal nerves of the cauda equina can be seen outlined by the CSF, usually lying posteriorly in the thecal space, except for those passing anteriorly from the exit foramina.

Other procedures

Before the advent of CT and MRI, the following procedures were sometimes used for evaluation of the vertebral canal and its contents:

- *Phlebography*: opacification of the epidural veins by injection of the lumbar veins via a lumbar approach;
- *Epidurography*: injection into the epidural space (between dura and the vertebral bone) either via a lumbar route or by injection from below into the sacral canal; and
- *Endomyelography*: injection of contrast into the spinal cord under general anaesthesia, usually for differentiation of cystic swelling and central canal expansion.

CHAPTER 4 *THE THORAX*

The thoracic cage

The diaphragm

The pleura

The trachea and bronchi

The lungs

Mediastinal divisions

The heart

The great vessels

The oesophagus

The thoracic duct and the mediastinal lymphatics

The thymus

The azygous system

Important nerves of the mediastinum

The mediastinum on the chest radiograph

Cross-sectional anatomy

THE THORACIC CAGE

The roof of the thoracic cage is formed by the suprapleural membrane and the diaphragm is its floor. The walls of the thoracic cage are made of the skeleton and attached muscles. The bones involved are: (i) 12 thoracic vertebrae (see section on vertebral column, p. 86); (ii) 12 ribs and their costal cartilages; and (iii) the sternum.

THE RIBS

There are 12 pairs of ribs — 7 true, 3 false and 2 floating. Occasionally a normal subject has only 11 pairs.

THE TYPICAL RIB (Fig. 4.1)

A typical rib has a head, neck, tubercle and shaft.

The head has two facets for articulation with vertebral bodies, for example the sixth rib articulates with the bodies of T5 and T6 vertebrae. These costovertebral joints are synovial joints.

The neck of the rib is attached by a ligament to the transverse process of the vertebra above.

The tubercle has a facet for articulation with its own transverse process. This costotransverse joint is also a synovial joint. The tubercle also has a nonarticular part for ligament attachment.

The shaft has a posterior angle and a much less prominent anterior angle. It has a subcostal groove that is much more prominent posteriorly. This lodges the intercostal vessels and nerves.

The intercostal space

This is bridged by the muscles — the external, internal and innermost intercostal muscles. The neurovascular bundle lies between the internal and innermost muscle layers.

ATYPICAL RIBS

First rib (Fig. 4.2)

This is the shortest, flattest and most curved rib. It articulates with T1 only. A tubercle on its inner border marks the attachment of the scalenus anterior muscle. It is grooved by the subclavian vein posteriorly. Anteriorly, another groove marks where the lowest trunk of the brachial plexus and the subclavian artery, that is, the nerve trunk and not the artery lies in contact with the bone.

Second rib

This is less curved and twice as long as the first rib. It has a tubercle on its external (lower) border, which is often well marked on a chest radiograph, at the site of attachment of the second head of the scalenus anterior muscle.

Tenth rib

This differs from the typical ribs by having only one articular facet on its head.

Eleventh rib

This also has only one articular facet on its head. It has no tubercle for articulation with the transverse process.

Twelfth rib

This has only one articular facet on its head; it has no tubercle and no subcostal groove.

COSTAL CARTILAGES

These are the unossified anterior ends of the ribs. They slope upwards to the sternum where they form synovial sternochondral joints (except the first, which forms a primary cartilaginous joint with the sternum). The joint between the rib and costal cartilage is a primary cartilaginous joint. The costal cartilages of the first seven ribs articulate with the sternum. The eighth to tenth ribs articulate with the costal cartilages of the rib above. The eleventh and twelfth costal cartilages have pointed ends and end in the muscles of the abdominal wall.

RADIOLOGICAL FEATURES OF THE THORACIC CAGE

These are as follows:

■ Normal variants: ribs may fuse or bifurcate, they may be splayed or hypoplastic. Variation is commoner in the upper ribs, especially the first;

■ On a PA chest radiograph the *subcostal groove* may appear as a fine line below the rib, especially posteriorly (not to be mistaken for a periosteal reaction). It may also appear as shallow indentation posteriorly near the neck (not to be mistaken for rib notching);

■ A prominence is often seen on the second rib on a chest radiograph, which is usually symmetrical right and left, this is due to insertion of part of the scalenus anterior muscle;

■ The costal cartilages may calcify or ossify from early adulthood, especially the first costal cartilage. In males the calcification is usually in marginal bands, and in females in a central tongue;

■ Cervical ribs: these are bony or fibrous bands between C7 vertebra and the first rib found in 1–2% of subjects. Of these, 50% are bilateral and often they are asymmetrical. They may be distinguished from the first rib by the orientation of the transverse process — that of C7 points downward while that of T1 is horizontal or points upward. A fibrous band is likely to be present if

Fig. 4.1 A typical rib.

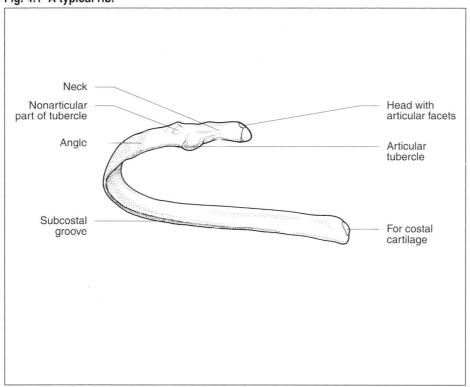

Fig. 4.2 (a) First rib; (b) structures crossing first rib.

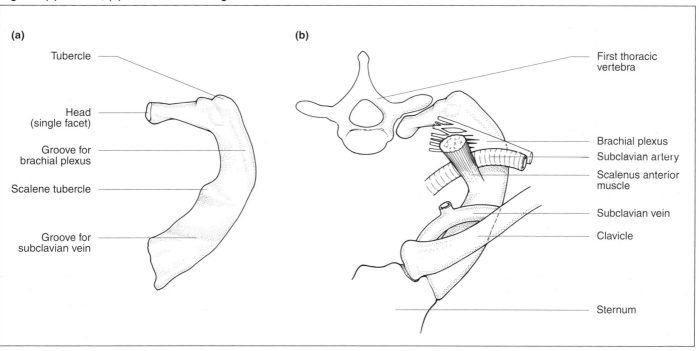

the anterior tubercle of the transverse process of C7 is prominent on a radiograph. The brachial plexus is likely to be prefixed (that is, arise from C4–C8 rather than C5–T1 if the cervical rib is well developed. This situation is less likely to cause neurological symptoms;

■ Lumbar ribs: the transverse process (which is the costal element of the lumbar vertebra), may fail to fuse with the vertebral body and retain a synovial joint with the neural arch. These are symptomless;

■ Ossification of the ribs: a bony centre arises at the angle of the rib in the eighth fetal week. Secondary centres occur at the head and at the tubercle at 15 years of age and fuse at 25 years of age.

THE STERNUM (see **Fig. 4.3**)

The sternum has:

■ A *manubrium* opposite T3 and T4 vertebrae, which articulates with the clavicle and with one-and-one-half costal cartilages;

■ A *sternal angle*, which is a secondary cartilaginous joint and lies opposite T4/5 disc space;

■ A *body* opposite T5–T9 vertebrae, made up of four stenebrae, which articulate with five-and-one-half costal cartilages; and

■ A *xiphoid process*, which remains cartilaginous well into adult life.

RADIOLOGICAL FEATURES OF THE STERNUM

Plain films

On a PA chest radiograph the manubrial borders may simulate mediastinal widening. The remainder of the sternum is not seen. Oblique views are necessary to project the sternum away from the heart. These project it over the lungs whose markings may cause confusing shadows. Lateral views are also helpful.

Variation in sternal configuration include: (i) depression of the lower end — known as pectus excavatum; and (ii) prominence of the mid portion — known as pectus carinatum.

Ossification of the sternum

Bony centres for the manubrium and stenebrae appear from above downwards from the fifth to the ninth fetal months. Stenebrae fuse from below upwards, between 15 and 25 years of age. The xiphoid process fuses with the body at 40 years of age and the body and manubrium fuse in old age, if at all.

Computed tomography

On CT images of the thorax the manubrium is usually angled with respect to the gantry and this may cause cortical unsharpness. The body of the sternum is usually perpendicular to the beam and well demarcated.

Fig. 4.3 The sternum.

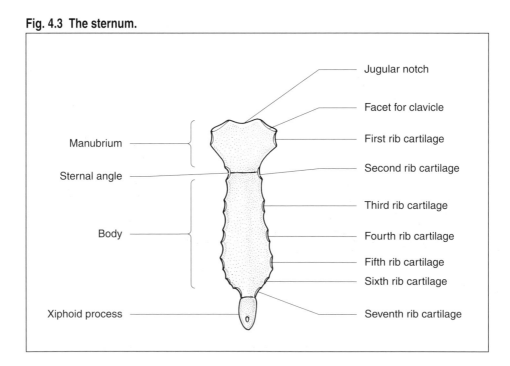

THE DIAPHRAGM (Fig. 4.4)

The diaphragm forms the highly convex floor of the thoracic cage. It arises from *vertebral, costal* and *sternal* origins and from the *central tendon.*

The *vertebral part* arises from the *crura* and *arcuate ligaments.* The right crus is attached to the bodies and discs of L1–L3 vertebrae. The smaller left crus arises from the vertebral body and disc of L1 and L2 vertebrae.

The *medial arcuate ligament* is a thickening of the fascia over the psoas muscle from the body of L2 to the transverse process of L1 lumbar vertebrae. The *lateral arcuate ligament* is a thickening of the fascia over quadratus lumborum from the transverse process of L1 vertebrae to the twelfth rib. The *median arcuate ligament* is the fibrous medial part of both crura behind which the aorta passes; no diaphragmatic muscle arises from this.

The *costal part* of the diaphragm arises in slips from the lower six costal cartilages.

The *sternal part* of the diaphragm arises in two small slips of muscle from the posterior surface of the xiphisternum.

The *central tendon* is, in fact, not central but closer to the sternum. Its midpart is fused with the pericardium and its right and left posterior parts extend towards the paravertebral gutters.

OPENINGS IN THE DIAPHRAGM

These are as follows:

- Aortic — at level T12: in fact the aorta passes behind the median arcuate ligament rather than through the diaphragm. The thoracic duct and the azygous vein pass with the aorta;
- Oesophageal hiatus — at level T10: this is to the left of the midline but is surrounded by fibres of the left crus. With the oesophagus it transmits the vagal trunks, branches of the left gastric artery, veins and lymphatics;
- Caval opening — at level T8: transmits the inferior vena cava whose adventitial wall is fused with the central tendon, and the right phrenic nerve;
- Behind the medial arcuate ligament — the sympathetic trunk;
- Behind the lateral arcuate ligament — the subcostal nerves and vessels; and
- Between sternal and costal origins — the superior epigastric vessels.

Fig. 4.4 Diaphragm: (a) view from below showing origin and openings; (b) crura and arcuate ligaments. (Courtesy of Prof. JB Coakley.)

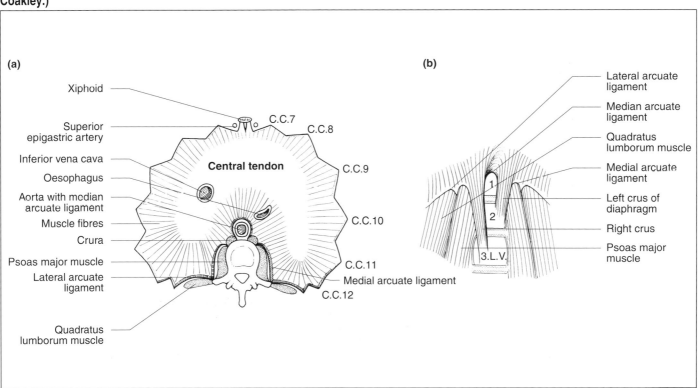

Fig. 4.5 PA chest radiograph.

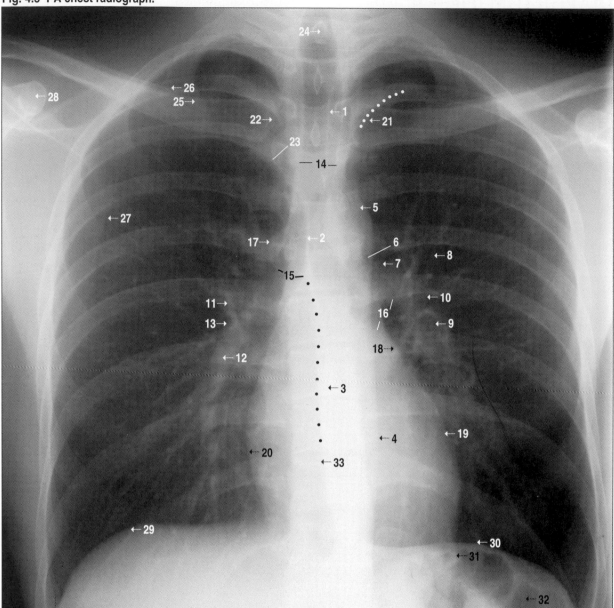

1. Posterior mediastinal line
2. Anterior mediastinal line
3. Azygo-oesophageal line
4. Left wall of descending aorta
5. Aortic knuckle
6. Aortopulmonary window
7. Pulmonary trunk/left pulmonary artery
8. Left superior pulmonary vein
9. Left inferior pulmonary artery
10. Left hilar point
11. Right superior pulmonary vein
12. Interlobar artery
13. Right hilar point
14. Trachea
15. Right main bronchus
16. Left main bronchus
17. Azygous vein and position of azygous node
18. Position of left atrial appendage
19. Left ventricle
20. Right atrium
21. Inferior aspect of left brachio cephalic vein
22. Medial end of right clavicle
23. Right lateral aspect of manubrium sterni
24. Spinous process of T1
25. Superior surface of clavicle
26. Companion shadow of clavicle
27. Medial aspect of right scapula
28. Coracoid process of right scapula
29. Dome of right hemidiaphragm
30. Dome of left hemidiaphragm
31. Stomach bubble
32. Gas in splenic flexure of colon
33. Intervertebral disc space: level of T9/T10

STRUCTURES THAT PIERCE THE DIAPHRAGM

The structures that pierce the diaphragm are as follows:

- The left phrenic nerve, which pierces the central tendon;
- The greater, lesser and least splanchnic nerves, which pierce each crus; and
- The lymph vessels between the abdomen and thorax, which pierce the diaphragm throughout, especially posteriorly.

BLOOD SUPPLY TO THE DIAPHRAGM

The diaphragm is supplied from its abdominal surface by the inferior phrenic arteries from the abdominal aorta. The costal margins are supplied by the intercostal arteries.

NERVE SUPPLY TO THE DIAPHRAGM

Right and left phrenic nerves from C3–C5 roots provide the motor supply of the diaphragm. Sensory impulses from the central part of the diaphragm pass with the phrenic nerves and those from the peripheral part with the intercostal nerves.

RADIOLOGICAL FEATURES OF THE DIAPHRAGM

PA chest radiograph (Fig. 4.5)

The highest point of the right dome is at the sixth intercostal space anteriorly (ranging from the fourth to seventh ribs); it is more accurate to count anterior rather than posterior ribs since the diaphragmatic dome is nearer to the anterior ribs and the film, and is therefore less subject to distortion by slight angulation of the patient or the beam.

The right dome is higher than the left by 2 cm but the left may be higher than the right in the normal subject, especially with swallowed gas in the colon.

The range of movement of the diaphragm with respiration is as follows:

- Quiet respiration: 1 cm; and
- Deep inspiration/expiration: 4 cm (wide range of normal).

In each case the left hemidiaphragm moves more than the right.

The variation of the diaphragm with posture is as follows:

- Supine: higher; and
- Lateral decubitus: dome on the dependant side is higher.

In dextrocardia, even if the liver is on the right side, the left dome of the diaphragm tends to be higher.

Partial reduplication of the diaphragm — known as accessory hemidiaphragm — may occur. This is much commoner on the right side.

Lateral chest radiograph (Fig. 4.6)

The following anatomical details help identify the domes of the diaphragm:

- The heart shadow obliterates part of the left dome;
- The inferior vena cava may be seen piercing the right dome; and
- Air within the gastric fundus lies under the left dome.

There is apparent thickness of the diaphragm on radiographs:

- With the pleura and peritoneum when there is air in the peritoneum: 2–3 mm thick; and
- With the pleura and fundal wall of stomach: 5–8 mm thick.

Curvature of the dome

The perpendicular height of the dome of the diaphragm from a line between costophrenic and cardiophrenic angles is 1.5 cm.

Ultrasound

The diaphragm is readily imaged by ultrasound, using the liver or spleen as an acoustic window. It is seen as an echogenic line outlining the upper surface of these organs. The diaphragmatic interdigitations may occasionally be pronounced to give the spurious impression of an echogenic mass on the surface of the liver.

Computed tomography

The diaphragm is not usually visible as a structure discrete from the liver or other abdominal organs, unless there is a lot of fat on its abdominal aspect.

The costal origins may be prominent with deep inspirations. The crura are usually visible on the anterior surface of the upper lumbar vertebrae. In young, muscular subjects the crura may be very thick or even nodular; however, their tubular nature and changes with respiration serve to distinguish these from lymph nodes. The right crus extends more inferiorly than the left.

The retrocrural space contains fat, the azygous and hemiazygous veins, the thoracic duct and lymph nodes and should not be greater than 6 mm wide.

Magnetic resonance imaging

This technique yields excellent sagittal and coronal images of the diaphragm as a thin muscular septum of intermediate signal intensity. The crura are elegantly displayed on coronal images.

Table 4.1 Lower limits of lung and pleura

	Visceral pleura and lung	Parietal pleura
Anterior	6th costal cartilage	6th costal cartilage
Mid-axillary line	8th rib	10th rib
Posterior	T10	T10

Fig. 4.6 Lateral chest radiograph.

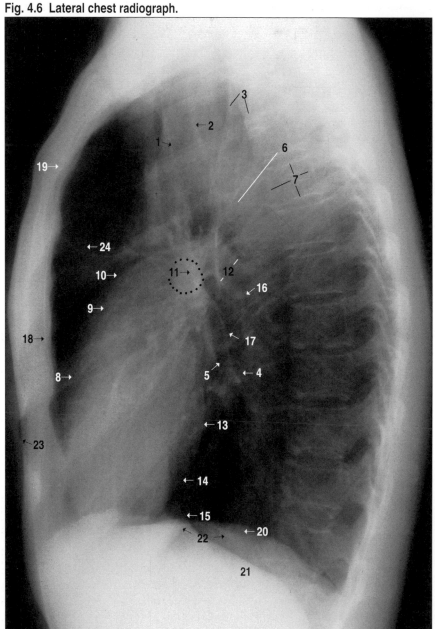

1. Anterior wall of trachea
2. Posterior tracheal stripe
3. Scapulae
4. Left lower-lobe bronchus
5. Right lower-lobe bronchus
6. Aorta (not well seen)
7. Vertebral body of T4
8. Anterior aspect of right ventricle
9. Pulmonary outflow tract
10. Main pulmonary artery
11. Right pulmonary artery
12. Left pulmonary artery
13. Left atrium
14. Left ventricle
15. Inferior vena cava
16. Horizontal (minor) fissure
17. Oblique (major) fissure
18. Deep surface of sternum
19. Manubriosternal joint
20. Left hemidiaphragm
21. Right hemidiaphragm
22. Stomach bubble
23. Lung projected anterior to sternum in intercostal space
24. Retrosternal airspace

THE PLEURA (Fig. 4.7)

The pleura is a serous membrane that: (i) covers the lung (i.e. the *visceral pleura*); and (ii) lines the thoracic cavity and mediastinum (i.e. the *parietal pleura*). Parts of the pleura are named according to site, for example costal, diaphragmatic, mediastinal and apical pleura.

The visceral and parietal layers are continuous with each other anterior and posterior to the lung root, but below the hilum the two layers hang down in a loose fold called the *pulmonary ligament*. This may extend to the diaphragm or have a free inferior border, and allows descent of the lung root in respiration and also distension of the pulmonary veins (note that these lie inferiorly in the lung root).

The pleura extends into *interlobar* and *accessory fissures*. At rest the parietal pleura extends deeper into the costophrenic and costomediastinal recesses than the lungs and visceral pleura do (see **Table 4.1** for lower limits of lungs and pleura).

RADIOLOGICAL FEATURES OF THE PLEURA

Plain films

On a chest radiograph, pleura is visible only if tangential to the beam and if fat or air is on each side of it. Thus pleura is visible in a normal subject at:

- Fissures;
- Sites where parietal pleura lies on extrapleural fat:
  — seen just below the second rib and
  — extending vertically upwards from the costophrenic recess; and
- Junctional lines (see **Figs 4.29**, **4.30** and **4.34**):
  — *anterior junctional line:* anterior to the arch of the aorta the two lungs may come in contact with one another, separated only by four layers of pleura This pleura is then seen as the anterior junctional line on a PA chest radiograph
  — *posterior junctional line:* if the lungs lie close to one another posteriorly, a posterior junctional line is seen on a PA chest radiograph, extending vertically downwards from the apices (approximately T1) for a variable distance. It disappears where the lungs envelope the aortic arch and may reform inferiorly. Where the junctional lines are seen well, a mass between the lungs in that area can be excluded.

Computed tomography

On axial CT the pleura cannot usually be distinguished from the thoracic wall or mediastinum unless it is thickened (see the section on fissures, p. 118). The pulmonary ligaments can be seen occasionally extending below the inferior pulmonary vein caudally and posteriorly to the diaphragm. The right pulmonary ligament lies close to the inferior vena cava (IVC), while the left pulmonary ligament lies close to the oesophagus.

Fig. 4.7 Pleura: (a) anterior view; (b) posterior view.

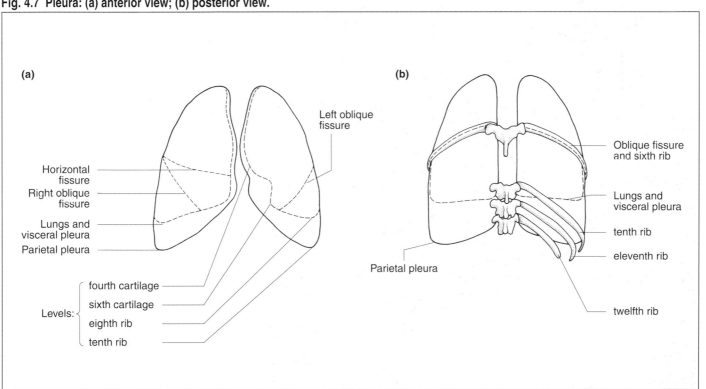

THE TRACHEA AND BRONCHI (Figs 4.8–4.12)

THE TRACHEA

The trachea begins at the lower border of the cricoid cartilage at the level of C6 vertebra. It extends to the *carina* at the level of the sternal angle (T5 level, T4 on inspiration and T6 on expiration). The trachea is 15 cm long and 2 cm in diameter and is made up of incomplete rings of cartilage that are bridged posteriorly by the trachealis muscle. The trachea is lined by ciliated columnar epithelium.

Relations of the trachea

Cervical (see Figs 1.34–1.36)

The anterior relations are as follows:

- Anterior:
  — Isthmus of thyroid: second, third and fourth rings
  — Inferior thyroid veins
  — Strap muscles: sternohyoid and sternothyroid muscles;
- Posterior: oesophagus and recurrent laryngeal nerves; and
- Lateral: lobes of thyroid gland
  — Common carotid artery.

Thoracic (see Figs 4.6, 4.15, 4.31 and 4.32)

The thoracic relations are as follows:

- Anterior:
  — Brachiocephalic and left common carotid arteries
  — Left brachiocephalic vein
- Posterior: oesophagus and left recurrent laryngeal nerve
- Left lateral:
  — Arch of the aorta
  — Left common carotid and left subclavian arteries; and
- Right lateral: right brachiocephalic artery
  — Right vagus nerve
  — Arch of the azygous vein
  — Pleura (in direct contact unlike the other side).

Blood supply of the trachea

The upper trachea is supplied by the inferior thyroid artery, while the lower part is supplied by branches of the bronchial artery.

Venous drainage is to the inferior thyroid venous plexus.

Fig. 4.8 Trachea and main bronchi: anterior relations.

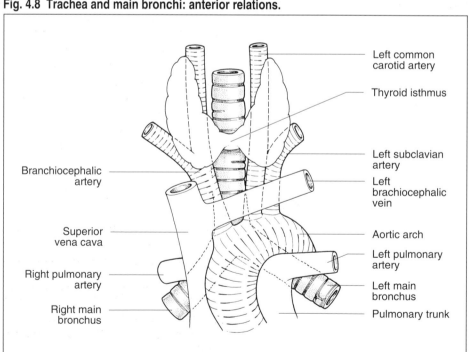

MAIN BRONCHI (see **Figs 4.9–4.12**)

Carina

This is the anteroposterior ridge at the junction of the main bronchi. It lies at T5 vertebral level (T4 on inspiration and T6 on expiration) and at the level of the sternal angle. The carinal angle measures approximately 65° — that is, 20° to the right of the midline and 40° to the left. This angle is slightly larger in children.

The right main bronchus (eparterial bronchus)

The right main bronchus lies at about 25° to the median plane. It is 2.5 cm long and 1.5 cm wide. It is thus wider, shorter and more vertical than the left main bronchus.

Relations

The relations of the right main bronchus are as follows:

■ Anterior:
— Superior vena cava
— Right pulmonary artery;
■ Posterior: azygous vein; and
■ Superior: arch of azygous vein.

The bronchus to the upper lobe arises almost immediately after the tracheal bifurcation, entering the hilum of the lung separately, thereafter dividing into anterior, apical and posterior bronchi. The right bronchus continues as the bronchus intermedius, which then divides into middle- and lower-lobe bronchi. The middle-lobe bronchus has medial and lateral divisions. The apical segment bronchus of the lower lobe comes off opposite the bronchus to the middle lobe. The lower-lobe bronchus divides into four basal segment bronchi — the posterior, lateral, anterior and medial basal segment bronchi.

Left main bronchus (hyparterial bronchus)

The left main bronchus lies at 40° to the median plane. It is 5 cm long and 1.2 cm in diameter.

Relations

The relations of the left main bronchus are as follows:

■ Anterior: pulmonary trunk;
■ Posterior
— Oesophagus
— Descending aorta; and
■ Superior:
— Aortic arch
— Pulmonary artery.

The left main bronchus divides into upper- and lower-lobe bronchi within the lung. The upper-lobe divisions are similar to the right. The posterior and apical segmental bronchi usually have a common apicoposterior bronchus, which then subdivides. The lingular lobe bronchus comes off the upper-lobe bronchus and has superior and inferior divisions. The lower-lobe bronchus has apical, lateral, anterior and posterior basal segments but no medial basal segment.

The anatomy of the bronchial tree is shown diagrammatically in **Fig. 4.10.** Naming basal bronchi laterally to medially is easier if the constant relationship of anterior, lateral and posterior bronchi (ALP) is remembered, with only the medial bronchus in the right lung changing its relative position (see **Table 4.2**).

Blood supply

While the lungs receive the entire output of the right heart, their own nutritive supply arises from the *bronchial arteries,* branches of the thoracic aorta.

The *bronchial veins* drain on the right to the azygous system and on the left to the hemiazygous system.

RADIOLOGICAL FEATURES

The radiological features of the trachea and bronchi are discussed in the following section on the lungs (see p. 120).

Fig. 4.9 Diagrammatic representation of normal anatomy: situs solitus.

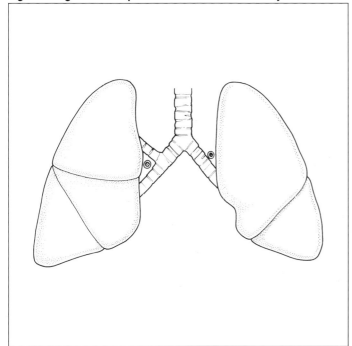

Fig. 4.10 Bronchial tree — main and segmental anatomy as seen on bronchography: (a) anterior view; (b) right lateral view; (c) left lateral view; (d) left oblique view.

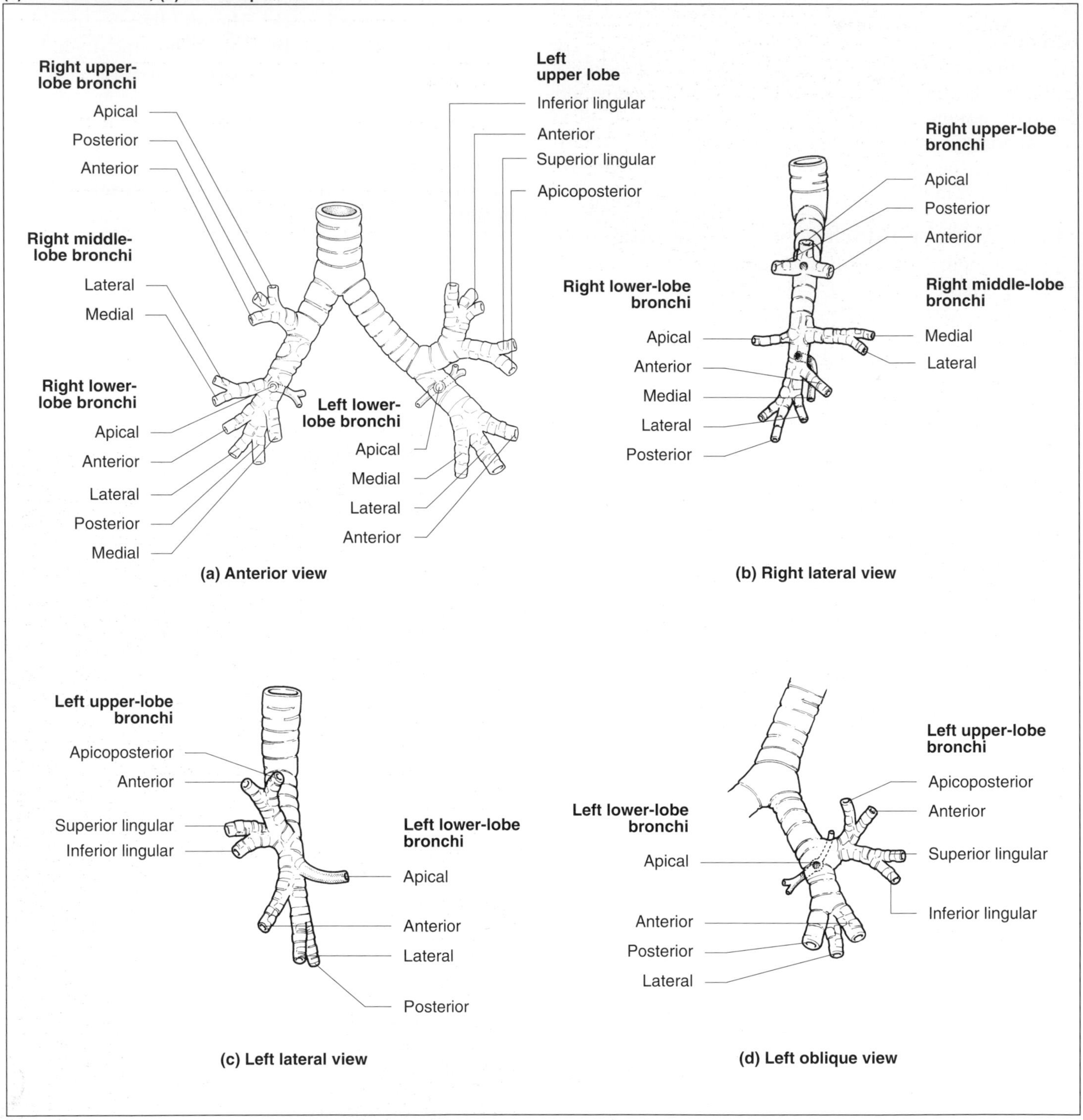

Right upper-lobe bronchi
Apical
Posterior
Anterior

Right middle-lobe bronchi
Lateral
Medial

Right lower-lobe bronchi
Apical
Anterior
Lateral
Posterior
Medial

Left upper lobe
Inferior lingular
Anterior
Superior lingular
Apicoposterior

Left lower-lobe bronchi
Apical
Medial
Lateral
Anterior

(a) Anterior view

Right upper-lobe bronchi
Apical
Posterior
Anterior

Right lower-lobe bronchi
Apical
Anterior
Medial
Lateral
Posterior

Right middle-lobe bronchi
Medial
Lateral

(b) Right lateral view

Left upper-lobe bronchi
Apicoposterior
Anterior
Superior lingular
Inferior lingular

Left lower-lobe bronchi
Apical
Anterior
Lateral
Posterior

(c) Left lateral view

Left lower-lobe bronchi
Apical
Anterior
Posterior
Lateral

Left upper-lobe bronchi
Apicoposterior
Anterior
Superior lingular
Inferior lingular

(d) Left oblique view

Fig. 4.11 Bronchogram: right lung, left anterior oblique view.

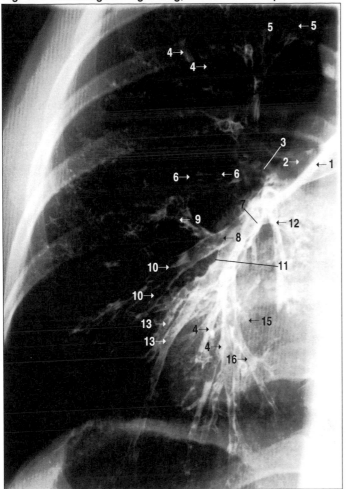

Table 4.2 Identification of the basal bronchi

	Right lung	Left lung
AP view	ALPM	ALP
45° oblique view	ALMP	ALP
Lateral view	AMLP	ALP

A=anterior; L=lateral; P=posterior; M=medial.

Fig. 4.12 Bronchogram: left lung, right anterior oblique view.

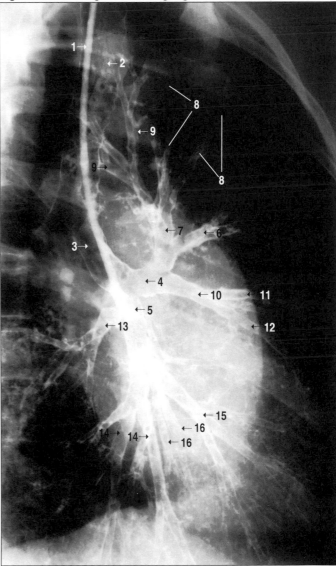

1. Catheter
2. Right main bronchus
3. Upper-lobe bronchus
4. Apical segmental bronchi
5. Posterior segmental bronchi
6. Anterior segmental bronchi
7. Bronchus intermedius
8. Middle-lobe bronchus
9. Lateral segmental bronchi
10. Medial segmental bronchi
11. Lower-lobe bronchus
12. Apical basal bronchi
13. Lateral basal bronchi
14. Posterior basal bronchi
15. Medial basal bronchi
16. Anterior basal bronchi

1. Catheter
2. Trachea
3. Left mainstem bronchus
4. Left upper-lobe bronchus
5. Left lower-lobe bronchus
6. Anterior segmental bronchus
7. Apicoposterior bronchus
8. Apical segmental bronchi
9. Posterior segmental bronchi
10. Lingular bronchus
11. Superior segmental bronchus
12. Inferior segmental bronchus
13. Apical basal bronchus
14. Posterior basal bronchi
15. Anterior basal bronchus
16. Lateral basal bronchi

THE LUNGS (Fig. 4.13; see Fig.4.9)

The lungs are described as having costal, mediastinal, apical and diaphragmatic surfaces. The right lung has three lobes and the left has two with the lingula of the left upper lobe corresponding to the right middle lobe.

INTERLOBAR FISSURES (see **Fig. 4.7**)

The depth of fissures varies from a superficial slit to complete separation of lobes.

The oblique (major) fissure

This is similar in the right and left lungs. It extends from T4/T5 posteriorly to the diaphragm anteroinferiorly. The left major fissure is more vertically orientated than the right. The fissures do not follow a straight plane from top to bottom but are undulating in their course. The medial aspect of each fissure passes through the hilum. The lateral aspect of each fissure is anterior to the medial aspect at the level of the hila and below. Above the hila, the relationship changes and the lateral aspect of the fissure is more posterior than the medial aspect.

The transverse (minor) fissure

This separates the upper and middle lobes of the right lung. It runs horizontally from the hilum to the anterior and lateral surfaces of the right lung at the level of the fourth costal cartilage. Its posterior limit is the right oblique fissure, which it meets at the level of the sixth rib in the mid-axillary line. It is anatomically complete in only one third of subjects and is absent in 10%.

ACCESSORY FISSURES

The azygous fissure

This is in fact a downward invagination of the azygous vein through the apical portion of the right upper lobe. It therefore has four pleural layers — two visceral and two parietal layers. The term 'azygous lobe' is inappropriate as there is no corresponding change in lobar architecture.

The superior accessory fissure

This separates the apical segment of the right lower lobe from other basal segments. It lies parallel and inferior to the transverse fissure and passes posteriorly from the right oblique fissure to the posterior surface of the lung. It is seen in 5% of PA chest radiographs.

The inferior accessory fissure

This separates the medial basal from other right lower-lobe segments. Called Twining's line, it is seen in 45% of post-mortem examinations but in only 8% of PA chest radiographs.

Left transverse fissure

This is found in 8% of post-mortem specimens but is rarely seen on chest radiographs.

BRONCHOPULMONARY SEGMENTS (see **Figs 4.10 and 4.13**)

Each lobe is subdivided into several bronchopulmonary segments each of which is supplied by a segmental bronchus, artery and vein. Each segment takes its title from that of its supplying bronchus.

Anatomy of segmental bronchi is subject to variation — the commonest being the origin of apical segmental bronchi, especially the right, from the trachea.

There is very little connection between segments except via:

- The *pores of Kohn*: openings in the alveolar walls connecting adjacent alveolar lumens; and
- The *canals of Lambert*: connections between terminal bronchioles and adjacent alveoli.

These allow gas and fluid transfer between segments but not between lobes. Ventilation of a segment is therefore possible when its segmental bronchus is occluded. This is called collateral air drift.

THE PULMONARY ARTERY (**Fig. 4.14**; see **Fig. 4.33**)

(See also section on the great vessels.)

The *pulmonary trunk* leaves the fibrous pericardium and bifurcates almost at once in the concavity of the aortic arch anterior to the left main bronchus.

The *right pulmonary artery* is longer than the left. It passes across the midline below the carina and comes to lie anterior to the right main bronchus. It bifurcates while still in the hilum of the right lung. An artery for the right upper lobe passes anterior to the right upper-lobe bronchus. The *interlobar artery* to the right middle and lower lobes passes with the bronchus intermedius.

The *left pulmonary artery* spirals over the superior aspect of the left main bronchus to reach its posterior surface. It is attached to the concavity of the aortic arch by the ligamentum arteriosum.

The pulmonary arteries further subdivide into segmental arteries that travel with the segmental bronchi. The pulmonary arteries supply only the alveoli (*cf.* the bronchial arteries, which supply the bronchi).

Fig. 4.13 Bronchopulmonary segments as seen on PA chest radiograph; (a) upper lobes; (b) middle lobes; (c) lower lobes.

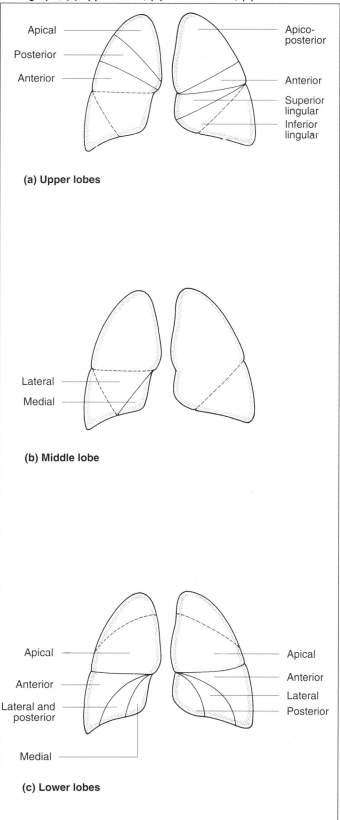

(a) Upper lobes

Apical

Posterior

Anterior

Apico-posterior

Anterior

Superior lingular

Inferior lingular

(b) Middle lobe

Lateral

Medial

(c) Lower lobes

Apical

Anterior

Lateral and posterior

Medial

Apical

Anterior

Lateral

Posterior

THE PULMONARY VEINS

These do not follow the bronchial pattern but tend to run in intersegmental septa. Two veins pass to each hilum — from lung tissue above and below each oblique fissure. These enter the mediastinum slightly below and anterior to the pulmonary arteries. Those on the right often unite and enter the right atrium as a single vessel. On the left side, the upper pulmonary vein enters the superolateral aspect of the left atrium and the lower pulmonary vein enters separately and more inferiorly.

THE BRONCHIAL ARTERIES

The bronchial arteries supply the bronchi, visceral pleura and the connective tissue of the lungs. They arise from the thoracic aorta in 90% of subjects; at T5 or T6 vertebral level in 80% of cases.

There are usually one right and two left bronchial arteries. When a second bronchial artery occurs on the right side it often arises from the third intercostal artery.

Bronchial arteries may also arise from the subclavian artery or from its internal thoracic branch.

Fig. 4.14 Pulmonary arteries.

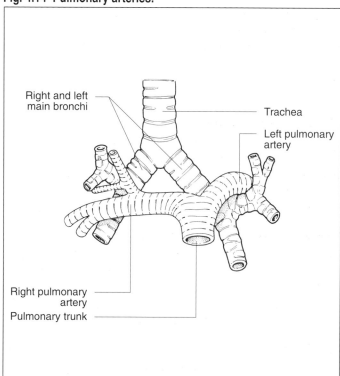

Right and left main bronchi

Trachea

Left pulmonary artery

Right pulmonary artery

Pulmonary trunk

Tissues supplied by bronchial arteries drain to pulmonary veins or bronchial veins.

BRONCHIAL VEINS

Bronchial veins drain to the azygous vein on the right side and to the accessory hemiazygous vein on the left side.

LYMPHATICS (Fig. 4.15)

Mediastinal lymph nodes that drain the lung are named according to their position. Bronchopulmonary nodes are found at the hilum, carinal nodes below the hilum and tracheobronchial nodes above the tracheobronchial junction.

The right lung and the lower half of the left lung drain via right paratracheal nodes to the right mediastinal lymph trunk and right subclavian vein. The upper half of the left lung drains via left paratracheal nodes to the left mediastinal lymph trunk and the thoracic duct, or directly to the left subclavian vein.

Fig. 4.15 Lymph nodes related to the trachea and main bronchi.

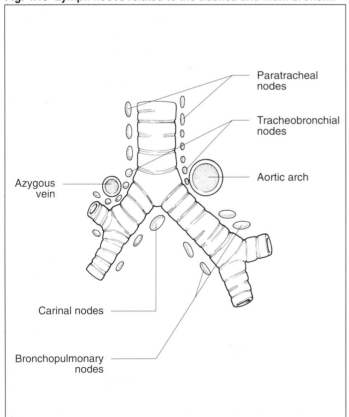

LUNG ROOTS (Fig. 4.16)

The roots of the lungs are formed by the structures that enter and emerge at the hila. They lie at vertebral levels T5–T7. The right lung root lies below the arch of the azygous vein and posterior to the superior vena cava and the right atrium. The left lung root lies below the arch of the aorta and anterior to the descending aorta.

RADIOLOGICAL FEATURES OF THE LUNG AND BRONCHIAL TREE

PA chest radiograph (see Fig. 4.5)

Fissures

Fissures are only seen if tangential to the beam and, because of curvatures in three dimensions, they are seldom seen in their entire length. The transverse fissure of the right lung is seen in 80% of dissection specimens but only 50% of chest radiographs. The azygous fissure is seen in 0.4% of radiographs with the 'tear-drop' shadow of the azygous vein in its lower end. The superior accessory fissure is seen in 5% of chest radiographs and, when present, is at a lower level than the transverse fissure. The inferior accessory fissure in 8% but the left transverse fissure is rarely seen.

Trachea

The trachea is seen as a midline translucency with a slight inclination to the right in its lower half. It lumen is 1.5–2 cm in diameter.

The right paratracheal stripe (normally <5 mm) is formed by the right wall of the trachea and the pleura outlined on both sides by air. The left side of the trachea is not seen separately from the mediastinal shadows.

A smooth indentation on the trachea is commonly seen just above the bifurcation on the left side. This is caused by the arch of the aorta.

Gross AP or side-to-side (usually to the right side due to the aortic arch) displacement may be normal in a *child*.

Bronchi

The bronchi contribute very little to the lung markings seen on plain films. The proximal bronchi may, however, be seen if outlined by the lungs.

On the frontal chest radiograph the bronchi to the anterior segments of the upper lobes are often seen end on, just above and lateral to the hila. Their corresponding pulmonary arteries may be seen accompanying the bronchi as circular densities of about the same size. The

Fig. 4.16 Lung roots: (a) right lung root; (b) left lung root.

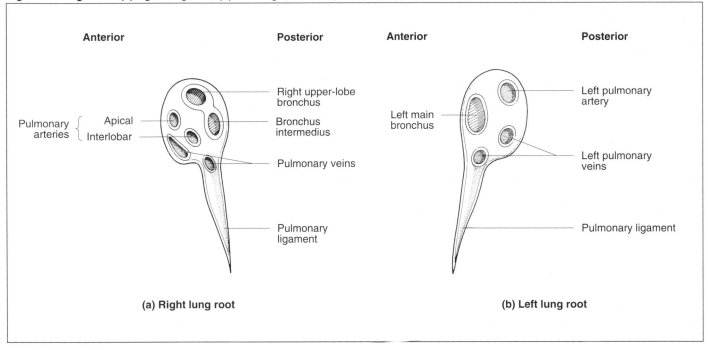

(a) Right lung root

(b) Left lung root

right pair are higher than the left as the upper-lobe bronchus comes off at a higher level on the right.

The right main bronchus is orientated more vertically than the left.

The bronchus intermedius can be identified to the right of the cardiac shadow and medial to the density of the interlobar artery. The lower-lobe bronchus on the left is not normally seen as it lies behind the heart shadow.

Bronchopulmonary segments
These are depicted in **Fig. 4.13.**

Pulmonary vasculature
The vessels account for most of the lung markings.

The pulmonary trunk forms part of the left border of the heart. The interlobar artery is seen lateral to the bronchus intermedius on the right. This should not measure more than 16 mm midway down its visible length.

Bronchi and arteries are seen together radiating out from the hila. Pulmonary veins enter the mediastinum lower than the arteries as they converge toward the posterior aspect of the left atrium. This means that:

- In the upper zone the veins are inferolateral to the arteries; and
- In the lower zone the veins are almost horizontal and the arteries almost vertical.

The inferior pulmonary veins drain anteriorly and superiorly from the lung bases to the left atrium. Owing to their more horizontal course, if seen end on the chest film they may simulate a pulmonary mass.

The *hilar point* is where the upper-lobe vein crosses the descending pulmonary artery. The right hilar point is projected over the sixth posterior interspace and is 1 cm lower than the left.

The *hilar angle* is the angle between the vessels at the hilar point — normally 120°.

Situs inversus
The identification of situs inversus (see **Fig. 4.9**) is helped by the appearance of the main bronchi on high-voltage chest radiographs or tomography. The morphological right lung, whether on the right or left side of the thorax, is trilobed, has a short main bronchus and has its bronchus above its pulmonary artery.

Lymphatics
Normal lymph nodes do not form discernible densities on plain radiographs.

Lateral chest radiograph (see Fig. 4.6)
Fissures
The left oblique fissure is more vertical and reaches the diaphragm more posteriorly than that on the right. The

left oblique fissure is at an angle of 60° to the horizontal, and the right at an angle of 50°. The anterior ends of the oblique fissures are 2–3 cm behind the anterior chest wall. Occasionally the upper end of the oblique fissure may reach T3. As the fissures are undulating, they may appear to be doubled in parts, and are often not seen in entirety. The posterior part of the transverse fissure may occasionally seem to cross the right oblique fissure for the same reason. Where there is a superior accessory fissure, this extends posteriorly from the oblique fissure.

Trachea

On a lateral chest radiograph (see **Fig. 4.6**) the trachea is seen to enter the thorax midway between the sternum and the vertebrae. Owing to some posterior inclination it ends closer to the vertebrae.

The *posterior paratracheal stripe* is formed by the posterior wall of the trachea and the pleura and is visible if the lung passes behind the trachea.

The *tracheo-oesophageal stripe* is formed by the posterior wall of the trachea and the anterior wall of the oesophagus. This is visible if there is air in the oesophagus.

Bronchi

On a lateral chest radiograph (see **Fig. 4.6**) the right main bronchus, being more horizontal, is seen as a circular structure. The left main bronchus is more vertical and is therefore tubular on this view. The left pulmonary artery is seen as a comma-shaped density passing backwards over the left main bronchus.

The posterior wall of the right main bronchus and its division into upper-lobe bronchus and bronchus intermedius are often visible as a thin stripe as they are in contact with the lung. On the left side, however, the pulmonary artery and its branches are posterior to the bronchus and thus obscure the view of its posterior wall.

The upper-lobe bronchi may be seen as two rounded radiolucencies projected over the lower end of the trachea, with the right being 1–2 cm higher than the left. The right upper-lobe bronchus is seen about half the time and the left in about 75% of cases. The left has more sharply

defined margins as the pulmonary artery lies superiorly and the superior pulmonary vein lies inferiorly.

The lower-lobe bronchi may be seen running in an inferoposterior course in many cases. The left lower-lobe bronchus is the more posterior, and has a curved configuration in its anterior aspect, merging with the orifice of the upper-lobe bronchus.

Vasculature

The pulmonary arteries may be seen at the hilum forming a conglomerate density with the pulmonary veins. The right pulmonary artery is seen end on and is oval in appearance. The left pulmonary artery is comma-shaped as it arches over the left main bronchus. They may each measure up to 3 cm in diameter.

The confluence of the pulmonary veins is seen below the oval density of the right pulmonary artery on the lateral film. The superior veins are more anterior than the inferior pulmonary veins.

Plain tomography

Tomography is sometimes used to see the trachea throughout its length. Owing to its posterior inclination, no single cut includes the entire trachea in the supine subject. Tomography in a prone subject may show the entire trachea and several branches, as the prone position causes the bronchial tree to fall forward into an almost horizontal position.

Tomography of the hila in both posterior oblique and lateral planes enhances visualization of the bronchi and their proximal divisions, and gives better demonstration of the hilar vascular structures.

Bronchography (see Figs 4.11 and 4.12)

This technique outlines the trachea, main bronchi and the bronchial tree. For the anatomy of the standard views see **Fig. 4.10**.

The naming of basal bronchi laterally to medially is easier if the constant relationship of anterior, lateral and posterior bronchi (ALP) is remembered, with only the medial bronchus in the right lung changing its relative position (see **Table 4.2**).

Pulmonary angiography

A catheter is inserted via the femoral vein to the IVC, right heart and pulmonary trunk. The pulmonary trunk inclines posteriorly as it leaves the heart and is best seen when the beam is angled at 45° to the anterior chest wall. The pulmonary arteries and branches are seen as described above. Pulmonary veins are seen in the venous phase.

Bronchial angiography

This is used in the diagnosis and embolic treatment of haemoptysis. The bronchial arteries are catheterized from the thoracic aorta if they arise from it. Owing to the variable origin of the bronchial arteries it may be necessary to catheterize the subclavian, internal thoracic or intercostal arteries.

Since spinal arteries also arise from these vessels (*cf.* Chapter 3) there is a risk of spinal ischaemia using this procedure.

Computed tomography (Figs 4.30–4.33)

(See also section on cross-sectional anatomy of the chest at the end of this chapter.)

Fissures

Fissures are less visible than on plain radiographs. They are seen as regions of relative avascularity on the outer cortex of the lobe where tapering vessels are less visible. Discrete lines are only seen if the vertical axis of the fissure is perpendicular to plane of the CT slice, which sometimes occurs in parts of the oblique fissure but not in the transverse fissure.

Bronchi

The bronchi may be seen depending upon their size and orientation. Narrow slices improve visualization.

The horizontally orientated bronchi, such as the anterior segment bronchus of the upper lobes, the superior segmental bronchi of the lower lobes and the proximal part of the middle-lobe bronchus, may be seen as tubular structures.

The vertically orientated bronchi such as the main bronchi, bronchus intermedius, lower-lobe bronchi and apical segmental bronchi may be seen as circular air-filled structures.

The posterior wall of the right main bronchus and its divisions into upper-lobe bronchus and bronchus intermedius should be outlined by lung as it invaginates into the azygo-oesophageal recess.

Occasionally, a pulmonary vein may pass behind the bronchus intermedius on its way to the left atrium, simulating a small mass, which is usually less than 1 cm in diameter.

The posterior walls of left main and upper-lobe bronchi are usually outlined by lung. Below the hilum, lung tissue may also be seen in contact with the posterior wall of the lower-lobe bronchus.

Vasculature

The vessels account for most of the lung markings seen on CT. The relationships of the pulmonary arteries and veins to the bronchi are best seen at hilar level. The right pulmonary artery is anterior to the right bronchus, and the right superior pulmonary vein may be seen anterior to this. The left pulmonary artery is seen anterior to the left main bronchus, and above it on a higher section. The lower-lobe artery is seen posterolateral to the lower-lobe bronchus. The left superior pulmonary vein is separated from the lower-lobe artery at hilar level by the left bronchus.

Magnetic resonance imaging

Since the lungs are of very low proton density they are poorly seen by this method. Third-order pulmonary arteries are visible as are pulmonary veins close to the hilum. Segmental bronchi and fissures are not seen. The axial anatomy as seen is the same as that of CT.

Isotope ventilation-perfusion scanning

A ventilation scan outlines the trachea and main bronchi in addition to the lungs. A gap is seen due to the mediastinum and a cardiac notch is seen in the anterior border of the left lung.

Perfusion scanning may show differential isotope distribution from apex to diaphragm due to variation in blood flow associated with this posture.

THE MEDIASTINAL DIVISIONS (Fig. 4.17)

The mediastinum is the space between the lungs and their pleura. It is arbitrarily divided into superior, middle, anterior and posterior sections; however, these divisions are not anatomical and are used to describe the location of pathological processes. The superior mediastinum is above a line drawn from the lower border of T4 to the sternal angle. Below this line are anterior, middle and posterior compartments. The middle mediastinum is occupied by the heart and its vessels. The anterior mediastinum is between the anterior part of the heart and the sternum. The posterior mediastinum is between the posterior part of the heart and the thoracic spine, extending down behind the posterior part of the diaphragm as it slopes inferiorly.

The superior mediastinum contains the:

■ Aortic arch and branches;
■ Brachiocephalic veins and superior vena cava;
■ Trachea;
■ Oesophagus;
■ Thoracic duct;
■ Lymph nodes; and
■ Nerves.

The anterior mediastinum contains the:

■ Thymus;
■ Mammary vessels; and
■ Lymph nodes.

The posterior mediastinum contains the:

■ Descending aorta;
■ Oesophagus;
■ Azygous venous system;
■ Thoracic duct; and
■ Para-aortic, oesophageal and paraspinal nodes.

The middle mediastinum contains the:

■ Heart and pericardium:
■ Nerves;
■ Lymph nodes; and
■ Great vessels.

Fig. 4.17 Mediastinal divisions. (Courtesy of Prof. JB Coakley.)

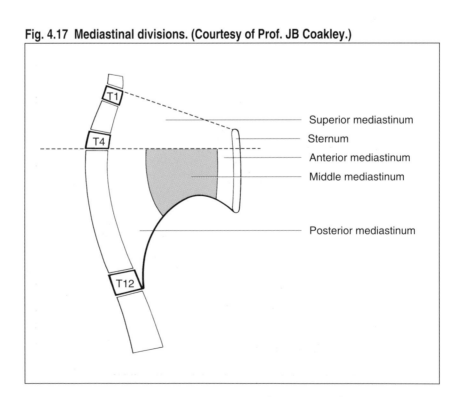

THE HEART

GROSS ANATOMY AND ORIENTATION (Figs 4.18–4.20; see Figs 4.5, 4.6 and 4.21):

The heart has a pyramidal shape and lies obliquely in the chest. Its square-shaped base points posteriorly and the elongated apex to the left and inferiorly. The left atrium forms the base or posterior part, with the superior and inferior pulmonary veins draining into its four corners. The right atrium forms the right border with superior and inferior venae cavae draining into its upper and lower parts. The apex and left border are formed by the left ventricle. The right ventricle forms the anterior part. The inferior (diaphragmatic) part of the heart is formed by both ventricles anteriorly and a small part of right atrium posteriorly where the IVC enters this chamber.

The oblique orientation of the heart causes the ventricles to lie anterior and inferior to the atria. The heart is also rotated in a clockwise fashion about its axis so that the right atrium and ventricle are at slightly higher level than their left counterparts. The interatrial and interventricular septa are said to lie in the left anterior oblique plane. This means that the long axis of the septa runs anteriorly to the left. The tricuspid and mitral valves, which separate the right and left atria and ventricles respectively, are roughly vertically oriented. The plane of the valves is also inclined inferiorly and to the left. This means that the transverse axis of the pair of valves runs to the right and anteriorly and they are said to lie in the right anterior oblique plane.

PERICARDIUM

This is a closed sac consisting of parietal and visceral layers that enclose a potential space. It is draped over the heart and great vessels. The visceral layer adheres to the myocardium and is also known as the epicardium. The parietal layer is free, except inferiorly, where it is bound to the central tendon of the diaphragm, and superiorly where it fuses with the covering of the great vessels. The pericardial reflections, which are really the boundaries of the closed sac, are found posteriorly around the IVC and pulmonary veins, and anterosuperiorly over the superior vena cava (SVC) and the aorta and pulmonary artery.

The pericardium extends superiorly for 2–3 cm over the ascending aorta and over the pulmonary artery almost to its bifurcation. It also extends for a short distance over the venae cavae and pulmonary veins. Some fat is present between the epicardium and myocardium.

Fig. 4.18 Heart: anterior view.

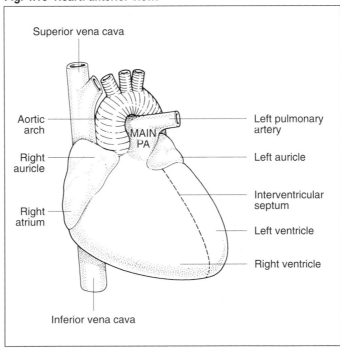

Fig. 4.19 Heart and mediastinum viewed from right. (Courtesy of Prof. JB Coakley.)

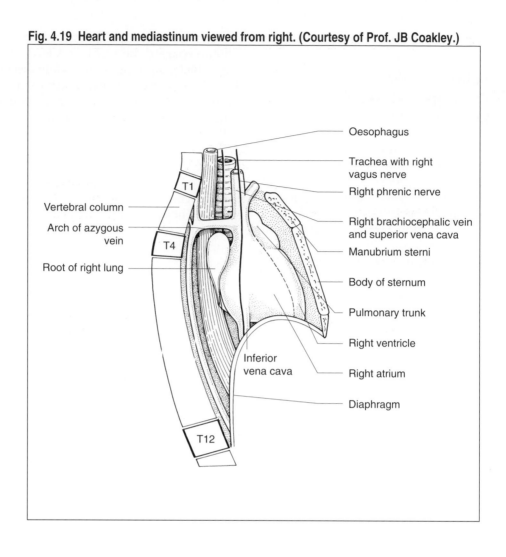

This increases with age. Fat is also present between the pericardium and mediastinal pleura, and it may be extensive in the anterior and lateral cardiophrenic angles where it is known as the pericardial fat pad.

CARDIAC CHAMBERS AND VALVES (Fig. 4.21; see Fig. 4.37)

Right atrium

This has a smooth posterior wall into which the great veins drain. The coronary sinus drains into the posterior wall between the orifice of the IVC and the tricuspid valve. The anterior wall has muscular ridges that are continuous with the muscular ridges of the atrial appendage. The interatrial septum bears an oval depression on its lower part — known as the fossa ovalis. This represents the closed foramen ovale through which oxygenated blood from the maternal circulation reached the left side of the heart in the fetus. A raised limbus surrounds the

fossa ovalis. The right atrial appendage is roughly triangular and projects upward and forward and to the left; it is the only part of the right atrium to contribute to the cardiac outline on the lateral view.

Right ventricle

This chamber is roughly triangular and flattened from front to back as the left ventricle bulges into it. The lower half of the right ventricle normally touches the lower part of the sternum on the lateral view. Viewed from the side it has a muscular inflow tract and a smooth outflow tract, separated by a muscular prominence or conus also known as the infundibulum. The outflow tract inclines superiorly, to the left and posteriorly to the pulmonary valve. The entrance to the right ventricle is the tricuspid valve. This has three leaflets or cusps, each attached to the papillary muscles of the ventricular wall by several tendinous cords — the cordae tendinae. The pulmonary valve has three semilunar cusps — right and left anterior

Fig. 4.20 Heart and mediastinum viewed from left.(Courtesy of Prof. JB Coakley.)

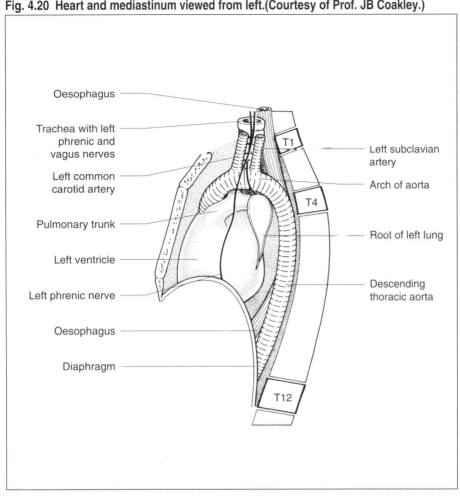

Oesophagus

Trachea with left phrenic and vagus nerves

Left common carotid artery

Pulmonary trunk

Left ventricle

Left phrenic nerve

Oesophagus

Diaphragm

T1

T4

T12

Left subclavian artery

Arch of aorta

Root of left lung

Descending thoracic aorta

Fig. 4.21 CT scan of thorax: axial section through heart. This image was obtained during infusion of contrast. The chambers of the heart are abnormally large.

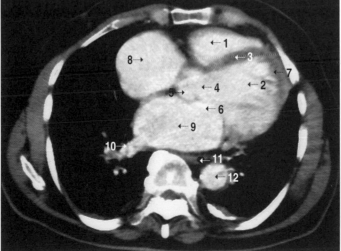

1. Right ventricle
2. Left ventricle
3. Interventricular septum
4. Left ventricular outflow tract and region of aortic valve
5. Root of aorta (note dilation of right posterior sinus)
6. Left ventricular inflow tract and region of mitral valve
7. Left ventricular wall
8. Right atrium
9. Left atrium
10. Left pulmonary vein
11. Oesophagus
12. Descending aorta

cusps and a posterior cusp. It faces to the left and slightly posteriorly. It is the most anterior and superior of all the cardiac valves.

Left atrium

This is square-shaped and smooth-walled and forms the upper posterior part of the heart on the lateral view. It receives the four pulmonary veins in its upper part. It has a long, narrow, trabeculated appendage that projects anteriorly on the left side of the pulmonary trunk, overlapping its origin. This is embedded in fat and is not seen on the frontal view unless enlarged.

Left ventricle

This is a thick-walled finely trabeculated cavity that is shaped like an elongated cone, being roughly circular in cross-section. It forms the lower half of the posterior part of the heart on the lateral view. The mitral valve separates it from the left atrium. This valve has two cusps — the anterior and posterior cusps — whose free margins are attached to the ventricular wall by chordae tendinae. Instead of a muscular conus as on the right, the larger anterior cusp of the mitral valve separates inflow and outflow tracts, and blood flows over both its surfaces. The mitral and aortic valves are in fibrous continuity. The aortic valve has three semilunar cusps — anterior, and right and left posterior. Above each cusp is a localized dilatation or sinus. These are known as the sinuses of Valsalva.

The right coronary artery arises from the anterior sinus and this is also known as the right coronary sinus. The left coronary artery arises from the left posterior sinus — also known as the left coronary sinus. No artery arises from the right anterior sinus, so this is also called the noncoronary sinus. The ventricles are separated by the interventricular septum, which is mostly thick and muscular. It has a short membranous part at the top and bulges into the right ventricle, causing this to have a flattened appearance from front to back, and giving the left ventricle a circular shape in cross-section.

THE CORONARY ARTERIES AND VEINS (Figs 4.22–4.25)

Right coronary artery (Figs 4.22 and 4.23)

The right coronary artery supplies the right ventricle and inferior wall of the left ventricle. It arises from the anterior (right) sinus of Valsalva and passes to the right between the pulmonary trunk and the right atrium to descend in the right atrioventricular groove as the *marginal artery*. On the inferior surface of the heart it anasto-

Fig. 4.22 Right coronary angiogram: (a) left anterior oblique projection; (b) right anterior oblique projection. The AV nodal branch is not seen.

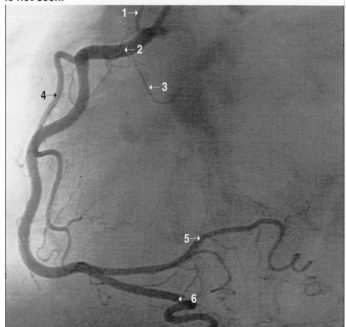

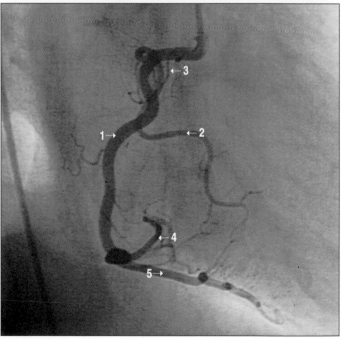

(a)
1. Sinus artery
2. Right coronary artery
3. Conus branch
4. Right ventricular branch
5. Posterolateral branch
6. Posterior descending artery

(b)
1. Right coronary artery
2. Right ventricular branch
3. Conus branch
4. Posterolateral branch
5. Posterior descending artery

moses with the left coronary artery in the region of the posterior interventricular groove.

Branches

The branches of the right coronary artery are as follows:

- Conus artery to the pulmonary outflow tract;
- Atrial and ventricular branches;
- Branch to sinoatrial node, which curves anti-clockwise around the SVC to reach the sinoatrial node;
- Acute marginal branches, which run anteriorly from the RCA to supply the right ventricle;
- Branch to atrioventricular node, which arises from the right coronary artery as it forms a characteristic loop at the region where it continues as the posterior interventricular artery; and
- Posterior interventricular artery, which runs anteriorly from the terminal part of the RCA in the posterior interventricular groove, and supplies the inferior surface of the left ventricle and the posterior two thirds of the interventricular septum.

Left coronary artery (Figs 4.23 and 4.24)

The left coronary artery arises from the left sinus of Valsalva and supplies the remainder of the left ventricle. It arises as the left main coronary artery and passes behind and to the left of the pulmonary trunk to reach the left part of the atrioventricular groove. It bifurcates early into the *left circumflex artery*, which continues laterally in the atrioventricular groove to anastomose with the right coronary artery, and the *anterior descending artery*, which descends in the interventricular groove.

Branches of the anterior descending artery

These are as follows:

- Septal branches;
- Diagonal branches that run over the anterolateral wall of the left ventricle supplying it; and
- A branch to the right ventricle (occasionally).

Branches of the left circumflex artery

These are as follows:

- Obtuse marginal branches, which supply the lateral wall of the left ventricle; and
- Atrial branches.

In general, the RCA supplies the right ventricle and the inferior part of the left ventricle. The left coronary artery supplies the remainder of the left ventricle. The interventricular septum is supplied by the left coronary anteriorly and the right coronary artery posteriorly. The atria have a variable supply. In more than 50% of cases, the sinoatrial node is supplied by the right coronary artery and, in 90%

Fig. 4.23 Left coronary angiogram: (a) right anterior oblique projection; (b) left lateral projection.

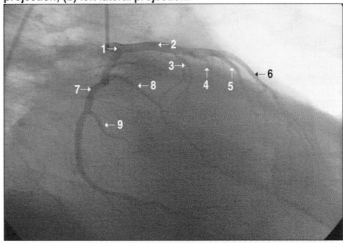

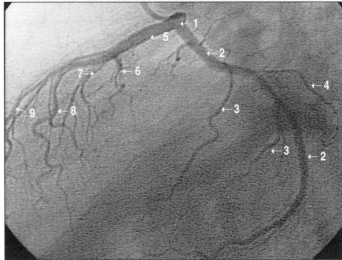

(a)
1. Left main coronary artery
2. Left anterior descending artery (LAD)
3. Septal branch
4. First diagonal branch
5. Second diagonal branch
6. Continuation of LAD
7. Circumflex artery
8. First obtuse marginal branch
9. Second obtuse marginal branch

(b)
1. Left main coronary artery seen end on
2. Circumflex artery
3. Obtuse marginals
4. Posterolateral branch
5. Left anterior descending artery (LAD)
6. Septal branch
7. First diagonal branch
8. Second diagonal branch
9. Continuation of LAD

Fig. 4.24 The coronary arteries.

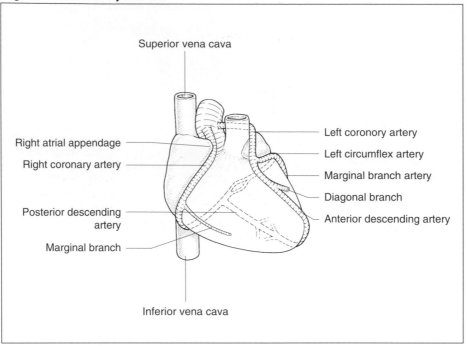

of cases, the right coronary artery supplies the atrioventricular node. *Coronary dominance* is determined by the vessel that supplies the inferior and lateral walls of the left ventricle. In right dominance (the usual situation), the right coronary artery gives rise to the posterior interventricular branch and continues around in the atrioventricular groove, giving branches to the posterolateral wall of the left ventricle. In left dominant situations, the right coronary artery is short, and the left circumflex supplies the posterolateral wall of the left ventricle and gives off the posterior descending artery.

THE VEINS OF THE HEART (**Fig. 4.25**)

Venous drainage of the heart is mainly via veins that accompany the coronary arteries and that drain via the coronary sinus. The coronary sinus lies in the posterior atrioventricular groove and drains into the posterior wall of the right atrium to the left of the orifice of the IVC. Its tributaries are:

■ The *great cardiac vein*, which ascends in the anterior interventricular groove and then runs to the left in the atrioventricular groove to become the coronary sinus;

■ The *middle cardiac vein*, which ascends in the posterior interventricular groove;

■ The *small cardiac vein*, which accompanies the marginal branches of the RCA on the inferior surface of the heart and then runs posteriorly in the right atrioventricular groove to enter the right side of the coronary sinus; and

■ The *left posterior ventricular vein*, which accompanies the obtuse marginals of the left coronary artery, running up the posterior aspect of the left ventricle to drain into the coronary sinus.

■ The *anterior cardiac veins* drain much of the anterior surface of the heart and drain into the anterior wall of the right atrium directly. Several small veins, the venae cordis minimae, drain directly into the cardiac chambers.

Fig. 4.25 The coronary veins.

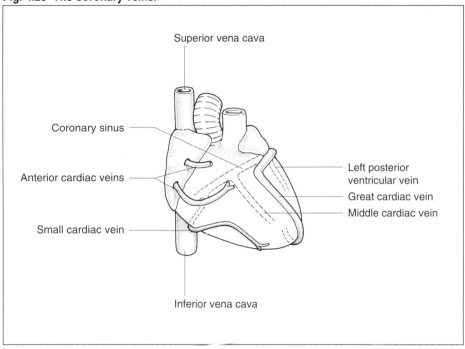

THE CONDUCTING SYSTEM OF THE HEART

The *sinoatrial node*, which is just to the right of the orifice of the SVC initiates the cardiac impulse. The impulse spreads through the musculature of the right atrium to the *atrioventricular node*, which lies in the interatrial septum. It is then conducted to the ventricles via the *atrioventricular bundle of His* (a specialized muscle that can conduct the electrical impulse). The bundle of His divides into right and left branches in the upper part of the interventricular septum, which activate the ventricular contraction.

RADIOLOGY OF THE HEART

Chest radiography

The *cardiac contour* is seen on the frontal and lateral chest film. Posteroanterior films are preferred to antero-

posterior ones as the heart, being anterior, is closer to the film and is not magnified to the same extent as with anteroposterior films. (For a description of the cardiac contour, see the section on the mediastinal contour, p. 139.)

The *coronary arteries* may be calcified in normal people.

The *position of the valves* may be deduced on PA and lateral films. The aortic and mitral valves are the most important to recognize, as these are most often affected by disease. On the PA film, if a line is drawn from the top of the left atrium to lowest part of the right heart border, the pulmonary, aortic and mitral valves lie above and just to the left of the line, from above downward. The aortic valve is projected over the middle third of the cardiac shadow. The tricuspid valve lies below the line and to just to the right of the line, below the pulmonary valve. On the lateral film, if a line is drawn from the middle of the oval density of the right pulmonary artery to the cardiac apex, the aortic valve lies in front and above the line and the mitral valve behind and below. The lower part of the aortic valve is in very close proximity to the anterior part of the mitral valve, being in fibrous continuity anatomically.

Fluoroscopy

The heart and its valves may be assessed by fluoroscopy. If the valves are calcified (usually pathologically), they may be distinguished by their characteristic motion as well as their location. The aortic valve has a to-and-fro motion in the plane of the ascending aorta, that is, upwards, backwards and to the right. The mitral valve has a circular as well as a to-and-fro motion in the left anterior oblique plane of the left atrium and ventricle.

Echocardiography

Two-dimensional echocardiography uses ultrasound to image the heart. A subcostal or intracostal window may be used and images may be obtained in any plane. Longitudinal images through the outflow tracts are usually obtained, as well as cross-sectional images through the valves and chambers. Ultrasound is probably the best modality for imaging the internal anatomy of the heart, the walls, chambers and valves. The movement of the walls and valves may also be assessed dynamically throughout the cardiac cycle.

Angiocardiography

This technique involves the injection of contrast directly into the heart chambers via a pigtail catheter, which is usually introduced through the femoral artery or vein for the left and right chambers respectively. The chambers are recognized by their position and characteristic configuration.

Coronary angiography

Coronary angiography involves selective catheterization of the coronary arteries. A small volume of contrast is injected and images may be obtained in lateral, anterior oblique and AP projections. There is individual variation in the branches of the coronary arteries, which are demonstrated from case to case. This is due both to anatomical variation and technical factors. The major arteries are demonstrated in **Figs 4.22** and **4.23.**

Nuclear medicine

Nuclear medicine studies are used mainly for functional assessment of the heart, which, in clinical practice, is often more important than the demonstration of the anatomy. ***Thallium-201*** and ***technetium-99m-labelled MIBI*** (2 methoxy isobutyrl isonitrile) are taken up by normally perfused myocardium, and images obtained by gamma camera show the heart. The use of SPECT (single photon emission CT) allows images to be constructed in any plane — usually with three sets of images — along the short cardiac axis (at right angles to the long axis of the heart), and along the vertical and horizontal long axes. It also improves the target:backround ratio, as neither radiopharmaceutical agent is taken up exclusively by the myocardium. Other functional information on ventricular filling, ejection fraction and so on may be obtained by blood-pool imaging using technetium 99m-labelled red blood cells and electrocardiogram (ECG)-gated acquisition of data.

Computed tomography (see Fig. 4.21)

CT scanning shows the heart and vessels in cross-section. The pericardium may be identified between epicardial and mediastinal fat. Dynamic scans obtained during intravenous infusion of contrast demonstrate the cardiac chambers and vessels to greater advantage. ECG gating allows images to be acquired during the same part of the cardiac cycle, thus reducing motion artefacts and providing better images.

Magnetic resonance imaging

The applications for MRI in cardiac radiology are steadily increasing. Acquisition of images is gated to the ECG to overcome motion artefact and faster scan times have improved image quality. The cardiac chambers, valves and major vessels may be imaged in any plane to give information previously only obtainable with cardioangiography and with the added advantage of demonstrating the soft tissues. The pericardium is shown as dark line of 1–2 mm thickness.

THE GREAT VESSELS (see Figs 4.8, 4.18, 4.20 and 4.30–4.33)

THE AORTA (see **Figs 4.8** and **4.26**)

The ascending aorta begins at the aortic valve at the level of the lower border of the third costal cartilage. It ascends to the right, arching over the pulmonary trunk to lie behind the upper border of the second right costal cartilage. The first few centimetres of the ascending aorta and the pulmonary trunk are enclosed in a common sheath of pericardium. At its origin it lies behind the outflow tract of the right ventricle and the pulmonary trunk, and the right atrial appendage overlaps it. It ascends anteriorly and to the right, passing over the right pulmonary artery and right main bronchus. The right lung and sternum are anterior. The coronary arteries arise from aortic sinuses — three localized dilatations above the cusps of the aortic valve.

The arch of the aorta passes posteriorly and from right to left. It passes anterior to the trachea and arches over the left mainstem bronchus and pulmonary artery to come to lie to the left of the body of T4. Anterior and to the left of the arch are the pleura and left lung. On its right side are the trachea, oesophagus, thoracic duct and body of T4 from front to back. Its inferior aspect is connected to the ligamentum arteriosum, the fibrous remnant of the ductus arteriosus. Superiorly are the three branches of the arch that are crossed anteriorly by the left brachiocephalic vein. The left superior intercostal vein runs down to the brachiocephalic vein, passing anterior to the aorta and occasionally causing a small bulge on the arch, which is visible on the chest radiograph. The branches of the arch of the aorta are the brachiocephalic artery, the left common carotid and the left subclavian arteries. The brachiocephalic and left common carotid arteries ascend on either side of the trachea in a 'V' shape to come to lie behind the sternoclavicular joints, at which point the brachiocephalic bifurcates into the right common carotid and subclavian arteries. From this point the common carotids ascend symmetrically into the neck.

The *aortic isthmus* is the junction of the arch of the aorta and the descending aorta. This area is relatively fixed and is thus prone to injury with shearing forces of blunt trauma.

The descending aorta passes inferiorly through the posterior mediastinum to the left of the spinal column. It passes through the diaphragm at the level of T12. On its left side are the pleura and left lung. Posteriorly are the vertebral column and the hemiazygous veins. At its highest point, the oesophagus lies to its right. The descending aorta then lies behind the oesophagus as the latter passes anteriorly, and the right lung and pleura lie to its right in contact with it. It passes behind the left main bronchus and pulmonary artery, the left atrium, the oesophagus and the posterior part of the diaphragm as it descends. To its right are the thoracic duct and the azygous vein.

The branches of the descending aorta are as follows:

■ Nine pairs of intercostal arteries and a pair of subcostal arteries arise from the posterior aspect of the descending aorta to run in the neurovascular grooves of the third to twelfth ribs;

■ Two to three bronchial arteries. The origin of these is variable. The right bronchial artery usually arises from the third posterior intercostal artery and the two left bronchial arteries from the aorta itself. The upper left usually arises opposite T5 and the lower left bronchial artery below the left main bronchus;

■ Four to five oesophageal branches arise from the front of the aorta. These ramify on the oesophagus forming a network with oesophageal branches of the inferior thyroid artery and ascending branches of the left phrenic and left gastric arteries;

■ Mediastinal branches;

■ Phrenic branches to the upper part of the posterior diaphragm; and

■ Pericardial branches to the posterior pericardium.

SUBCLAVIAN ARTERY (see **Fig. 1.42**)

The right subclavian artery arises from the bifurcation of the brachiocephalic trunk behind the right sternoclavicular joint. The left subclavian artery arises from the arch of the aorta in front of the trachea at the level of the T3/T4 disc space. It ascends on the left of the trachea to behind the left sternoclavicular joint. From this point, both arteries have a similar course. The scalenus anterior muscle (which passes from the transverse processes of the upper cervical vertebrae to the inner border of the first rib) divides the artery into three parts. The first part arches over the apex of the lung and lies deeply in the neck. The second part passes laterally behind the scalenus anterior muscle, which separates it from the subclavian vein. The third part passes to the lateral border of the first rib, from where it becomes the axillary artery (see Chapter 1 for branches).

PULMONARY ARTERIES (see **Figs 4.14** and **4.18**)

(See also pulmonary arteries in the lung.)

The pulmonary trunk begins at the pulmonary valve and is approximately 5 cm long. At first it lies anterior to the aorta, then passes posteriorly and to its left to lie in the concavity of the arch, where it bifurcates into right and left main pulmonary arteries. The entire pulmonary artery is covered by the pericardium in a common sheath with the ascending aorta.

The right and left atrial appendages and the right and left coronary arteries surround the base of the pulmonary trunk. Anterior and to the left it is in contact with the left lung and pleura.

The right pulmonary artery runs horizontally and to the right, passing behind the ascending aorta and SVC in front of the right main bronchus. It is crossed anteriorly by the right superior pulmonary vein as this drains to the left atrium.

The left pulmonary artery runs to the left, running anterior to the left main bronchus and arching over this structure as it gives off the upper-lobe bronchus. It has a slightly higher position in the chest and is slightly shorter and smaller than the right pulmonary artery. It is crossed anteriorly by the left superior pulmonary vein. It is attached to the concavity of the aortic arch by the ligamentum arteriosum.

GREAT VEINS (see **Figs 4.8** and **1.44**)

The brachiocephalic veins are formed by the union of internal jugular and subclavian veins at either side, behind the medial end of the clavicles. On the right, the brachiocephalic vein runs inferiorly behind the right border of the manubrium, anterolateral to the brachiocephalic artery. The left brachiocephalic vein is longer. It descends obliquely behind the manubrium, crossing the origins of the left common carotid and subclavian arteries. It joins with the right brachiocephalic vein to form the superior vena cava behind the junction of the first right costal cartilage with the manubrium.

The *superior vena cava* runs inferiorly behind the right border of the manubrium to enter the right atrium at the level of the third costal cartilage. Its only tributary is the azygous vein, which enters its posterior aspect just above the upper limit of its covering sheath of pericardium.

Tributaries of the brachiocephalic veins

These are as follows:

- Internal thoracic (mammary) veins, which drain into the inferior aspect of the brachiocephalic veins;
- Inferior thyroid veins, which arise in the thyroid gland, and form a plexus anterior the trachea. From here, left and right veins drain into the corresponding brachiocephalic vein, close to their confluence; and the
- Left superior intercostal vein, which drains the left second and third posterior intercostal veins and passes obliquely down anterior to the aortic arch to drain into the left brachiocephalic vein.

RADIOLOGY OF THE GREAT VESSELS

The great vessels may be imaged by two-dimensional echocardiography, angiography, CT or MRI. Using MRI one can image in any plane without the need for contrast. A sagittal oblique plane is particularly useful for imaging the thoracic aorta. With two-dimensional echocardiography, the aortic root and sinuses, ascending and descending aorta may be visualized using an anterior approach. The arch of the aorta and its branches are occasionally well visualized from a suprasternal approach.

THE OESOPHAGUS
(Fig. 4.26; see Figs 4.34–4.38)

This begins at the level of C5/C6 or the lower border of the cricoid cartilage as the continuation of the oropharynx (see also Chapter 1). Its upper limit is defined by the cricopharyngeus muscle, which encircles it from front to back. It descends behind the trachea and thyroid, lying in front of the lower cervical vertebrae. It then inclines slightly to the left in the neck and upper mediastinum before returning to the midline at the level of T5 from where it passes to the left again before sweeping forward to pass through the diaphragm. In the chest it passes behind the trachea, left main bronchus, left atrium and upper part of left ventricle from above downward; it then passes behind the posterior sloping part of the diaphragm before traversing this at the level of T10.

On its left side, where is found the origin of the left subclavian artery, it is grooved by the arch of the aorta. Below this level, its left side lies on left lung and pleural tissue. On its right side, it is crossed by the termination of the azygous vein at the level of T4. Below this, the azygous vein lies behind and to its right and it is in contact with right lung and pleura. Posteriorly are the thoracic vertebrae and thoracic duct, the azygous vein and tributaries and the right posterior intercostal arteries as these cross the vertebral column from the descending aorta. The descending aorta lies to its left side initially. Then as the oesophagus passes forwards and to the left, it becomes anterior to this vessel in the mid thorax and anterior and to its left as it passes through the diaphragm. In its terminal part in the abdomen it is retroperitoneal. It enters the stomach at the oesophagogastric junction.

BLOOD SUPPLY

The blood supply is organized in thirds (with free anastomosis between each third) as follows:

- Branches of the inferior thyroid artery supply the upper third;
- Branches from the descending aorta supply the middle third; and
- Branches from the left gastric artery supply the lower third.

Fig. 4.26 Posterior mediastinum. (Courtesy of Prof. JB Coakley.)

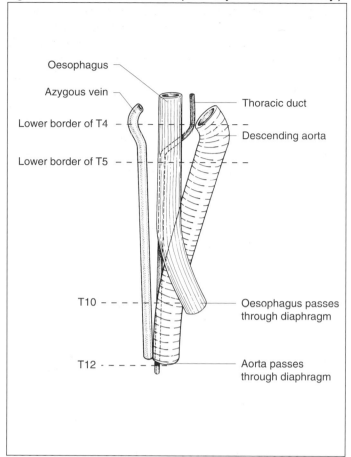

Venous drainage is also found in thirds: to the inferior thyroid veins, the azygous system and to the portal system via the left gastric vein. Thus there is communication of the systemic and portal venous systems in the oesophagus.

LYMPH DRAINAGE

This is via a rich paraoesophageal plexus to posterior mediastinal nodes, draining from here to supraclavicular nodes. The lower part drains to left gastric and coeliac nodes.

Fig. 4.27 Barium-swallow technique showing the oesophagus:(a) upper oesophagus and oropharynx, lateral view; (b) mid-oesophagus, right anterior oblique view; (c) distal oesophagus.

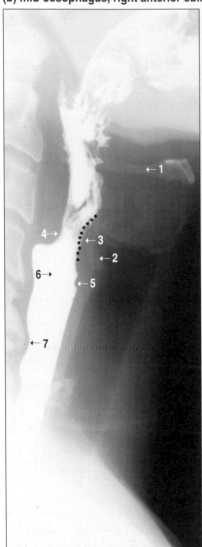

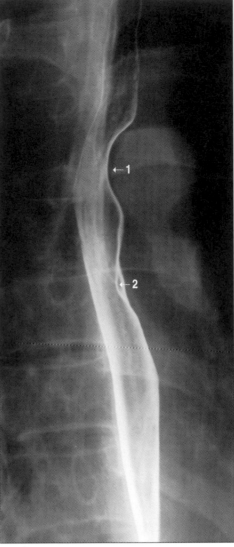

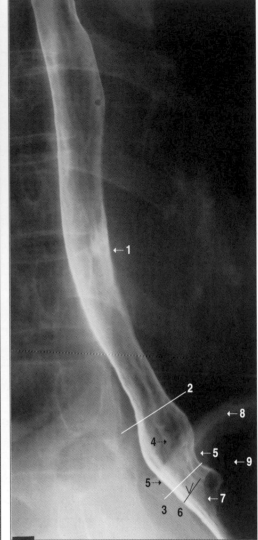

(a)
1. Hyoid bone
2. Cricoid cartilage
3. Cricoid impression
4. Cricopharyngeus muscle impression
5. Postcricoid venous plexus
6. Oesophagus
7. Impression caused by osteophytes

(b)
1. Impression of aortic arch
2. Impression of left main bronchus

(c)
1. Cardiac impression (mainly left atrium)
2. A ring: upper limit of ampulla (vestibule)
3. B ring (Schatzki ring): lower limit of ampulla
4. Ampulla (oesophageal vestibule)
5. Diaphragmatic hiatus
6. Oesophageal mucosal folds
7. Oesophagogastric junction (Z-line)
8. Diaphragm
9. Air in fundus of stomach

RADIOLOGY OF THE OESOPHAGUS (Fig. 4.27)

Plain films

The right wall of the oesophagus and azygous vein is outlined by lung, which may be seen on the frontal film as the azygo-oesophageal line. Above the level of the arch of the azygous (at T4 level), the right wall is sometimes seen a the pleuro-oesophageal line. If the oesophagus contains air, the posterior aspect of the anterior oesophageal wall may be seen on the lateral film, behind the trachea. This is known as the 'posterior tracheal stripe'.

Barium studies

The main radiological method of assessing the oesophagus is the barium-swallow technique. Here the oesophagus is outlined by barium. Gas is usually swallowed in addition to give a double-contrast examination and to distend the oesophagus. The use of a paralysing agent such as intravenous hyoscine butylbromide (Buscopan) stops intrinsic oesophageal contraction, allowing better appreciation of oesophageal anatomy.

On the frontal view, the oropharynx may be examined. The piriform fossae are outlined by barium and the epiglottis and base of the tongue show as filling defects in the midline. The cervical oesophagus is seen to curve slightly to the left.

On the lateral view, the tongue base and epiglottis are seen from the side, with the vallecula between. A posterior indentation caused by the contraction of cricopharyngeus muscle to initiate deglutition indicates the commencement of the oesophagus proper. Just above this, on the anterior wall of the oesophagus, a small impression may be made by a submucosal plexus of veins. The cervical oesophagus is seen to lie on the anterior surface of the vertebral bodies of the cervical spine.

In the chest, the oesophagus is best demonstrated with the subject rotated slightly off lateral — usually in the right posterior oblique position. Three major impressions are seen anteriorly. These are made by the aortic arch, the left main bronchus and the left heart chambers (mainly left atrium) from above down. In this position the oesophagus can be seen to curve anteriorly in its distal part to enter the stomach.

On the frontal view, the oesophagus has a left-sided indentation from the aortic arch. The left main bronchus also makes an impression on its left side and may make a linear impression as it indents the anterior wall. The lower oesophagus curves to the left to enter the stomach. The course of the oesophagus may be altered by unfolding of the aorta in elderly people.

The lower end of the oesophagus has a fusiform dilatation just above the oesophagogastric junction. This is called the oesophageal vestibule. On barium examination, the upper part of the vestibule is defined by a transiently contractile ring known as the 'A ring'. The lower limit of the vestibule is defined by another transiently contractile ring known as the 'B ring', 'Schatzki ring' or 'transverse mucosal fold'. The vestibule corresponds to the manometrically measurable zone of increased pressure that is felt to represent the lower oesophageal sphincter. The upper oesophageal sphincter is formed by cricopharyngeus. In young people, the vestibule may span the diaphragm. In this case only the upper ring may be identified radiologically. As the oesophagus passes through the diaphragm, the latter makes an indentation on it.

The oesophageal mucosa is arranged in longitudinal folds that are best seen when the oesophagus is not distended. These measure approximately 3 mm in width. The thicker folds of the stomach are seen distally indicating the oesophagogastric junction. This may rise into the thorax on swallowing in normal people.

Cross-sectional imaging

The oesophagus may also be imaged by CT and MRI. On cross-section its relationship to the other structures of the thorax is appreciated (see **Figs 4.30 and 4.31**). Its visualization is improved if it contains air. When collapsed it is seen as a narrow, thin-walled structure in the posterior mediastinum. Appreciation of the areas in which air-containing lung is adjacent to the oesophagus provides an understanding of the mediastinal lines seen on the frontal chest radiograph.

THE THORACIC DUCT AND MEDIASTINAL LYMPHATICS (see Figs 4.15 and 4.26)

The thoracic duct arises from a saccular lymphatic reservoir called the 'cysterna chyli', which lies behind the right crus of the diaphragm, anterior to the bodies of L1 and L2. Lymph from the abdomen and lower limbs passes from here into the thoracic duct, which runs superiorly into the posterior mediastinum, passing through the aortic opening in the diaphragm. The thoracic duct ascends anterior to the vertebral column with the descending aorta to its left and the azygous vein to its right. The right posterior intercostal arteries run across the vertebral column behind the duct, and the terminal parts of the hemiazygous and accessory azygous veins cross behind it to enter the azygous vein. It ascends behind the oesophagus coming to lie to the left of this at T5 and then running superiorly on its left side into the neck. It then passes laterally behind the carotid vessels and at the level of C7, the duct arches anteriorly over the left lung, rising 3–4 cm above the clavicle. It then descends to drain into the left subclavian vein at the jugulosubclavian junction. It receives lymph drainage from the entire thorax as well as the left side of the head and neck and the left subclavian trunk, which drains the left arm.

The right lymphatic duct drains the right side of the head and neck and receives the right subclavian trunk. It drains into the right jugulosubclavian junction. It is about 1 cm long.

The mediastinum contains numerous lymph-node groups, which may enlarge in disease states. The anterior mediastinal nodes comprise the internal mammary chain, accompanying the internal mammary vessels, and a preaortic group lying anterior to the ascending aorta. The tracheobronchial nodes lie centrally around the trachea and its bifurcation. They comprise:

- Right and left paratracheal nodes on either side of the trachea;
- The azygous node in the right tracheobronchial angle;
- Pretracheal nodes anterior to the trachea;
- Aortopulmonary node between the concavity of the aortic arch and the pulmonary artery; and
- Subcarinal nodes inferior to the carina.

The posterior mediastinal lymph nodes are found along the aorta and oesophagus and also anterior to and on either side of the spinal column. They take their name from their location, for example paraspinal, para-aortic and so on. Normal nodes are not appreciated on the plain chest radiograph. Nodes may be seen on CT; if they measure more than 1 cm in diameter, they are likely to be pathological.

THE THYMUS

This organ is part of the lymphatic system and lies in the anterior mediastinum. It has two lobes that extend down so far as the fourth costal cartilage in infancy. It is a soft structure and is moulded into the sternum and ribs anteriorly, and the pericardium, great vessels and trachea posteriorly. It is extremely variable in size and shape even in the same subject at different times. It is visible on the chest radiograph within 24 hours of birth, gradually involuting after the age of 2 years of age. It is rarely seen of the chest radiograph after 8 years of age but may be identified into early adulthood on CT as a small triangular structure in the anterior mediastinum, rarely measuring greater that 1 cm in diameter.

THE AZYGOUS SYSTEM (Fig. 4.28; see Figs 4.19, 4.26, 4.32 and 4.33)

These veins are found in the posterior mediastinum. The system consists of the azygous vein on the right and the hemiazygous and accessory hemiazygous azygous veins on the left.

The azygous vein commences variably anterior to the L2 vertebra, either as a branch of the inferior vena cava or as a confluence of the right ascending lumbar vein and right subcostal vein. It ascends to the right of the aorta and thoracic duct, anteriorly to the bodies of T12 to T5 and the right posterior intercostal arteries, which cross behind it. The right lung and pleura are to its right. It usually passes behind the right crus of the diaphragm to enter the thorax (see **Fig. 4.4**). At the level of T4, the azygous vein arches anteriorly, passing over the hilum of the right lung with the trachea and oesophagus medially from the posterior side to the anterior side. The azygous vein drains into the superior vena cava just above the upper limit of the pericardium, behind the third costal cartilage.

The azygous vein receives all but the first intercostal vein on the right. The second, third and fourth intercostal veins usually drain via a common channel — the right superior intercostal vein. The hemiazygous and accessory azygous veins drain into it at mid-thoracic level. The right bronchial veins drain into the azygous vein near its termination. It also receives tributaries from the oesophagus, pericardium and mediastinum.

The hemiazygous vein commences in a similar manner to the azygous vein on the left side of the aorta. Its origin may communicate with the left renal vein, and it ascends anterior to the vertebral column to the mid-thoracic level, then passes behind the aorta to drain into the azygous vein. It receives the left ascending lumbar and lowest four posterior intercostal veins, as well as mediastinal and oesophageal veins.

The accessory hemiazygous vein receives the fourth to the eighth posterior intercostal veins. (The first to third posterior intercostal veins drain into the left brachiocephalic vein.) It may also receive the left bronchial veins. It descends on the left side of the vertebral column to the mid-thoracic level, then crosses to the right behind the aorta to drain into the azygous vein. The hemiazygous and accessory hemiazygous veins may drain into the azygous vein separately or via a common trunk.

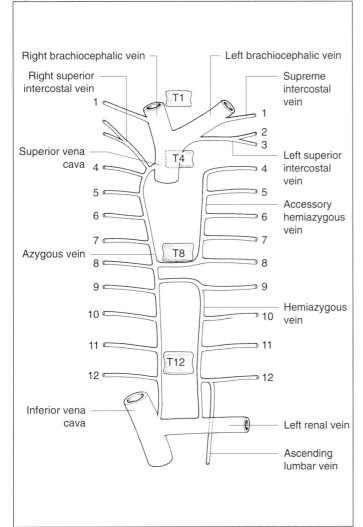

Fig. 4.28 Azygous system. (Courtesy of Prof. JB Coakley.)

Right brachiocephalic vein
Right superior intercostal vein
Left brachiocephalic vein
Supreme intercostal vein
T1
1
1
2
3
Superior vena cava
T4
Left superior intercostal vein
4
4
5
5
6
6
Accessory hemiazygous vein
7
7
Azygous vein
T8
8
8
9
9
10
Hemiazygous vein
10
11
11
T12
12
12
Inferior vena cava
Left renal vein
Ascending lumbar vein

IMPORTANT NERVES OF THE MEDIASTINUM

The *vagus nerves* are the tenth cranial nerves and pass through the neck in the carotid sheath. Composed of motor and sensory fibres, the vagus nerve enters the superior mediastinum posterior to the internal jugular vein and brachiocephalic veins. It passes behind the main bronchi, forming a posterior pulmonary plexus; branches then pass to the oesophagus, forming anterior and posterior oesophageal plexi, which continue into the abdomen through the oesophageal hiatus as anterior and posterior vagal trunks. The *recurrent laryngeal nerves* arise from the vagi. On the right the recurrent laryngeal nerve winds around the subclavian artery, on the left it winds around the aortic arch.

The *phrenic nerves* arise from the third to fifth cervical nerves and are the motor supply to the diaphragm. They enter the chest anterior to the subclavian artery and deep to the vein. The right phrenic nerve runs down in front of the superior vena cava, over the right heart border and inferior vena cava to reach the diaphragm. The left phrenic nerve runs down over the aortic arch and left superior intercostal vein, in front of the left hilum and runs on the left heart border to reach the diaphragm.

The *sympathetic trunk* runs inferiorly in the posterior mediastinum in the paraspinal gutters, coming to lie in front of the bodies of T11 and T12 before passing through the diaphragm behind the medial arcuate ligament to continue as the lumbar sympathetic trunk. It is distributed to the thoracic viscera and forms the splanchnic nerves to the abdominal viscera.

THE MEDIASTINUM ON THE CHEST RADIOGRAPH

MEDIASTINAL CONTOUR ON THE FRONTAL CHEST RADIOGRAPH (see **Fig. 4.5**)

The heart and great vessels form a characteristic contour on the frontal chest radiograph. The right side of the mediastinal contour is formed from above downward by the brachiocephalic vein and the SVC. The SVC forms a shallow angle with the right atrium, which forms the right heart border. The terminal part of the IVC may be seen just medial to the cardiophrenic angle, which is usually sharp. Occasionally a fibrofatty pad displaces the right pleura laterally, obscuring the cardiophrenic angle.

The left side of the mediastinal contour is formed by the composite shadow of the subclavian vessels superiorly. The artery is lower and actually forms the contour. This fades out laterally and is usually indistinct. Below this the aortic prominence is termed the 'aortic knuckle' or 'knob'. This is formed by the posterior part of the arch. It may be indistinct in young people and very prominent in older people, especially if there is aortic unfolding. Sometimes a small 'nipple' may be seen projecting from the aortic knuckle. This is caused by the left superior intercostal vein as it crosses the aorta to drain into the left brachiocephalic vein. In older people, the left side of the descending aorta may be visible descending from the aortic knuckle. Below the aortic knuckle is an air space called the aortopulmonary window. Failure to identify this clear space indicates pathology. Below the aortopulmonary window is the main pulmonary artery, which has a straight upper border, and below this is the left ventricle. The left atrial appendage lies embedded in fat below the pulmonary artery but is not contour-forming unless enlarged. The left cardiophrenic angle is not so sharp as the left. In deep inspiration, air-filled lung may be seen under the apex of the left ventricle. Occasionally, a fat pad is present in the left cardiophrenic angle.

The pulmonary arteries and veins form the densities of the hila on the frontal chest radiograph (see radiological features of the lung, p. 120).

MEDIASTINAL CONTOURS ON THE

LATERAL CHEST RADIOGRAPH (see **Fig. 4.6**)

The heart shadow lies behind the lower third of sternum. The anterior border is formed by the right ventricle and outflow tract. Higher up the lungs are in contact with each other behind the sternum and in front of the ascending aorta forming the retrosternal air space. The posterior contour of the heart shadow is formed by the left atrium above and the left ventricle below. The IVC may be identified as a triangular structure crossing the diaphragm to enter the right atrium, which lies in a more anterior plane that the left atrium.

The aorta

The aorta may be invisible in young people but is usually seen, at least in part, in middle-aged subjects. The ascending aorta is indistinct. The arch curves evenly from front to back and the descending aorta is seen anterior to the vertebral column. Its walls should be parallel. In older people, unfolding may cause it to overlie the vertebral bodies.

MEDIASTINAL LINES (**Figs 4.29** and **4.30**; see **Figs 4.5** and **4.6**)

Wherever air-filled lung outlines a linear soft-tissue structure, the difference in density is detected by the plain radiograph as a *line*. If air outlines two sides of a thin

Fig. 4.29 Cross-sectional anatomy: level T3.

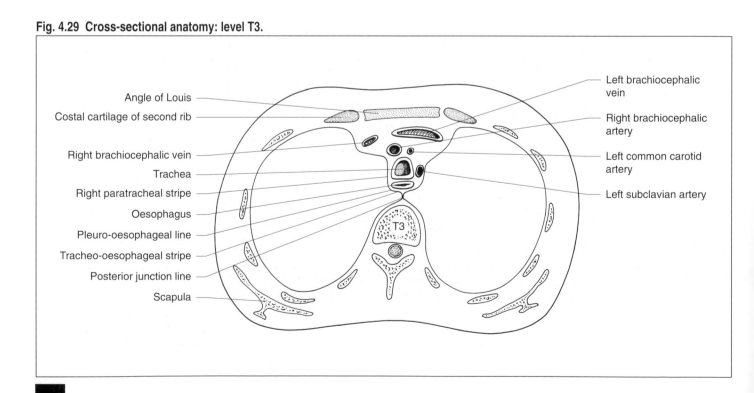

Angle of Louis
Costal cartilage of second rib
Right brachiocephalic vein
Trachea
Right paratracheal stripe
Oesophagus
Pleuro-oesophageal line
Tracheo-oesophageal stripe
Posterior junction line
Scapula

T3

Left brachiocephalic vein
Right brachiocephalic artery
Left common carotid artery
Left subclavian artery

Fig. 4.30 CT scan of thorax: upper T4 level showing mediastinal lines.

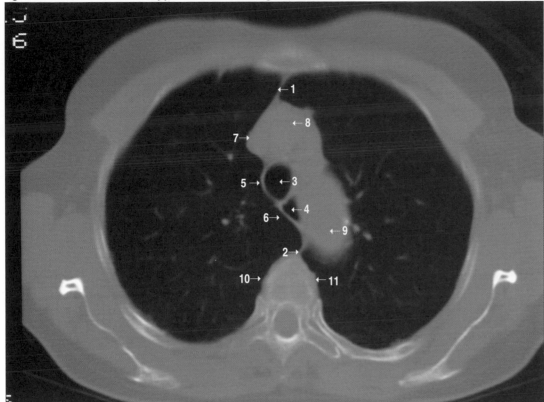

1. Anterior junction line
2. Posterior junction line
3. Air-filled trachea
4. Air-filled oesophagus
5. Right paratracheal stripe
6. Pleuro-oesophageal stripe (the azygous vein has drained into the superior vena cava at the T4 level)
7. Superior vena cava
8. Ascending aorta
9. Descending aorta
10. Right paraspinal line
11. Left paraspinal line

Fig. 4.31 CT scan of thorax: level T3.

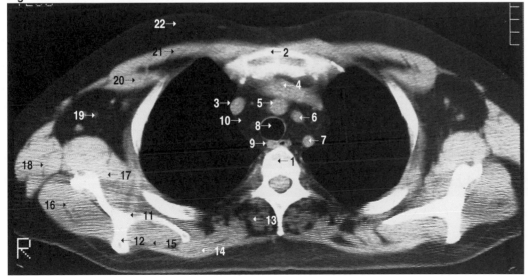

1. Body of T3
2. Body of manubrium sterni
3. Right brachiocephalic vein
4. Left brachiocephalic vein
5. Brachiocephalic trunk
6. Left common carotid artery
7. Left subclavian artery
8. Trachea
9. Oesophagus
10. Mediastinal fat
11. Right scapula
12. Spine of scapula
13. Erector spinae muscle
14. Trapezius muscle
15. Supraspinatus muscle
16. Infraspinatus muscle
17. Subscapularis muscle
18. Deltoid muscle
19. Fat in axilla
20. Pectoralis minor muscle
21. Pectoralis major muscle
22. Subcutaneous fat

Fig. 4.32 CT scan of thorax: level T4 .

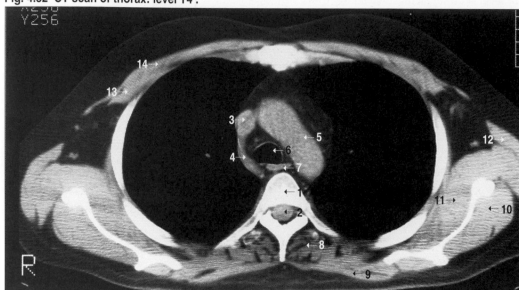

1. Body of T4
2. Thecal sac and spinal cord
3. Superior vena cava
4. Azygous vein
5. Arch of aorta
6. Trachea
7. Oesophagus
8. Erector spinae muscle
9. Trapezius muscle
10. Infraspinatus muscle
11. Subscapularis muscle
12. Deltoid muscle
13. Pectoralis minor muscle
14. Pectoralis major muscle

Fig. 4.33 CT scan of thorax: lower T5 level.

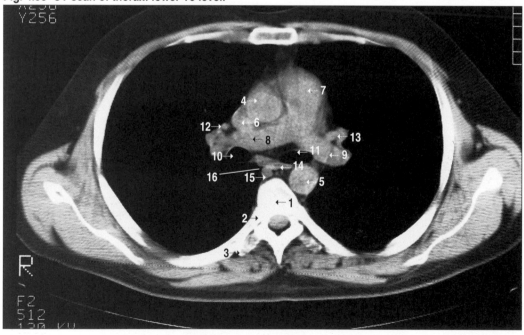

1. Lower part of body of T5
2. Right fifth rib and costovertebral joint
3. Right transverse process of T5 and costotransverse joint
4. Ascending aorta
5. Descending aorta
6. Superior vena cava
7. Main pulmonary trunk
8. Right pulmonary artery
9. Left pulmonary artery
10. Right main bronchus
11. Left main bronchus
12. Right superior pulmonary vein
13. Left superior pulmonary vein
14. Oesophagus
15. Azygous vein
16. Azygo-oesophageal recess

structure the soft-tissue density is seen as a *stripe*. This relationship may be appreciated on CT scans (see **Fig. 4.30**).

Right paratracheal stripe (Fig. 4.29)

The lung is in contact with the trachea from the level of the clavicles to the azygous vein in the right tracheo-bronchial angle. As the trachea is air-filled, the right tracheal wall is seen as a stripe, which should not measure more than 3 mm (the left tracheal wall is separated from lung by the aorta and great vessels and is not seen).

Posterior junction line (Fig. 4.29)

This is formed by the apposition of the two lungs posteriorly. It extends from well above the clavicles vertically downwards to the arch of the aorta. The aortic arch separates the lungs and the line disappears. It may reform below the arch. The line represents the four layers of pleura between the posterior part of the lungs seen from the front.

Anterior junction line (see Fig. 4.34)

This line is formed by the apposition of the lungs anteriorly. It begins below the clavicles and runs inferiorly and to the left. Its oblique course is because of the differing anterior extent of the two lungs. It always ends at the right ventricular outflow tract.

Pleuro-oesophageal line (Fig. 4.29)

This is formed by the right lung outlining the right wall of the oesophagus above the level of the azygous vein. If the oesophagus happens to be distended with air, the pleuro-oesophageal stripe is seen. The thickness of this represents the thickness of the oesophageal wall and pleura and should not exceed 2 mm.

Azygo-oesophageal line (see Fig. 4.35)

The azygous vein is closely related to the right posterolateral aspect of the oesophagus in the posterior mediastinum. The right lung abuts the two structures forming the azygo-oesophageal line, tucking in behind them in the azygo-oesophageal *recess*. On the frontal chest film, the line curves to the right as the azygous vein crosses to gain the right tracheobronchial angle before draining into the SVC.

Paraspinal lines (Fig. 4.35)

These are outlined by lung apposing the spinal column. The right line is sharper than the left as the descending aorta tends to reflect the pleura off the thoracic spine on the left, making the line more indistinct. The distance from the lateral border of the spine to the line may vary with body habitus and may be 1 cm on the left in obese people with paraspinal fat deposits.

Aortopulmonary mediastinal stripe

This is the reflected pleura from the aortic arch to the pulmonary trunk and left pulmonary artery. It defines the lateral boundary of the aortopulmonary window.

Posterior tracheal stripe

This is seen on the lateral view and represents the posterior wall of the trachea outlined on either side by air. It measures 2–3 mm. If the collapsed oesophagus is apposed to the posterior trachea, the stripe may measure 1 cm If there is air in the oesophagus, the stripe represents posterior tracheal and anterior oesophageal walls.

CROSS-SECTIONAL ANATOMY

(Refer to **Figs 4.29** and **4.34–4.38** for this section.)

LEVEL T3 (Fig. 4.29)

This is the superior mediastinal level. The trachea is seen in the midline with the great vessels anteriorly and the oesophagus behind. The brachiocephalic veins are anterior and lateral to the arteries and unite to form the superior vena cava at about this level. The left brachiocephalic vein is seen passing anteriorly to the branches of the aortic arch.

LEVEL T4 (see Fig. 4.34)

This plane passes through the lower border of T4 and the sternal angle. Above this plane is the superior mediastinum. At this level is the lower part of the aortic arch to the right of the trachea, and the arch of the azygous vein to the left, crossing the left hilum to drain into the posterior aspect of the superior vena cava. The oblique fissure, although demonstrated on these figures, is not always seen on CT as a line.

LEVEL T5 (Fig. 4.35)

This plane is at, or just below, the tracheal bifurcation. The main pulmonary artery is seen dividing into right pulmonary artery, which runs anteriorly to its bronchus, and left pulmonary artery, which arches superiorly out of the plane to pass over the left bronchus. The descending lower-lobe artery is seen lying posterolateral to the bronchus.

The superior pulmonary veins are seen anteriorly. On the right this is anterior to the interlobar artery. On the left it is separated from the lower-lobe artery by the left bronchus.

Fig. 4.34 Cross-sectional anatomy: level T4.

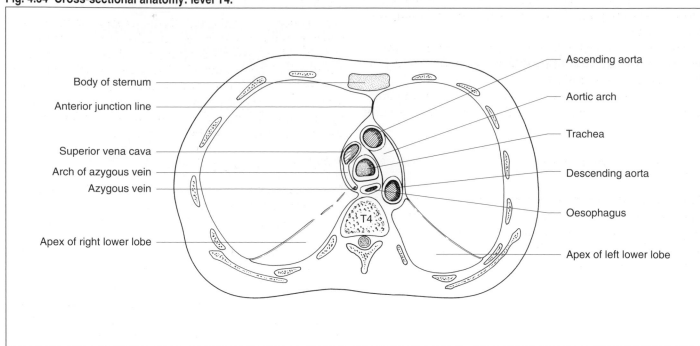

Fig. 4.35 Cross-sectional anatomy: level T5.

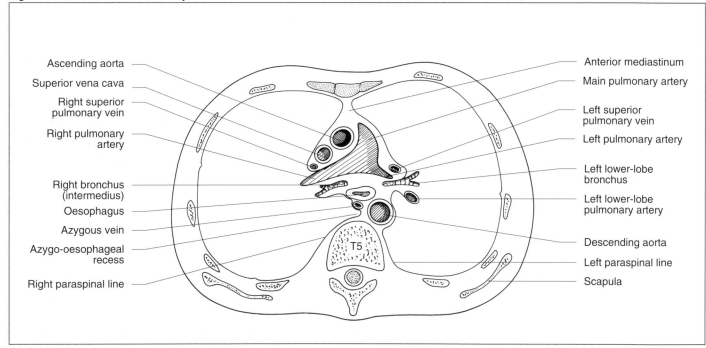

The ascending aorta is seen in cross-section, lying in a more posterior plane than the origin of the main pulmonary artery.

Anterior to this is the junction of the anterior pleurae of the lungs, which forms the anterior junction line on the frontal chest radiograph.

The oesophagus, azygous veins and descending aorta are seen in the posterior mediastinum. The azygo-oesophageal recess may be seen.

LEVEL T6 (**Fig. 4.36**)

This section passes through the upper part of the heart. The right atrial appendage may be seen overlapping the origin of the aorta. The coronary arteries come off the aorta at this level. The right ventricular outflow tract is seen anterior to the origin of the aorta. The relationship of the oesophagus to the left atrium is seen.

LEVEL T8 (**Fig. 4.37**)

This section passes through the heart and shows the relationship of the chambers to each other. The left ventricular inflow and outflow tracts are separated from each other by the anterior leaflet of the mitral valve. The aortic sinuses are seen as localized bulges. Note that the right heart border is formed by the right atrium, the anterior border is formed by the right ventricle, the left border by the left ventricle and the posterior border by the left atrium.

LEVEL T10 (**Fig. 4.38**)

At this level, part of the abdominal cavity is also seen as the dome of the diaphragm reaches the level of T9 approximately. The oesophagus traverses the diaphragm at this level, in a relatively anterior position, through the oesophageal hiatus and joins the stomach at the oesophagogastric junction. The fundus of the stomach and part of the spleen and liver are seen. The inferior vena cava is situated slightly anteriorly; on higher cuts it enters the right atrium. The descending aorta with azygous and hemi azygous veins on its right and left are posterior.

Fig. 4.36 Cross-sectional anatomy: level T6.

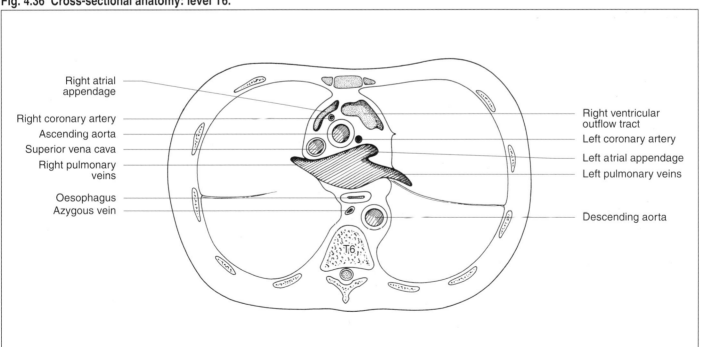

Fig. 4.37 Cross-sectional anatomy: level T8.

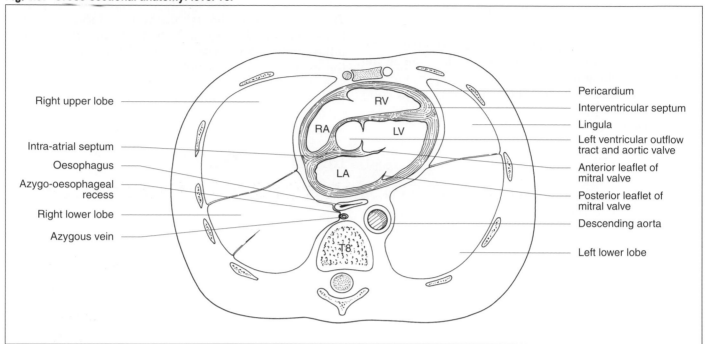

Fig. 4.38 Cross-sectional anatomy: level T10

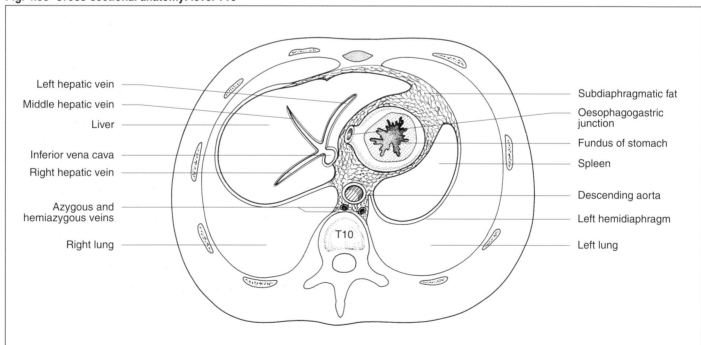

CHAPTER 5 *THE ABDOMEN*

Anterior abdominal wall

Stomach

Duodenum

Small intestine

Ileocaecal valve

Vermiform appendix

Large intestine

Liver

Biliary system

Pancreas

Spleen

Portal venous system

Kidneys and ureter

Adrenal glands

Abdominal aorta

Inferior vena cava

Veins of the posterior abdominal wall

Lymphatic drainage of the abdomen

Peritoneal spaces of the abdomen

Cross-sectional anatomy of the abdomen

THE ANTERIOR ABDOMINAL WALL

Deep to the skin and subcutaneous fat of the lower anterior abdominal wall is a fibrous layer called Scarpa's fascia. This extends to the penis and scrotum (or labia majora) as Colles' fascia, which is attached to the posterior border of the perineal membrane and the pubic rami.

MUSCLE LAYERS

The *external oblique muscle* arises on the anterior surface of the lower ribs and is inserted into the linea alba, pubic crest, inguinal ligament and iliac crest.

The *internal oblique muscle* arises from the lumbar fascia, iliac crest and the lateral two-thirds of the inguinal ligament and is inserted into the linea alba and the costal margin.

The *transversus abdominis muscle* arises from the lower ribs, interdigitating with the diaphragm, the lumbar fascia, the iliac crest and the lateral half of the inguinal ligament and is inserted into the linea alba.

The *rectus abdominis muscle* is a thick ribbon of muscle on either side of the midline from the costal cartilages to the pubic crest. It has three to four tendinous intersections at intervals along its length, which adhere to the anterior rectus sheath. The rectus sheath is formed by the aponeuroses of the other abdominal wall muscles as they surround the rectus muscle to attach to the linea alba.

Fig. 5.1 Plain film of abdomen.

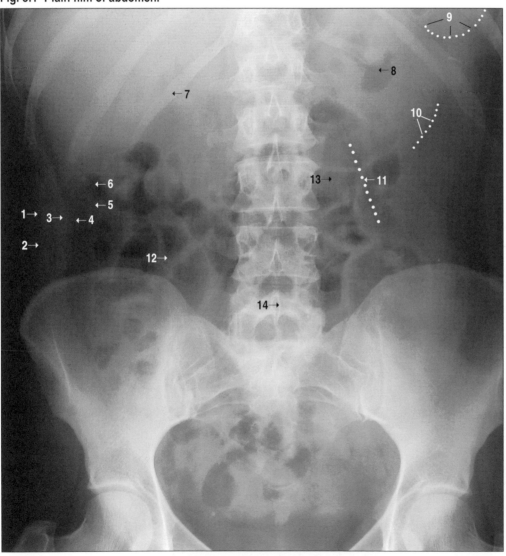

1. Internal oblique muscle
2. Fat between internal oblique muscle and transversus abdominis muscle
3. Transversus abdominis muscle
4. Properitoneal fat line (extraperitoneal fat layer)
5. Inferior border of right lobe of liver
6. Gas in hepatic flexure
7. Right twelfth rib
8. Gas in transverse colon
9. Inferior border of spleen
10. Left kidney
11. Left psoas muscle outline
12. Right psoas muscle outline
13. Left transverse process of L3
14. Spinous process of L5

THE STOMACH (Figs 5.5–5.8)

The stomach is 'J'-shaped but varies in size and shape with the volume of its contents, with erect or supine position and even with inspiration and expiration. The size and shape of the stomach also varies considerably from person to person, differing especially with the build of the subject.

The stomach has two *orifices* — the cardiac orifice (so named because of proximity through the diaphragm to the heart) at the oesophagogastric junction, and the pylorus. It has two curvatures — the greater and lesser curves. The *incisura* is an angulation of the lesser curve.

The part of the stomach above the cardia is called the *fundus*. Between the cardia and the incisura is the *body* of the stomach and distal to the incisura is the gastric antrum. The lumen of the pylorus is referred to as the *pyloric canal*.

The stomach is lined by mucosa, which has tiny nodular elevations called the *areae gastricae* and is thrown into folds called *rugae*. Longitudinal folds paralleling the lesser curve are called the *'magenstrasse'*, rugae elsewhere in the stomach are random and patternless.

There are three *muscle layers* in the wall of the stomach: (i) an outer longitudinal; (ii) an inner circular; and (iii) an incomplete, innermost, oblique layer. The circular layer is thickened at the pylorus as a sphincter but not at the oesophagogastric junction. Fibres of the oblique layer loop around the notch between the oesophagus and the fundus and help to prevent reflux here. The oblique fibres are responsible for the 'magenstrasse' and can pinch off the remainder of the stomach and allow fluids to pass directly from oesophagus along the lesser curve to the duodenum.

Peritoneum coats the anterior and posterior surface of the stomach and is continued between the lesser curve and the liver as the lesser omentum and beyond the greater curve as the greater omentum.

ANTERIOR RELATIONS OF THE STOMACH

The upper part of the stomach is covered by the left lobe of the liver on the left and by the diaphragm on the right. The fundus occupies the concavity of the left dome of the diaphragm. The remainder of the anterior of the stomach is covered by the anterior abdominal wall.

Fig. 5.5 The stomach.

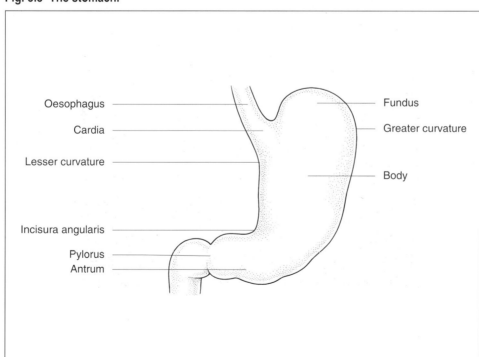

Oesophagus

Cardia

Lesser curvature

Incisura angularis

Pylorus

Antrum

Fundus

Greater curvature

Body

POSTERIOR RELATIONS OF THE STOMACH (see **Fig. 5.6**)

Posterior to the stomach lies the lesser sac. The structures of the posterior abdominal wall that are posterior to this are referred to as the stomach bed. The pancreas lies across the mid-portion of the stomach bed with the splenic artery partly above and partly behind it, and the spleen at its tail. Above the pancreas is the aorta and its coeliac trunk and surrounding plexus and nodes, the diaphragm, the left kidney and adrenal gland. Attached to the anterior surface of the pancreas is the transverse mesocolon, which forms the inferior part of the stomach bed.

ARTERIAL SUPPLY OF THE STOMACH (see **Fig. 5.7**)

Arteries reach the stomach along its greater and lesser curve from branches of the coeliac trunk as follows:

- The left gastric artery from the coeliac trunk supplies the lesser curve;
- The right gastric artery from the hepatic artery supplies the lesser curve;
- The short gastric arteries from the splenic artery supply the greater curve and fundus;
- The left gastroepiploic artery from the splenic artery supplies the greater curve; and
- The right gastroepiploic artery from the gastroduodenal branch of the hepatic artery also supplies the greater curve.

The left gastric artery also supplies branches to the lower oesophagus.

The arteries of the stomach anastomose freely within the stomach wall, unlike the arteries of the small and large intestine where the vessels that enter the gut wall are end arteries.

Fig. 5.6 **Posterior relations of the stomach.(Courtesy of Prof. JB Coakley.)**

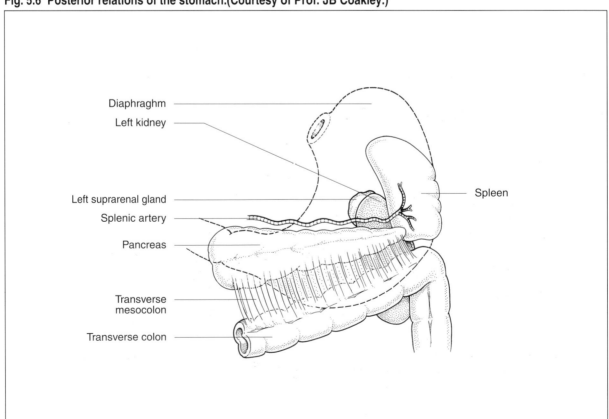

THE VENOUS DRAINAGE OF THE STOMACH (see **Fig. 5.8**)

The venous drainage of the stomach follows a similar pattern to the arterial supply:

■ The left and right gastric veins drain to the portal vein;

■ The short gastric and left gastroepiploic veins drain to the splenic vein; and

■ The right gastroepiploic vein drains to the superior mesenteric vein.

Fig. 5.7 Arterial supply of the stomach.(Courtesy of Prof. JB Coakley.)

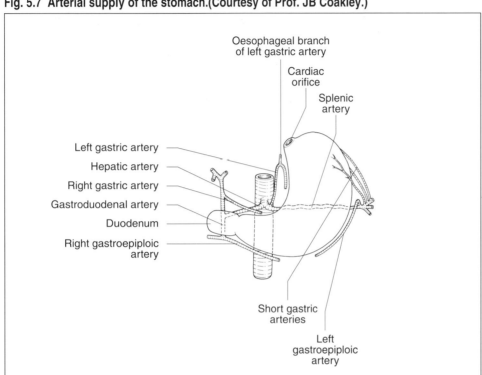

Fig. 5.8 Venous drainage of the stomach.

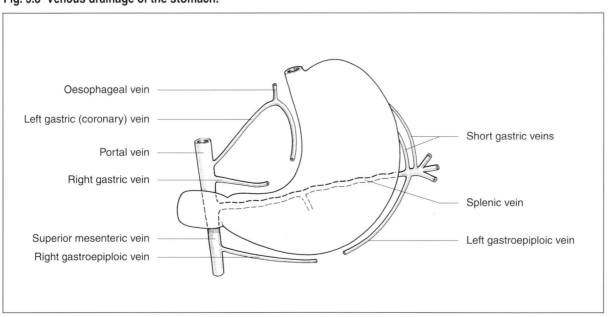

The left gastric vein, also known as the coronary vein, receives blood from the lower third of the oesophagus.

LYMPH DRAINAGE OF THE STOMACH

Lymph drainage also follows the arterial pattern and drains to nodes around the coeliac trunk:

- With the left gastric artery draining directly to coeliac nodes;
- With the right gastric artery draining via retro-duodenal nodes;
- With the short gastric and left gastroepiploic arteries draining via nodes in the splenic hilum and behind the pancreas; and
- With the right gastroepiploic artery draining via retroduodenal nodes.

The coeliac nodes drain to the cisterna chyli.

THE VAGAL SUPPLY TO THE STOMACH

The *anterior (left) vagal trunk* supplies parasympathetic nerves to the lesser curve and cardia and gives a hepatic branch, which, in turn, supplies a pyloric branch — the nerve of Latarjet.

The *posterior (right) vagal trunk* is bigger. It supplies the anterior and posterior body of the stomach; however, most of the nerve becomes the coeliac branch, which passes with the left gastric artery to the coeliac plexus from where it is distributed to the pancreas and to the gut to mid-transverse colon.

RADIOLOGICAL FEATURES OF THE STOMACH

Plain film of the abdomen (see Fig. 5.1)

If taken in the erect posture, a long fluid level is seen in the fundus. This is because the antrum and body contract when empty and a relatively small amount of fluid and gas in the fundus can produce a long fluid level.

In a supine view, the gas in the rugae on the anterior wall of the stomach gives a linear pattern. On intravenous urography (IVU) studies these rugal patterns should not be interpreted as a renal mass lesion.

Double-contrast barium-meal examination (Fig. 5.9)

Features of the stomach such as the greater and lesser curves, the incisura, the cardia, fundus, body, antrum and pylorus can be seen. The change in position of these

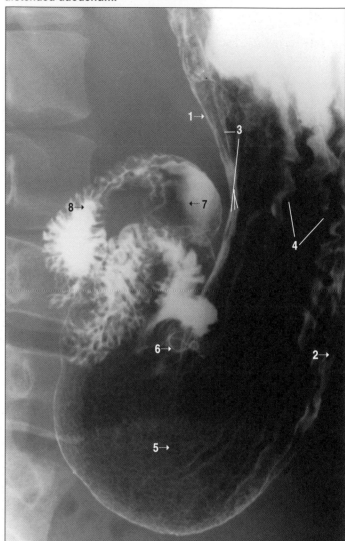

Fig. 5.9 Barium-meal technique. This film demonstrates the various rugal and mucosal folds in the stomach and in the non-distended duodenum.

1. Lesser curve of stomach
2. Greater curve of stomach
3. Longitudinal mucosal folds(magenstrasse)
4. Gastric rugae
5. Areae gastricae
6. Incisura
7. Duodenal cap (partially gas-distended)
8. Mucosal patter of non distended duodenum

with posture and respiration can be appreciated on fluoroscopy.

The areae gastricae can be seen as small nodular elevations of 2–3 mm in diameter. The rugae are 3–5 mm in thickness. These are effaced by gastroparetic agents such as glucagon or hyoscine butylbromide (Buscopan). The long rugae of the 'magenstrasse' paralleling the lesser curve can also be seen.

Compression views can only be obtained of that part of the stomach with the anterior abdominal wall as an anterior relation, that is, the lower body and the antrum.

Computed tomography

The relationship of the stomach to the structures of the stomach bed such as the pancreas, the aorta, the spleen and the left kidney and adrenal can be seen on CT at the level of T10–T12 (**Figs 5.10 and 5.11**; see **Fig**. 5.2).

Close to the gastro-oesophageal junction the stomach is attached to the liver by the gastrohepatic ligament. If the left lobe of the liver is large, part of the stomach may run transversely and, on axial sections, cause an appearance of pseudomass here in 25–30% of normal CT studies.

Fig. 5.10 CT scan: level T10.

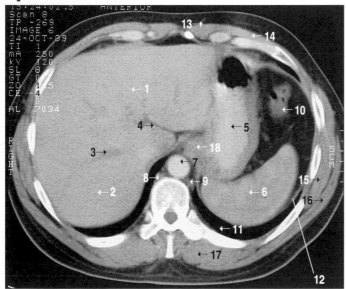

Fig. 5.11 CT scan: level T11.

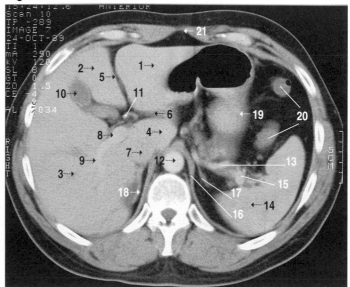

1.	Left lobe of liver	10.	Splenic flexure
2.	Right lobe of liver	11.	Left lung
3.	Right branch of portal vein	12.	Left diaphragm
4.	Fissure for ligamentum venosum	13.	Rectus abdominis muscle
5.	Contrast medium in stomach	14.	External oblique muscle
6.	Spleen	15.	Serratus anterior muscle
7.	Descending aorta	16.	Latissimus dorsi muscle
8.	Azygous vein	17.	Erector spinae muscle
9.	Hemiazygous vein	18.	Oesophagogastric junction

1.	Left lobe of liver: lateral segment	11.	Hepatic artery
2.	Left lobe of liver: medial segment	12.	Abdominal aorta
3.	Right lobe of liver	13.	Splenic artery
4.	Caudate lobe of liver	14.	Spleen
5.	Fissure for ligamentum teres	15.	Splenic vein
6.	Fissure for ligamentum venosum	16.	Left crus of diaphragm
7.	Inferior vena cava	17.	Left adrenal gland
8.	Portal vein	18.	Right adrenal gland
9.	Right branch of portal vein	19.	Stomach
10.	Gall bladder	20.	Splenic flexure
		21.	Linea alba (aponeurosis of rectus sheath)

Ultrasound studies of the abdomen

These are limited by the presence of intraluminal gas in the stomach and bowel. Structures in the stomach bed cannot be seen through the stomach if this is filled with gas. If gas-free then the pancreas and the aorta and coeliac trunk can be well seen.

In the infant, ultrasound is used in the study of the pylorus in cases of suspected pyloric stenosis. The mucosa of the pyloric canal is echogenic and surrounded by thickened echo-poor muscle. Pyloric muscle thicknesses greater than 4 mm and muscle lengths greater than 18 mm are considered abnormal.

Angiography of the coeliac trunk (Fig. 5.12)

This is used to image the vessels that supply the stomach. The stomach can be filled with gas to eliminate confusing rugal patterns.

Fig. 5.12 Coeliac axis angiogram.

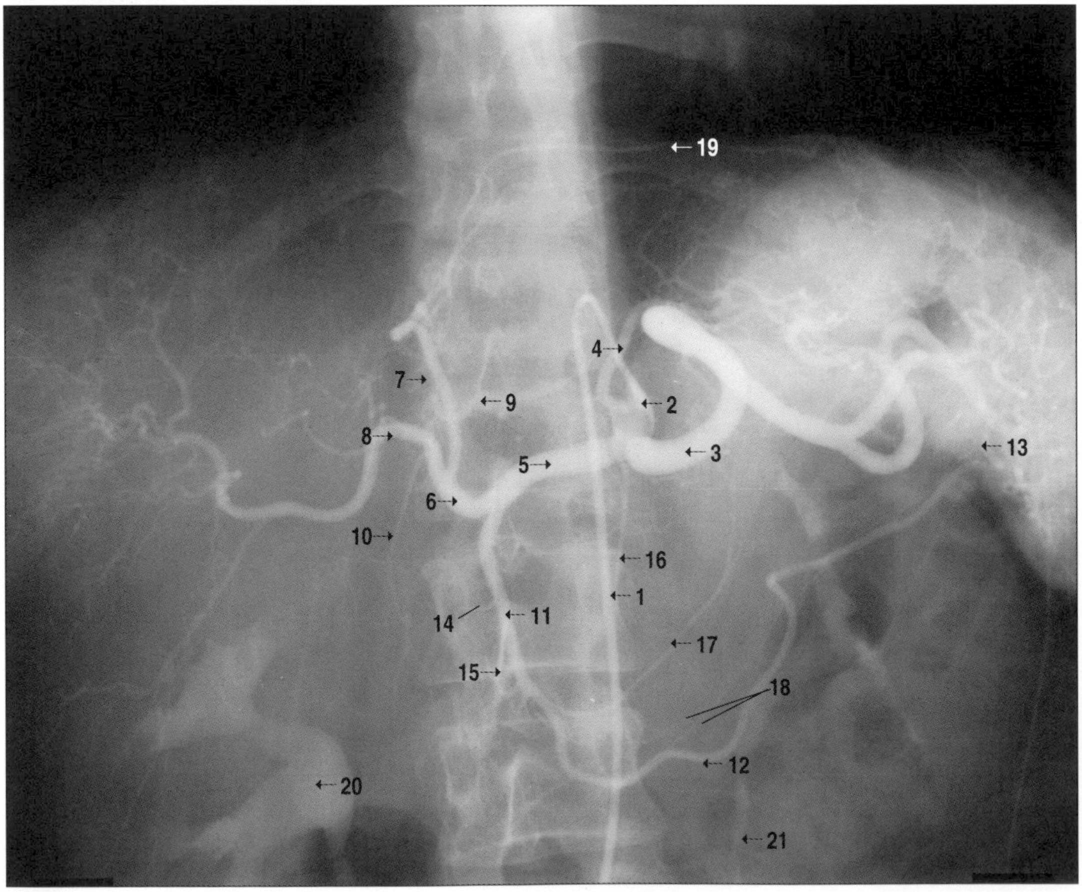

1. Catheter in aorta
2. Catheter tip in coeliac trunk
3. Splenic artery
4. Left gastric artery
5. Common hepatic artery
6. Hepatic artery proper
7. Left hepatic artery
8. Right hepatic artery
9. Right gastric artery
10. Cystic artery
11. Gastroduodenal artery
12. Right gastroepiploic artery
13. Left gastroepiploic artery
14. Posterior superior pancreaticoduodenal artery
15. Anterior superior pancreaticoduodenal artery
16. Dorsal pancreatic artery
17. Transverse pancreatic artery
18. Gastric branches of gastroepiploic artery
19. Phrenic branch of left hepatic artery
20. Contrast in right renal pelvis
21. Left ureter

Fig. 5.13 Duodenum: (a) anterior relations; (b) posterior relations. (Courtesy of Prof. JB Coakley.)

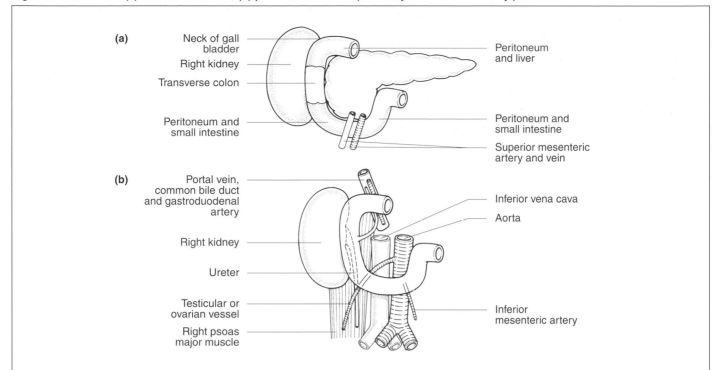

THE DUODENUM (Fig. 5.13)

The duodenum extends from the pylorus to the duodeno-jejunal flexure, where transition to the small bowel proper is marked by the assumption of a mesentery. The first 2.5 cm of duodenum, like the stomach, is attached to the greater and lesser omentum. The remainder of the duodenum is retroperitoneal and, as a result, less mobile than the small intestine. Its anterior surface is covered by peritoneum, except where the second part is crossed by the transverse mesocolon and the third part by the superior mesenteric vessels in the root of the mesentery .

The duodenum is 25 cm long and curves in a 'C' shape around the head of the pancreas. It is described as having four parts — the first (or superior), second (or descending), third (or horizontal) and fourth (or ascending) parts. The length of each part in inches is easily remembered being 2, 3, 4, and 1 inch respectively. The first part is at the level of L1 lumbar vertebra; the second at L2; the third at L3; and the fourth ascends again to L2 level.

The *first part*, called the duodenal cap, passes superiorly and posteriorly from the pylorus. It is overlapped anteriorly by the liver and gall bladder. The latter may indent the cap on barium examinations. The common bile duct, the portal vein and the gastroduodenal artery pass behind the first part of the duodenum and separate it from the inferior vena cava (IVC). Inferiorly it is in contact with the pancreatic head.

The *second part* of the duodenum has an opening half way down on its posteromedial aspect for the pancreatic and common bile ducts, variously called the duodenal papilla or ampulla of Vater. This is guarded by the sphincter of Oddi. An accessory pancreatic duct (of Santorini), if present, opens 2 cm proximal to this.

This part of the duodenum is crossed by the transverse mesocolon anteriorly. As a result, its upper half is supracolic and has the liver as an anterior relation. Its lower half is infracolic and has loops of jejunum anteriorly. Its posterior relations are the right kidney and adrenal gland and it is in contact with the pancreatic head medially.

The *third part* of the duodenum curves anteriorly around L3 vertebra and the IVC and aorta. Its posterior relations also include the right psoas muscle, ureter and gonadal vessels of the posterior abdominal wall. Anteriorly it is crossed by the root of the mesentery and the superior mesenteric vessels. The head of the pancreas is in contact with its superior border.

The *fourth part* of the duodenum passes upwards and to the left on the left side of the aorta, on the left psoas muscle and posterior to the stomach. It raises a peritoneal fold called the ligament of Treitz at the origin of the small bowel mesentery. The inferior mesenteric vessels raise another peritoneal fold lateral to the fourth part of the duodenum. The paraduodenal fossa lies between these.

ARTERIAL SUPPLY

The first 2.5 cm of the duodenum is supplied by the *right gastric and the right gastroepiploic arteries* like the adjoining stomach.

The *superior pancreaticoduodenal artery* supplies from beyond this to midway along the second part. This arises from the gastroduodenal branch of the hepatic artery, which passes behind the first part of the duodenum.

The remainder of the duodenum is supplied by the *inferior pancreaticoduodenal artery,* the first branch of the superior mesenteric artery. At the midpoint of the second part of the duodenum, therefore, there is a transition from supply by the coeliac trunk to supply by the superior mesenteric artery representing a transition from foregut to midgut.

VENOUS DRAINAGE

The first 2.5 cm of the duodenum drains to the prepyloric vein (of Mayo), which lies of the anterior surface of the pylorus. The remainder is drained by veins that correspond to the arteries and drain to the portal and superior mesenteric veins.

LYMPHATIC DRAINAGE

Pancreaticoduodenal nodes drain to pyloric nodes and to coeliac nodes.

1. Body of stomach
2. Fundus of stomach (undistended)
3. Gastric rugal fold
4. Lesser curvature of stomach
5. Greater curvature of stomach
6. Antrum
7. Second (descending) part of duodenum
8. Longitudinal duodenal fold: marks position of ampulla and vater
9. Third (horizontal) part of duodenum (a longitudinal impression may be seen here due to the superior mesenteric vessels and spinal column)
10. Fourth (ascending) part of duodenum (the duodenojejunal flexure is obscured by barium in the stomach)
11. Jejunum: normal 'feather-like' pattern of mucosal folds
12. Ileum: relatively featureless mucosal pattern in the collapsed state

RADIOLOGICAL FEATURES OF THE DUODENUM

Barium studies of the duodenum (Fig. 5.14; see Fig. 5.9)

The duodenum is usually examined as part of a double-contrast barium-meal examination (see **Fig. 5.9**). *Hypotonic duodenography* may be performed by swallowing the barium or by intubation of the duodenum. Anatomical features are similar on all methods.

Since the first part of the duodenum passes posteriorly as well as superiorly, it is foreshortened in AP views. The

Fig. 5.14 Barium follow-through study of the small bowel.

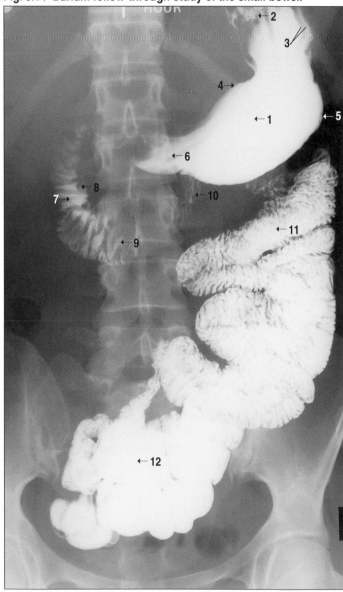

best air-filled views are obtained with the right side raised in a right anterior oblique view.

The duodenal cap may be indented by the normal gall bladder.

The cap has thin mucosal folds that are parallel, or parallel in spiral, from base to apex. These folds are effaced by hypotonic agents. Circular valvulae conniventes proper begin in the second part of the duodenum and are constant, despite distension or hypotonic agents.

The ampulla is visualized in two-thirds of normal examinations and an opening of an accessory pancreatic duct in less than one-quarter. The accessory duct opens more anteriorly than the main pancreatic duct. The ampulla is identified with the help of distinctive folds — a hooded fold superiorly and a distal longitudinal fold. An oblique fold extending inferolaterally from the ampulla is also occasionally seen.

Computed tomography (see Figs 5.3 and 5.4)

The junction of the stomach and duodenum is marked by increased thickness of the pyloric muscle posterior to the left lobe of the liver. The gastroduodenal artery may be seen posterior to the first part of the duodenum. The second part of the duodenum is seen between the liver and gall bladder laterally and the pancreatic head medially in CT at the level of L2. The fourth part of the duodenum or the duodenojejunal flexure is visible, also at this level.

Angiography

For full angiographic assessment of the duodenum, both the coeliac trunk and the superior mesenteric arteries must be visualized.

Ultrasound

Gas in the duodenum may hinder visualization of other organs — particularly the common bile duct, which runs behind the first part.

THE SMALL INTESTINE

The small intestine begins where the intestine assumes a mesentery at the duodenojejunal flexure and ends at the ileocaecal junction. It varies in length from 3–10 m with an average length of 6 m. The root of its mesentery extends from the left of L2 to the right sacroiliac joint and is only 15 cm long (**Fig. 5.15**). The small intestine is very mobile and lies in mobile coils in the central abdomen. The proximal two-fifths of the small intestine is called the

Fig. 5.15 Posterior abdominal wall showing the peritoneal attachment of mesentery.

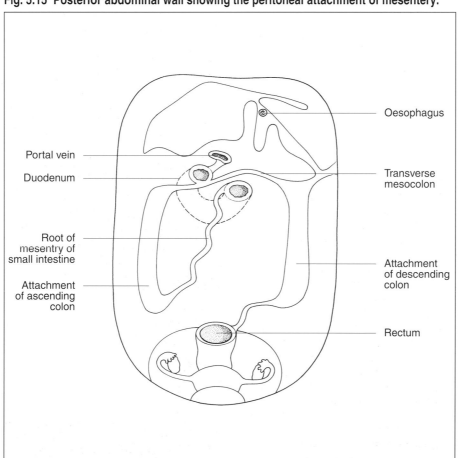

jejunum and the distal three-fifths the ileum, although the boundary between these is not well defined.

The circular mucosal folds — known as valvulae conniventes or plicae semilunaris — are seen in the duodenum and continued in the small intestine although they are less prominent distally and may be absent in distended views on barium studies.

Lymphoid follicles found in the mucous membrane throughout the intestinal tract become increasingly more numerous along the length of the small intestine. In the distal ileum they become aggregated together into patches called Peyer's patches. They are oval in shape and found on the antimesenteric border of the ileum.

Differences between jejunum and ileum are outlined in **Table 5.1.**

ARTERIAL SUPPLY OF THE SMALL INTESTINE (see **Fig. 5.42**)

The entire small intestine is supplied by the superior mesenteric artery, which arises from the aorta at the L1 vertebral level. Jejunal and ileal branches arise from the left of the main trunk. These branches link with one another in a series of arcades, which are single in the jejunum but number up to five in the distal ileum. The arteries that enter the intestinal wall, the vasa recta, are end arteries.

VENOUS DRAINAGE

Veins from the small intestine drain to the superior mesenteric vein, which in turn, drains to the portal vein.

MECKL'S DIVERTICULUM

This is a diverticulum that projects from the antimesenteric border of the lower ileum. It represents the persistent proximal part of the vitellointestinal duct, which connects the yolk sac to the primitive digestive tube in early fetal life and is found in about 2% of subjects.

Meckl's diverticulum is said to be 2 inches (5 cm) long and situated 2 feet (60 cm) from the ileocaecal valve. In fact, its length is very variable and may be merely a bulge on the ileal wall or be up to 15 cm long. Its distance from the caecum may also vary from 15 cm–3.5 m.

The apex of the diverticulum may be adherent to the umbilicus or attached to it by a fibrous cord. It may have gastric, hepatic or pancreatic tissue at its apex.

The vitellointestinal duct may also persist as a fistula from the small intestine to the umbilicus; as a cyst along the path of the duct or as a raspberry tumour of the umbilicus which is the pouting red mucosa of the persistent extremity of the duct.

Table 5.1 Comparison between jejunum and ileum

	Jejunum	Ileum
Diameter:	Wider (3.0–3.5 cm)	Narrower (2.5 cm)
Wall thickness	Thicker	Thinner
Position	Left upper abdomen	Right lower abdomen
Valvulae conniventes	Thicker and more prominent	Thinner and less prominent
Payer's patches	Fewer and bigger	More numerous
Arterial arcades	Single	Four to five present

RADIOLOGICAL FEATURES OF THE SMALL INTESTINE

Plain films of the abdomen

Gas and fluid levels are often visible in normal loops of small intestine. Up to five fluid levels in loops of 2.5 cm diameter or smaller, or two loops wider than this, may be seen in a normal radiograph.

Jejunal loops are distinguished from ileal loops by their position with the former being in the left upper abdomen, while the ileal loops tend to be in the lower abdomen and the right iliac fossa.

In radiographs of intestinal obstruction, the central position of dilated, small-bowel loops helps distinguish these from loops of dilated colon. Other identifying features of small-intestinal loops include the circular valvulae conniventes, as distinct from the incomplete septa formed by colonic haustra (see also the section on the colon).

Barium studies of the small intestine (see Fig. 5.14)

The small intestine may be imaged using a variety of contrast techniques. In a *barium follow-through* examination the barium is taken orally and imaged as it passes through to the caecum. In a *small-bowel enema (or enteroclysis)* a tube is passed to the duodenojejunal flexure and barium is passed directly into the small intestine. Since the transverse colon is an anterior relation of the jejunum, better visualization of the small intestine may be achieved by introduction of air into the colon per rectum when the barium is in the small intestine (a *pneumocolon technique*).

Normal upper limits of diameter are higher for the distended bowel than for the relaxed state. Thus diameters of up to 4 cm in the jejunum and 3 cm in the ileum are normal in small-bowel enemas. Normal valvulae conniventes may be up to 2 mm thick in the jejunum and

1 mm in the ileum. The valvulae conniventes may be absent in the ileum when distended, giving this a feature-less appearance.

Computed tomography (see Fig. 5.3)

As with all the intestine, oral contrast is used to distin-guish normal loops of small intestine from abdominal masses. Loops of small intestine fill most of the middle abdomen and the upper pelvis. When adequately filled with oral contrast, the thin wall of normal jejunum is almost imperceptible. Fine, transversely thickened areas due to the valvulae conniventes may be seen. These are seldom seen in the ileum. The mesentery and its vessels and also fat may be easily seen. Lymph nodes are visible if greater than 5 mm in diameter.

THE ILEOCAECAL VALVE (Fig. 5.16)

The distal ileum opens into the medial and posterior aspect of the large intestine at the junction of the caecum and the ascending colon. Two horizontal crescentic folds of mucosa and circular muscle project into the lumen on the colonic side. These folds are extended laterally as the frenula of the valve. Some thickening of the circular mus-cle of the ileum at the junction acts as a sphincter.

RADIOLOGICAL FEATURES OF THE ILEOCAECAL VALVE

Plain films of the abdomen

Gaseous distension of the colon is seen proximal to a site of colonic obstruction. In some of these cases, the ileocae-cal valve remains competent so that marked distension of the caecum can occur with or without distension of the small intestine. In other patients, the valve is incompetent and there is distension of both large and small intestine without excessive distension of the caecum.

Barium-enema examinations

The ileocaecal valve may present a filling defect in the posteromedial wall of the caecum. This may be polypoid or bilabial depending on the state of contraction of the valve. In the contracted valve, barium may fill a narrow slit between the folds like a linear ulcer.

The valve is at the site of the first completely transverse haustral cleft. The thickened posterior ends of this haus-tra are the frenula of the valve and should not be greater than 3 mm in diameter.

Computed tomography

Fat accumulation around the ileocaecal valve makes it easily visible in many abdominal CT scans.

Fig. 5.16 Internal view of the caecum showing the ileocaecal valve.

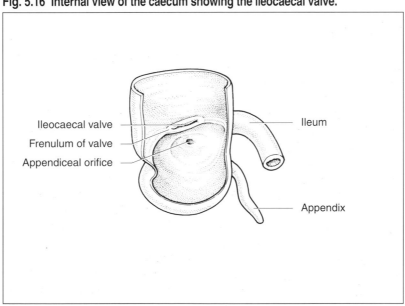

THE VERMIFORM APPENDIX
(see Fig. 5.16)

The appendix arises at the convergence of the taenia coli on the posteromedial wall of the caecum about 2 cm below the ileocaecal valve. Its length is very variable between 12 and 24 cm long. It has its own mesentery, a triangular fold from the lower border of the ileum and is, as a result, mobile. Its position is variable with the incidence of the commonest positions as follows:

■ Retrocaecal — 75%;
■ Subcaecal/pelvic — 20%; and
■ Pre- or postileal — 5%.

The lumen of the appendix is wide in the infant and obliterated after mid-adult life. Acute appendicitis, which is usually caused by obstruction of the lumen, is therefore rare in the extremes of life.

The appendix is supplied by the *appendicular artery,* which reaches it in the mesoappendix from the ileocolic artery. This is the sole supply and, if infection causes thrombosis of this artery, gangrene and perforation of the appendix results (compare with the gall bladder, which receives a rich collateral supply from the liver in the gall-bladder bed and gangrene and perforation are rare).

RADIOLOGICAL FEATURES OF THE APPENDIX

Plain abdominal film

Faecaliths or fluid levels of the appendix may be visible on plain films of the abdomen in the right iliac fossa.

Ultrasound

The appendix is identified as a blind-ended tube arising from the posterior aspect of the caecum. Unlike nearby loops of ileum, it does not display peristalsis. Its position is variable, with the subcaecal appendix being least likely to be obscured by caecal gas. If in a retrocaecal position, visualization of the appendix is aided by compression of the caecum.

Barium enema

If the lumen of the appendix is patent, it may fill on barium-enema examination. The lumen is often obliterated in patients past mid-adulthood. To fill the appendix the patient should be supine because its orifice is on the posterior aspect of the caecum. Some elevation of the head is also helpful.

Appendiceal abscess

Since the appendix is on a mesentery and mobile, pus from an infected appendix may cause *abscess formation*

in a variety of locations. Pus may travel inferiorly to the pelvic peritoneum to the rectovesical (or rectouterine) pouch. Pus may also travel superiorly in the right paracolic gutter to the infrahepatic spaces (see section on the peritoneum).

THE LARGE INTESTINE
(Figs 5.17 and 5.18)

(See also rectum and anus in the section on the pelvis.)

The length of the large intestine is very variable with an average length of 1.5 m. It is wider in diameter than the small intestine with maximum diameter of the caecum at 9 cm and the transverse colon at 5.5 cm.

The colon so far as the rectum is marked by *taeniae coli.* These are three flattened bands of longitudinal muscle that represent the longitudinal muscle layer of the colon. The taeniae converge on the appendix proximally and the rectum distally and these structures have a complete longitudinal muscle layer. The taeniae coli are about 1 foot (30 cm approx.) shorter than the colon and cause the formation of sacculations along the length of the colon. These give rise to the appearance of incomplete septa, called haustra, on radiographs.

Scattered over the free surface of the large intestine, except the caecum and rectum, are fat-filled peritoneal tags called *appendices epiploicae.* These are especially numerous in the sigmoid colon. Arteries supplying these perforate the muscle wall. Mucous membrane may herniate through these vascular perforations giving rise to diverticulosis.

PERITONEAL ATTACHMENTS OF THE COLON (see **Fig. 5.15**)

The ascending and descending parts of the colon are usually retroperitoneal. The peritoneal spaces lateral to these are called the paracolic gutters and may act as a route of spread of pus in peritoneal infection. Occasionally the ascending colon has a mesentery. The caecum may or may not have a mesentery giving rise to a retrocaecal space of variable degree of development.

The transverse colon, however, always has a mesentery, the mesocolon, on which it hangs in a loop between the hepatic and splenic flexures, which are fixed points. The convexity of the greater curve of the stomach lies in the concavity of the loop of transverse colon with the gastrocolic omentum attached between them. This continues below the transverse colon as the greater omentum (see the section on the peritoneum).

The sigmoid colon also has a mesentery. This is attached to the posterior abdominal wall to the left of the midline in an inverted 'V' shape whose limbs diverge

Fig. 5.17 Posterior relations of the colon.

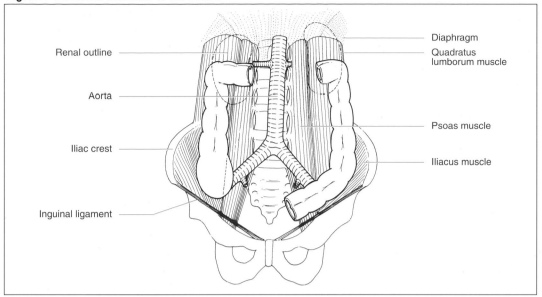

from the bifurcation of the common iliac artery over the sacroiliac (SI) joint at the pelvic brim.

The rectum has peritoneum laterally in its upper third and over its anterior surface in the upper two-thirds. The lower third of the rectum is below the pelvic peritoneum.

RELATIONS OF THE COLON
(see **Fig. 5.17**)

The parts of the colon that are retroperitoneal have as their *posterior relations* the structures of the posterior abdominal wall, that is, the psoas and iliac muscles, the quadratus lumborum muscles and the kidney. The more mobile transverse and sigmoid colon are related posteriorly to loops of small intestine.

The colon is an anterior structure in the abdomen (*cf.* development) and has the anterior abdominal wall as an *anterior relation,* particularly when full. The liver, gall bladder and spleen overlap superiorly and the sigmoid and rectum are related anteriorly to the bladder and retrovesical structures in the male and the uterus in the female.

1. Rectum
2. Valve of Houston (lateral mucosal fold)
3. Sigmoid colon
4. Descending colon
5. Splenic flexure
6. Transverse colon
7. Hepatic flexure
8. Ascending colon
9. Caecum
10. Caecal pole
11. Base of appendix
12. Tip of appendix

Fig. 5.18 Barium enema study (double-contrast with tube removed) of the colon.

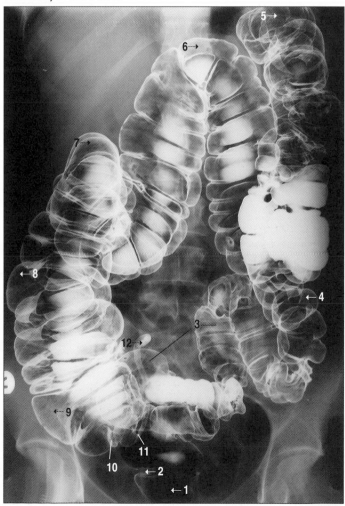

THE ARTERIAL SUPPLY OF THE COLON (Figs 5.19 and 5.20)

(See also rectum in pelvic section and superior and inferior mesenteric arteries.)

That part of the colon derived from the midgut (i.e. to the mid-transverse colon) is supplied by the *superior mesenteric artery* as follows:

- The ileocolic artery (a continuation of the main trunk of the superior mesenteric artery) supplies the caecum, appendix and the beginning of the ascending colon;
- The right colic artery supplies the remainder of the ascending colon; and
- The middle colic artery supplies the transverse colon to its midpoint.

Fig. 5.19 Superior mesenteric angiogram. The inferior pancreaticoduodenal artery (not shown) also arises from the proximal superior mesenteric artery and runs superiorly.

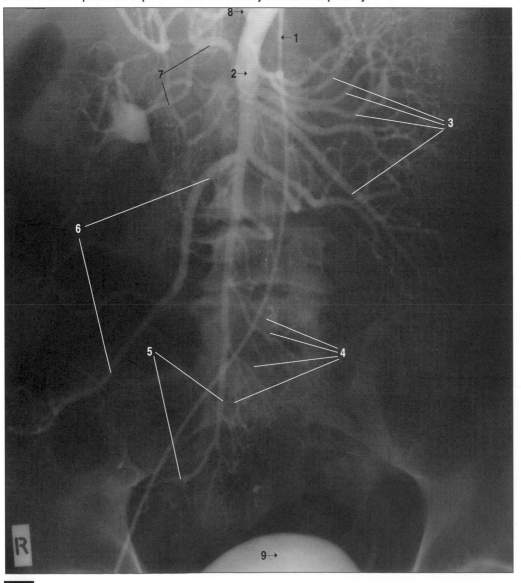

1. Catheter in aorta
2. Superior mesenteric artery
3. Jejunal branches
4. Ileal branches
5. Terminal superior mesenteric artery
6. Ileocolic artery
7. Right colic artery
8. Middle colic artery running superiorly
9. Contrast-filled bladder

The *inferior mesenteric artery* supplies the colon so far as the upper rectum as follows:

- The left colic artery to the descending colon;
- The sigmoid artery to the sigmoid colon; and
- The superior rectal (superior haemorrhoidal) artery to the upper rectum.

Each of these vessels anastomoses with its neighbour forming a *marginal artery* (of Drummond) close to the colon. The vessels that enter the bowel are, however, end arteries.

VENOUS DRAINAGE OF THE COLON

Veins corresponding with the arteries drain to the superior and inferior mesenteric veins.

Fig. 5.20 Inferior mesenteric angiogram.

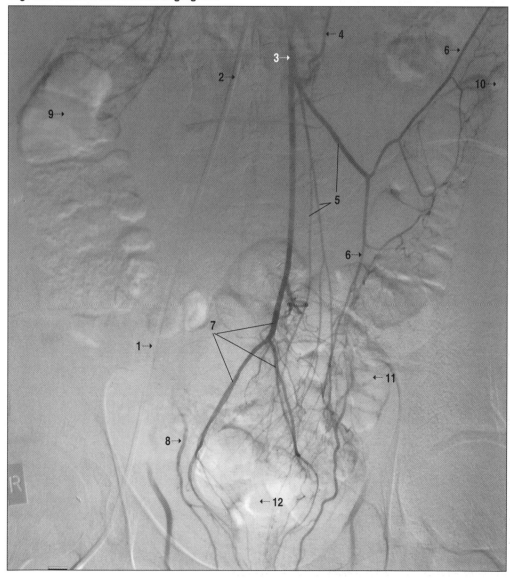

1. Catheter in right common iliac artery
2. Catheter in aorta
3. Inferior mesenteric artery
4. Left colic artery
5. Sigmoid arteries
6. Marginal artery of Drummond
7. Superior rectal artery and branches
8. Middle rectal artery (filling by reflux: a branch of the internal iliac artery)
9. Gas in ascending colon
10. Descending colon
11. Sigmoid colon
12. Rectum

LYMPHATIC DRAINAGE OF THE COLON

Lymph drains to nodes near the bowel wall, which drain to nodes in the mesentery. These, in turn, drain to nodes at the origin of the superior and inferior mesenteric arteries at the aorta and from there to the cisterna chyli.

DEVELOPMENT OF THE COLON

In the fifth fetal week, the midgut herniates into the umbilical cord with the vitellointestinal duct at the apex of the hernia. At the tenth week, the loops of gut return to the abdominal cavity, proximal bowel before distal and rotating 270° anticlockwise as it does so. This results in the jejunum being to the left and deeper than the colon, and the caecum being to the right and superficial.

In *malrotation* the bowel returns without twisting and the small intestine lies of the right and the colon on the left. The small intestinal mesentery is very short and is prone to volvulus.

In *exomphalos,* midgut herniation at the umbilicus persists at birth.

RADIOLOGICAL FEATURES OF THE COLON

Plain films of the abdomen (see Fig. 5.1)

Gas within the colon outlines the colon or parts of it. The sacculation of the colon by the taeniae coli give rise to septa called haustra. These are fixed anatomical structures in the proximal colon but, in the distal colon, require active contraction for their formation. Haustra may be absent distal to the mid-transverse colon.

The upper limit of normal diameter of the transverse colon on plain films is taken to be 5.5 cm, and of the caecum, 9 cm. Beyond these limits, in the right clinical setting, there is a risk of caecal perforation. Numerous gas-fluid levels may be normal and 18% of normal films have fluid levels in the caecum.

As it has a mesentery, the transverse colon is mobile and may interpose itself between the liver and the right hemidiaphragm in the normal subject. The resulting intracolic gas seen between the liver and diaphragm on an abdominal radiograph mimics a pneumoperitoneum. This is called **Chilaiditis syndrome** and is commoner in patients with chronic lung disease.

In intestinal obstruction, distinguishing dilated loops of small intestine from dilated loops of colon is based on several anatomical features (see **Table 5.2**).

Table 5.2 Anatomical features of small and large intestine in intestinal obstruction

	Small intestine	Colon
Position of loops	Central	Peripheral
Septa	Incomplete (haustra)	Complete (valvulae conniventes)
Number of loops	May be several	Few
Diameter	Up to 5 cm	>5 cm
Solid faeces	Absent	May be present

Double-contrast barium-enema examination (see Fig. 5.20)

The entire colon and appendix may be outlined. The technique for filling the colon with barium and air requires an understanding of anatomy. Since the transverse colon, for example, hangs anteriorly between the relatively posteriorly positioned splenic and hepatic flexures, this is easiest to fill when the patient is prone. Resumption of a supine position allows filling of the hepatic flexure and the ascending colon with barium. The junction of the caecum with both the appendix and the ileum are posterior and these therefore fill with barium in the supine position.

Visualization of the sigmoid colon may require oblique views and caudally angled views to overcome the problem of overlapping loops. Similarly, views of the ileocaecal area are best obtained with the patient's left side raised because of the posteromedial position of this junction.

The haustra can be seen well on double-contrast views of the colon. Gaseous distension may obliterate these distally so far as the midtransverse colon.

Small mucous glands in the mucosa of the colon (**crypts of Lieberkuhn**) may fill with barium on good double-contrast views. These are up to 1 mm deep and perpendicular to the colonic wall on tangential views and on 'en-face' views are seen as thin, transverse, parallel lines with short intercommunicating branches called *innominate lines.*

Lymphoid follicles are visible in 13% of adults on double-contrast barium studies. These are low elevations of 1–3 mm in diameter. These are larger in the rectum and are considered normal up to 4 mm in diameter.

A barium enema is used sometimes in children to diagnose **malrotation** of the bowel (a barium meal is also used). The caecum may be high in partial defects or on the left side of the abdomen in complete malrotation.

Angiography

For full evaluation of the blood supply of the colon both superior and inferior mesenteric arteries must be shown (see **Figs 5.19** and **5.20**).

Computed tomography of the abdomen (see Figs 5.2–5.4 and 5.11)

The caecum and ascending colon can be seen anterior to the muscles of the posterior abdominal wall on the right side. The right paracolic gutter is best seen if distended with pus or fluid. The hepatic flexure can be seen lateral to the second part of the duodenum and its relationship to the gall bladder to which it is attached by the hepatico-colic ligament, can be appreciated.

The transverse colon varies in its position because of its variable length and its mobility. Fat, blood vessels and lymph nodes may be seen in the mesocolon. The splenic flexure is seen behind the greater curvature of the stomach and the anterior splenic tip. The descending colon is seen on the muscles of the posterior abdominal wall on the left side. Loops of sigmoid colon are distinguished from small intestinal loops by the presence of solid faecal matter. Contrast material introduced by enema may also be helpful.

THE LIVER (Fig. 5.21)

The liver, the largest organ in the body, is found in the right upper quadrant of the abdomen. It is relatively much larger in the fetus and child. The liver assumes the

Fig. 5.21 Liver: (a) anterior view; (b) posterior view; (c) visceral surface; (d) structures seen through the liver. (Courtesy of Prof. JB Coakley.)

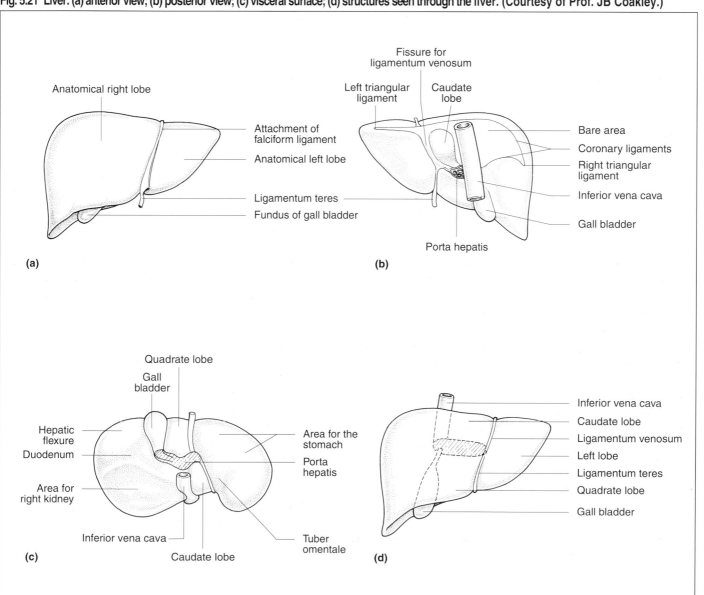

shape of the cavity it occupies, a shape that is unrelated to its function. Thus it has two surfaces — the diaphragmatic surface and the visceral surface.

The diaphragmatic surface is smooth and flat posteriorly and has a smooth, rounded upper surface with a large dome for the right hemidiaphragm and a smaller dome for the left hemidiaphragm. A depression between these marks the site of the central tendon and the overlying heart.

The diaphragmatic surface ends anteriorly in the inferior border of the liver. This lies at the costal margin laterally to within about 4 cm from the midline, the site of the gall-bladder notch. Medial to this, the inferior border ascends less obliquely than the costal margin and lies below it as it crosses the midline to meet the costal margin of the left side at approximately the eighth costal cartilage. The lateral extent of the left lobe is variable — it may extend only to the midline or may surround the stomach or spleen to reach the left lateral abdominal wall.

In addition to the notch for the gall bladder, the inferior border is marked by a notch for the ligamentum teres. This ligament is the obliterated remnant of the left umbilical vein, which carries blood from the placenta to the fetus. It passes, with small paraumbilical veins, from the umbilicus to the inferior border of the liver in the free edge of a crescentic fold of peritoneum called the falciform (meaning 'sickle-shaped') ligament. This meets the liver just to the right of the midline. The site of attachment of the falciform ligament is used as an anterior marker of the sagittal plane of division of the liver into anatomical left and right lobes.

The posteroinferior, or visceral, surface of the liver is marked by an 'H'-shaped arrangement of structures (see **Fig. 5.21c**). The crossbar of the 'H' is made by the horizontal hilum of the liver called the porta hepatis. This is the entry site of the right and left hepatic arteries and portal veins, and also the exit of the right and left hepatic ducts. There are also autonomic nerves and lymph vessels.

The gall bladder in its bed together with the IVC in a deep groove or tunnel form the right vertical part of the 'H'. These are separated by the caudate process, which connects the caudate lobe with the right lobe of the liver.

The left vertical part of the 'H' is formed by the ligamentum teres so far as its attachment to the left portal vein in the left extremity of the porta hepatis. This is continuous with the fissure for the ligamentum venosum, a deep fissure lined by peritoneum. At its base lodges the ligamentum venosum, the obliterated remnant of the ductus venosus, which shunts blood in the fetus from the left umbilical vein to the IVC, bypassing the liver. At the upper end of the fissure, the ligamentum venosum curves laterally to attach to the left hepatic vein or the IVC.

The visceral surface of the liver lies in contact with, and is slightly moulded by:

- The oesophagus, stomach and lesser omentum on the left;
- The pancreas (through the lesser omentum) and the duodenum in the midline; and
- The right kidney and adrenal and the hepatic flexure of the colon on the right.

The peritoneal attachments of the liver determine the distribution of free gas and of pus in this part of the peritoneal cavity and are discussed in the section on the peritoneum.

LOBES OF THE LIVER (Fig. 5.22)

The liver is described anatomically as having a large right lobe and a small left lobe, which are separated anteriorly by the attachment of the falciform ligament and on the visceral surface, by the grooves for the ligamenta teres and venosum. Two further lobes are described — the caudate lobe posteriorly between the IVC and the fissure for the ligamentum venosum, and the quadrate lobe anteroinferiorly between the gall-bladder bed and the fissure for the ligamentum teres. These are part of the anatomical right lobe.

Occasionally the lower border of the right lobe, a little to the right of the gall bladder, may project downwards for a considerable distance as a broad tongue-like or bulbous process called Reidel's lobe. This is not a true lobe.

The anatomical division into right and left lobes has no morphological significance. If instead the liver is divided according to the area of supply of the right and left hepatic arteries then *true morphological left and right lobes* are found, each is supplied by the right or left portal vein and drained by the right or left hepatic duct. There is little or no anastomosis between right and left branches of these structures. The plane of division between these lobes, called the *principal plane,* is marked on the visceral surface by the IVC and the gall-bladder bed. There is no external marking of this plane on the anterosuperior surface, but it lies parallel to and about 4 cm to the right of the attachment of the falciform ligament. The central hepatic vein lies in the principal plane and drains from both lobes.

Further subdivision into *segments* is also based on branches of the right and left hepatic arteries. Knowledge of these segments is important in assessment of extent of hepatic pathology prior to segmentectomy. Segments are numbered in the Couinaud system in an anticlockwise direction starting at the caudate lobe. In the Healey and Schroy classification, essentially similar segments are named rather than numbered (see **Fig. 5.22**).

The functional subunit of the liver is the microscopic *lobule*, which has a central vein and, in spaces between the lobules, has portal canals or triads — each with a branch of the hepatic artery, portal vein and bile duct.

Fig. 5.22 Segmental anatomy of the liver.

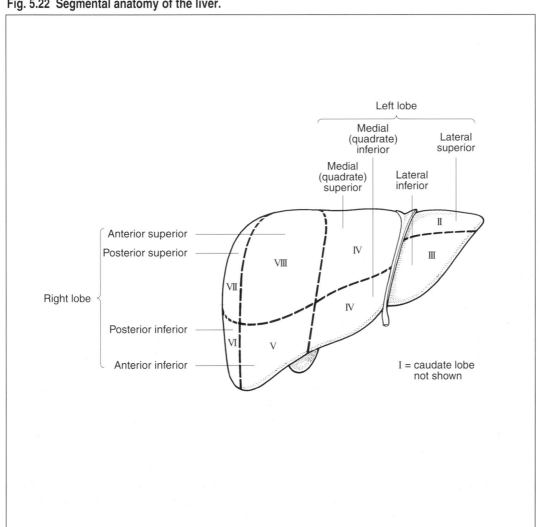

THE ARTERIAL SUPPLY OF THE LIVER

The hepatic artery, one of the three branches of the coeliac trunk, supplies the right gastric and gastroduodenal arteries before approaching the liver in the free edge of the lesser omentum, anterior to the portal vein and medial to the bile duct. It divides into approximately equal-sized right and left hepatic arteries before entering the liver at the porta hepatis. The right hepatic artery usually supplies the cystic artery to the gall bladder. Within the liver, the left hepatic artery supplies the anatomical left lobe, the quadrate lobe and most of the caudate lobe (see the description of the morphological left lobe already mentioned) and the right artery supplies the remainder of the right lobe, supplying a variable small amount of the caudate lobe.

Variations in arterial supply to the liver

These are common. The entire liver (2.5%) or part (6%) or all (10%) of the right lobe may be supplied by the superior mesenteric artery. When it does it passes posterior to the portal vein lateral to the common bile duct.

The left gastric artery may rarely replace the common hepatic artery or, less rarely, the left hepatic artery.

The common hepatic artery may divide early or trifurcate with the gastroduodenal artery. The hepatic artery may arise separately from the aorta rather than the coeliac trunk.

PORTAL VEIN

The portal vein passes in the free edge of the lesser omentum posterior to the bile duct and the hepatic artery to the porta hepatis, where it divides into right and left branches to the morphological right and left lobes.

The portal system is much less prone to anatomical variation than the hepatic artery. Occasionally the portal vein is double, caused by nonunion of the superior mesenteric and splenic veins (*cf.* section on portal system).

VENOUS DRAINAGE OF THE LIVER

The liver is drained by hepatic veins, which drain upwards and backwards to the IVC without an extrahepatic course. (These veins also assist in the stabilization of the liver.) The distribution of the hepatic veins differs from that of the hepatic artery, the portal vein and the bile ducts. A right, middle and left hepatic vein drain corresponding thirds of the liver. The middle hepatic vein lies in the principal plane and may unite with the left hepatic vein and have a common final course to the IVC.

A lower group of small veins drain directly to the IVC from the lower parts of the right and caudate lobes. Hepatic veins have no valves.

LYMPHATIC DRAINAGE OF THE LIVER

Lymph from the liver drains to nodes in the porta hepatis and from there via retropyloric nodes to the coeliac nodes. There is some communication with lymph vessels of the thorax via the diaphragm.

RADIOLOGICAL FEATURES OF THE LIVER

Plain films of the abdomen (see Fig. 5.1)

The margins of the liver are visible where they are outlined by fat; thus the lateral border can be seen where it is flanked by properitoneal fat. Intraperitoneal and omental fat lie near the inferior border. This border is best seen in the obese whose visceral surface tends to be less steep and more tangential to the beam on AP views. Air in the lungs outlines the pleura and diaphragm over the upper limit of the liver but gas in the stomach may give a misleading impression of the position of the inferior border of the liver since the stomach may pass posterior to this border.

Computed tomography (see Figs 5.2–5.4, 5.10 and 5.11)

The relationship of the liver to the diaphragm, pleura and lungs can be seen on CT. The relations of the visceral surface can be seen on lower cuts, that is, the lesser curve and stomach on the left, the pancreas and duodenum posteriorly in the midline and the right kidney and adrenal on the right.

The IVC can be seen in a tunnel or groove near the dome of the liver posteriorly with the hepatic veins draining into it. The structures at the porta hepatis and the gall bladder can also be seen. The position of the lobes and of segments are deduced from a knowledge of their relationship to these structures and their blood supply. Thus the caudate lobe is to the left of the IVC and posterior to the hilum and the quadrate lobe is to the left of the gall bladder.

The caudate lobe is connected to the remainder of the right lobe by the *caudate process*, which can be seen passing between the IVC and the portal vein. A projection of the caudate lobe to the left of the portal vein, called the *papillary process*, may mimic a porta hepatis mass on CT if its continuity with the liver is not appreciated. Fat within fissures including incomplete accessory fissures on the smooth diaphragmatic surface may also mimic a mass.

The hepatic veins lie between the following segments:

- The middle hepatic vein lies between the morphological right and left lobes;
- The left hepatic vein lies between medial and lateral segments of the left lobe; and
- The right hepatic vein lies between anterior and posterior segments of the right lobe.

Ultrasound

As a solid organ, the liver is particularly suitable for ultrasound examination (**Fig. 5.23**) and it is seldom covered by gas-containing bowel. Furthermore, the liver is used as an acoustic window for visualization of other structures including the right kidney and adrenal gland and the pancreas. Vessels and bile ducts of the liver are particularly well seen on ultrasound studies. Anatomical features are as for CT.

Magnetic resonance imaging

On MRI the liver is of equal signal intensity as the pancreas and higher on T1- and lower on T2-weighted images than the spleen. Normal hepatic vessels are seen as areas of signal void. The major hepatic veins and the secondary branches of the portal veins are visible. Hepatic arteries are less well seen and the intrahepatic

biliary radicals are not usually seen. On T2-weighted images the ligamentum venosum and the ligamentum teres are of low intensity but the fat within their fissures is of high intensity. As with CT and ultrasound, the hepatic veins and these fissures aid in identification of segments and lobes of the liver. An intravenous injection of a colloidal suspension of iron oxide, which is phagocytosed by the reticuloendothelial system has been used as a contrast agent.

Hepatic arteriography (see Fig. 5.12)

This is achieved via the aorta and the coeliac trunk with greater selectivity if the contrast agent is injected distal to the origin of the gastroduodenal artery. The frequency of variation in the arteries may make injection of the superior mesenteric or left gastic arteries also necessary.

Embolization of the hepatic artery

This is sometimes undertaken in symptomatic tumours of the liver. Embolization of the hepatic artery branches, which are end arteries, does not result in infarction because of the dual supply to the liver with the portal venous system also bringing blood to the liver. Radiographic demonstration of the patency of the portal system is essential prior to embolization. When the right lobe is being embolized it is preferable if the catheter tip is beyond the origin of the cystic artery.

Fig. 5.23 Ultrasound of upper abdomen: axial image.

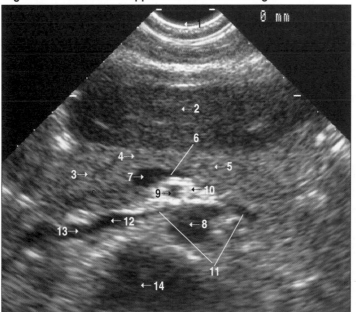

1. Skin surface
2. Left lobe of liver
3. Head of pancreas
4. Neck of pancreas
5. Body of pancreas
6. Splenic vein
7. Confluence of splenic and superior mesenteric veins to form portal vein
8. Aorta
9. Superior mesenteric artery
10. Fat around superior mesenteric artery
11. Left renal vein
12. Inferior vena cava (collapsed)
13. Right renal vein
14. Vertebral body

Portal venography

This may be achieved by many routes (see the section on the portal vein). Within the liver, the left portal vein passes anteriorly before turning left and oblique views are therefore necessary to view this part of the vein. Before turning left, a recurrent branch passes to the right to the quadrate lobe. This must not be mistaken for a right portal vein if the actual right vein is obstructed.

Hepatic venography

This is achieved via the inferior vena cava with catheterization of each of the three main hepatic veins in turn. The right vein may enter separately and the middle and left vein may be seen to unite as a common trunk. This approach may also be used to achieve radiographically directed hepatic venous pressure measurements or transjugular hepatic biopsy.

Venous drainage of the caudate lobe

Since the caudate lobe is drained by small veins that enter the inferior vena cava directly more inferiorly, this lobe may be spared in diseases that occlude the main hepatic veins (e.g. the Budd Chiari syndrome). As a result, it may undergo hypertrophy, which, if extensive, may itself obstruct the IVC.

Hepatic scintigraphy

On anterior views in hepatic scintigraphy, an indentation is seen in the inferior border of the liver at the site of the gall bladder and another at the site of the ligamentum teres. A photon-poor area is seen above the latter at the attachment of the falciform ligament. A defect is seen superiorly at the site of the entry of the hepatic veins into the IVC and another centrally at the porta hepatis. Superimposition of the breast and of the bowel (especially after barium studies) can cause false defects.

On lateral views, the liver is seen as elliptical with the renal fossa posteriorly and the gall-bladder fossa anteriorly and a central defect for the porta hepatis.

THE BILIARY SYSTEM
(Figs 5.24 and 5.25)

THE GALL BLADDER

The gall bladder is a pear-shaped sac that is attached to the extrahepatic bile ducts by the cystic duct. It measures up to 10 cm long and 3 cm wide and has a capacity of

Fig. 5.24 The biliary system and its relations (Courtesy of Prof. JB Coakley.)

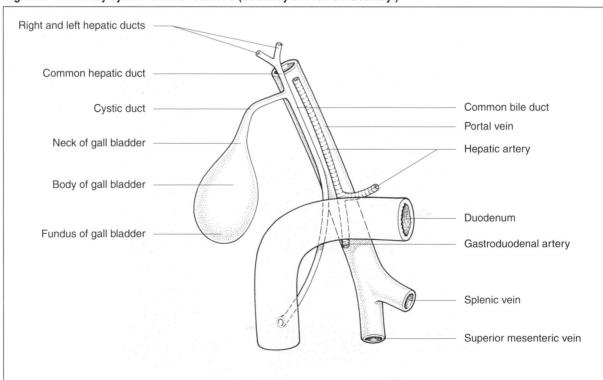

Right and left hepatic ducts

Common hepatic duct

Cystic duct

Neck of gall bladder

Body of gall bladder

Fundus of gall bladder

Common bile duct

Portal vein

Hepatic artery

Duodenum

Gastroduodenal artery

Splenic vein

Superior mesenteric vein

about 50 cm³. It is described as having a fundus, body and neck and it hangs on its bed on the visceral surface of the liver, with its neck lying superiorly and its fundus inferiorly. A pouch called Hartmann's pouch on the ventral surface just proximal to the neck, which is seen when the gall bladder is dilated in disease, is probably not a normal anatomical feature.

The gall bladder is covered by peritoneum on its fundus and inferior surface. Occasionally, it may have a mesentery and hang free from the inferior surface of the liver.

The mucosa lining the gall bladder is smooth except at the neck and the cystic duct where it forms folds that are arranged spirally and called valves of Heister.

The relations of the gall bladder

These are as follows:

- Anterosuperiorly:
  — The gall-bladder bed of the liver
  — The fundus is related to the anterior abdominal wall at the point where the lateral edge of the right rectus muscle meets the ninth costal cartilage; and
- Posteroinferiorly:
  — The neck: lesser omentum
  — The body: first part of the duodenum
  — The fundus: transverse colon.

Normal variants

These are as follows:

- Septated;
- Fundus folded back on itself — known as the Phrygian cap;
- Diverticula may occur anywhere, commonest at the fundus;
- Retrohepatic or suprahepatic;
- Intrahepatic (normal in the fetus up to 2 months);
- Left-sided:
  — Under the left lobe or;
  — Herniated through the epiploic foramen or;
  — As part of transposition of the viscera;
- Absent — very rare (0.05%) associated with other congenital abnormalities; and
- Double — even rarer (0.025%), if double they usually share a duct.

ARTERIAL SUPPLY

The gall bladder is supplied by the cystic artery, a branch of the right hepatic artery and by branches that supply it directly from the liver in the gall-bladder bed.

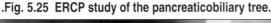

.Fig. 5.25 ERCP study of the pancreaticobiliary tree.

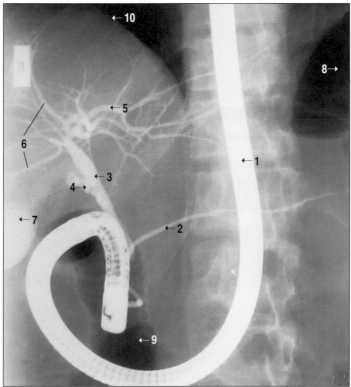

1. Endoscope
2. Pancreatic duct
3. Common hepatic duct
4. Cystic duct
5. Left hepatic duct
6. Right hepatic ducts
7. Gall bladder
8. Gas in fundus of stomach
9. Gas in duodenum
10. Right hemidiaphragm

VENOUS DRAINAGE

Blood from the gall bladder drains via small veins to the liver from the gall-bladder bed. Sometimes a cystic vein is formed that drains to the portal vein.

BILE DUCTS

Intrahepatic bile ducts follow the same pattern of distribution as the hepatic arteries. As with the arteries, a knowledge of the segmental anatomy is especially important in assessment prior to segmentectomy. Bile ducts from segments unite to form right and left hepatic ducts (with a normal diameter of up to 3 mm each), which in turn unite outside the liver in the porta hepatis to form the common hepatic duct. This duct measures up to 7 mm in diameter and is soon (3.5 cm later) joined by the cystic duct (itself 3.5 cm long) to form the common bile duct.

The common bile duct has a supraduodenal third where it lies in the free edge of the lesser omentum, with the hepatic artery on its left and the portal vein posteriorly. It also has a retroduodenal part where it passes behind the first part of the duodenum with the gastroduodenal artery, and a retropancreatic third where it passes behind the pancreas in a tunnel or groove towards the midpoint of the second part of the duodenum. The common bile duct usually unites with the pancreatic duct in a common dilated terminal ampulla (of Vater) and empties into the duodenum at the papilla 8–10 cm from the pylorus.

Variation in the biliary ducts

This is as follows:

■ Variation in the *intrahepatic ducts* may occur in up to 47% of cases. These vary more often than the extrahepatic ducts;

■ *Accessory hepatic ducts* may arise in the liver particularly in the right lobe and join the main hepatic duct or rarely the gall bladder;

■ The right and left ducts may fail to unite giving rise to a *'double' hepatic duct*;

■ The *cystic duct* may:
— Be absent so that the gall bladder joins the hepatic duct
— Join the hepatic duct on its left rather than its right side
— Join the right hepatic duct or
— Join the hepatic duct anywhere between the porta hepatis and the duodenum. Where the cystic duct is long it passes close to and usually behind the hepatic duct. Compression of the hepatic duct by calculi in such a cystic duct results in a syndrome is known as *Mirrizzi's syndrome*;

■ The *common bile duct* and the pancreatic duct may have separate openings close to each other in up to 40% of cases and widely separate from each other in 4% of cases; and

■ The *papilla* may be positioned as far proximally as the stomach or as far distally as the third part of the duodenum.

Fig. 5.26 Ultrasound of the portal vein and common bile duct.

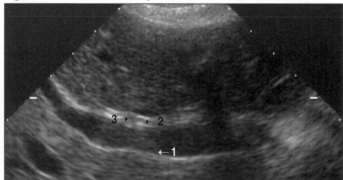

1. Portal vein
2. Common bile duct
3. Hepatic artery

RADIOLOGICAL FEATURES OF THE BILIARY SYSTEM

Plain films of the abdomen

The normal gall bladder or biliary system are not visible. Gas may be seen in the extrahepatic ducts in the elderly where the ampullary tone is low.

Ultrasound examination of the biliary system (Fig. 5.26)

Intrahepatic bile ducts are seen with portal vein radicles. The union of the right and left hepatic ducts can be seen in the porta hepatis. The upper limit of normal for diameter of the hepatic duct can be measured at 8 mm (up to 10 mm in the postcholecystectomy case).

The gall bladder can be visualized between the liver and the right kidney. Its wall thickness varies with the degree of distension. The size of the gall bladder varies also between the fed and fasting states but can be up to 10 cm long and 3 cm wide. The position of the fundus can be as low as the pelvis.

The spiral valves of Heister in the gall-bladder neck and the cystic duct may cast acoustic shadows that must not be confused with calculi.

The hepatic and common bile ducts can sometimes be visualized throughout their course but part of the common bile duct is often obscured by gas as it passes posterior to the first part of the duodenum.

Contrast examinations

A variety of contrast examinations of the gall bladder and biliary tree are possible, depending on the clinical circumstances. Some such as intravenous cholangiography and, to a great extent, oral cholecystography have been replaced by ultrasound. Others such as peroperative, T-tube, transhepatic and retrograde cholangiography (ERCP) are still in use (see **Fig. 5.25**). These show the union of the right and left hepatic ducts, the common hepatic and the common bile duct. Some show the cystic duct and gall bladder.

Anatomical points to note

These include:

■ Some intrahepatic ducts, particularly those to the left lobe have an anterior course and to fill these in transhepatic cholangiography, for example, a patient must be turned from a supine to a prone position. To view anteriorly or posteriorly directed ducts oblique views are taken. The ducts to the quadrate lobe (segment IV) and to the inferior segment of the left lobe (segment III) are most commonly used as afferent ducts to bypass hilar biliary tumours and their patency should be established in preoperative assessment of these patients;

■ The gall bladder is directed anteroinferiorly and to the right and the cystic duct usually joins the hepatic duct on its right side. These facts dictate patient manoeuvres to fill these organs. Owing to the variation in the position of the normal gall bladder, films of the entire abdomen may be necessary when there is difficulty locating it in contrast studies;

■ The extrahepatic bile ducts are anterior to the vertebral column and oblique views are necessary to view these away from the bones; and

■ Peroperative cholangiography during cholecystectomy is important not only to identify possible calculi in the bile ducts but also to show any anatomical variation to reduce the risk of surgical damage to anomalous ducts.

Computed tomography of the liver

The intrahepatic bile ducts are seen with the portal veins. These are distinguished from one another by the enhancement of the veins with intravenous contrast agents. Ducts are usually anterior to the portal vein radicles.

On CT at the level of T11 and T12 (see **Figs 5.2** and **5.10**) the gall bladder is seen between the right lobe and the quadrate lobe. The common bile duct is also seen at this level anterior to the portal vein.

On lower-level CT slices, the common bile duct may be seen in a groove or a tunnel posterior to the head of the pancreas. The body of the gall bladder is seen anterior to the duodenum. On these slices the fundus of the gall bladder is seen between the transverse colon and the anterior abdominal wall.

Scintigraphy of the biliary system using Tc^{99m} HIDA

This accumulates in the liver parenchyma and is excreted by the biliary system outlining the intrahepatic right and left ducts, the extrahepatic ducts, the gall bladder and the cystic duct. Radioactive material excreted into the duodenum is also seen on the scan.

THE PANCREAS (Figs 5.27–5.30)

The pancreas is situated on the posterior abdominal wall at approximately L1 level. It is described as having a head, neck, body and tail. It is retroperitoneal with the exception of the tail, which lies in the lienorenal ligament. It is over 15 cm long and lies transversely and slightly obliquely with the tail higher than the head.

The head of the pancreas lies in the curve of the duodenum, with the pylorus and the duodenal cap overlapping it slightly on its upper surface. The uncinate process projects posteriorly and to the left from its lower part to lie posterior to the superior mesenteric vessels. The remainder of the pancreatic head lies anterior to the vessels of the posterior abdominal wall, that is, the vena cava and renal veins, the aorta and its coeliac and superior mesenteric branches. The common bile duct passes posterior to the head of the pancreas in a groove or tunnel towards its termination in the second part of the duodenum.

The neck of the pancreas extends from the upper part of the anterior portion of the head. It lies anterior to the union of the splenic vein and the superior mesenteric vein to form the portal vein.

The body of the pancreas curves over the vertebrae and great vessels to reach the left paravertebral gutter. The splenic vein passes posterior to the body where it receives the inferior mesenteric vein. The splenic artery runs along the upper surface of the pancreas in a sinuous course that is intermittently above and behind the pancreas. The body lies anterior to the left kidney and adrenal.

The tail of the pancreas is related to the splenic hilum. Here it lies in the lienorenal ligament.

The lesser sac is anterior to the pancreas and anterior to this lies the stomach and part of the lesser omentum.

THE PANCREATIC DUCTS (see Fig. 5.28)

The pancreatic duct begins in the tail by the union of ductules (the trifurcation seen at ERCP) and passes transversely towards the head closer to the anterior than the posterior surface of the gland. It receives smaller ducts along its length at right angles and increases in size as it approaches the head. At the neck the duct turns inferiorly, somewhat posteriorly and to the right, and joins the bile duct to form a terminal, common, dilated portion called the ampulla (of Vater) before entering the duodenum at the papilla.

An accessory duct (of Santorini) arises in the lower part of the head, which it drains and passes upwards anterior to the main duct to which it is connected by a communicating duct and drains to the duodenum about 2 cm proximal to the papilla. This duct is occasionally absent.

Fig. 5.27 Pancreas: (a) anterior relations; (b and c) posterior relations.(Courtesy of Prof. JB Coakley.)

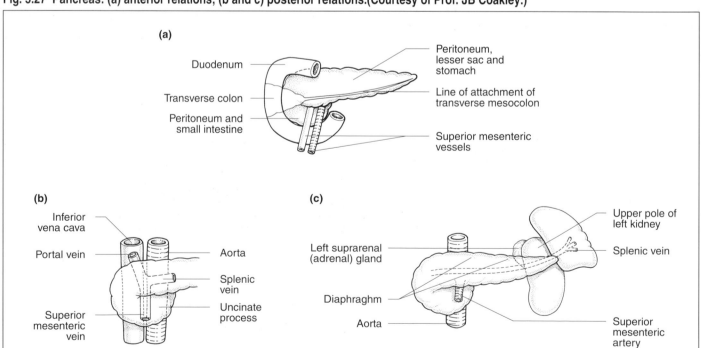

Fig. 5.28 Pancreatic ducts. (Courtesy of Prof. JB Coakley.)

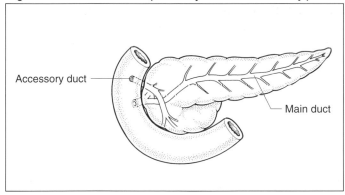

THE DEVELOPMENT OF THE PANCREAS (see **Fig. 5.29**)

The pancreas arises from the junction of the primitive foregut and midgut as a larger dorsal division and two smaller ventral buds. The ventral buds arise in common with the biliary duct. The left ventral bud atrophies and the right ventral bud swings posteriorly to unite with the inferior aspect of the dorsal division, trapping the superior mesenteric vessels between divisions. The duct of the smaller ventral portion becomes the main duct while the proximal part of the duct of the larger dorsal division becomes the accessory duct.

VARIATIONS IN PANCREATIC ANATOMY

These are as follows:

- *Annular pancreas*: this is pancreatic tissue surrounding the duodenum and occurs when part of the ventral bud fails to atrophy;
- *Pancreas divisum*: failure of fusion of the dorsal and ventral moieties results in the anterosuperior part of the head and the body and tail draining via the accessory papilla, while the posteroinferior part of the head drains to the ampulla;
- *Agenesis of the dorsal pancreatic moiety*: this results in a pancreas with a head but no body or tail and is very rare;
- *Left-sided pancreas* is an effect of age with laxity of the suspensory fascia of an otherwise normal gland; and
- *Accessory nodules* of pancreatic tissue may occur in the wall of the stomach, the duodenum, the small intestine or within a Meckl's diverticulum. The most common site is in the wall of the duodenum closest to the pancreas and close to the opening of the pancreatic duct.

Fig. 5.29 Development of the pancreas: (a) appearance of two ventral and one doral pancreatic bud; (b) development of one ventral and one dorsal bud; (c) fusion of the ventral and dorsal buds.

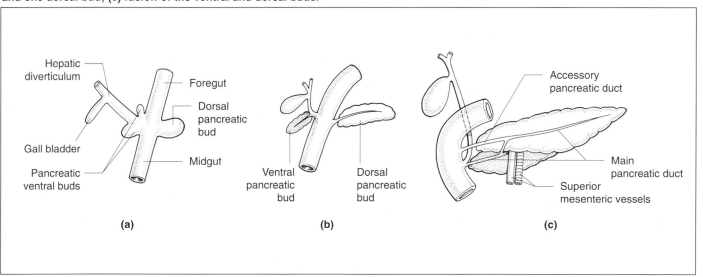

ARTERIAL SUPPLY OF THE PANCREAS (Fig. 5.30)

The pancreas is supplied by branches of the coeliac and superior mesenteric arteries. The coeliac supplies branches via its hepatic and splenic arteries. The gastroduodenal artery, arising from the hepatic artery, divides into the right gastroepiploic artery and the superior pancreaticoduodenal artery. This latter artery divides early into an anterior branch that lies in the groove between the pancreas and the duodenum and a posterior branch that passes posterior to the head of the pancreas.

The splenic artery passes along the upper surface of the pancreas and supplies many small branches to it. One of these is sometimes larger than the others and is called the pancreatica magna artery. The dorsal pancreatic artery arises close to the origin of the splenic artery (or separately from the coeliac artery or from the superior mesenteric artery) and passes vertically downwards behind the pancreas. It divides at right angles into a left branch, which passes towards the tail of the pancreas as the transverse pancreatic artery, and a right branch, which passes between the neck and the uncinate process to anastomose with arteries on the anterior surface of the gland.

The inferior pancreaticoduodenal artery arises from the right side of the superior mesenteric artery. It divides early into anterior and posterior branches that anastomose with those of the superior pancreaticoduodenal artery.

VENOUS DRAINAGE OF THE PANCREAS

The neck, body and tail of the pancreas drain to the splenic vein while the head drains to the superior mesenteric and portal veins.

LYMPHATIC DRAINAGE

Lymphatic drainage is to nodes along the course of the supplying arteries.

RADIOLOGICAL FEATURES OF THE PANCREAS

Plain films of the abdomen

The pancreas is not visible unless calcified. If calcification is distributed throughout the gland it is seen as a transverse structure at L1 level, with a larger head on the right side and a body and tail extending to the left and upwards.

Fig. 5.30 Arterial supply of the pancreas.

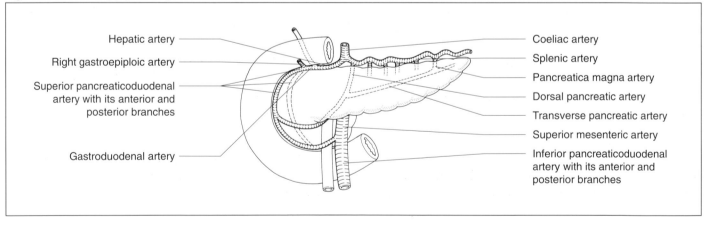

Hepatic artery

Right gastroepiploic artery

Superior pancreaticoduodenal artery with its anterior and posterior branches

Gastroduodenal artery

Coeliac artery

Splenic artery

Pancreatica magna artery

Dorsal pancreatic artery

Transverse pancreatic artery

Superior mesenteric artery

Inferior pancreaticoduodenal artery with its anterior and posterior branches

When the pancreas is inflamed it may cause ileus formation in the nearby duodenum and proximal jejunum, which is visible on plain films. It may also cause fluid collection in the lesser sac (pseudocyst formation), which causes displacement of the stomach gas anteriorly, which is visible on a lateral film of the abdomen.

Hypotonic duodenography

This technique for assessment of the pancreas by visualization of its effects on the closely related duodenal loop has been replaced by other imaging.

Ultrasound of the pancreas

This is possible when it is not obscured by overlying stomach and transverse colonic gas. The entire gland is seen well in only 60% of studies. It is identified on transverse sections by the presence of the splenic vein posteriorly (see **Fig. 5.23**). The coeliac artery division into hepatic and splenic arteries at right angles can easily be identified on ultrasound sections just above the pancreas. The head of the pancreas can be visualized through the left lobe of the liver and the bile duct is seen posterior to it. The tail is viewed by oblique views through the spleen.

The pancreatic duct is seen within the gland closer to its anterior surface. It may measure up to 4 mm in the pancreatic head.

Computed tomography (see Figs 5.2 and 5.3)

As a result of its oblique position, the pancreas is seldom seen on a single axial slice on CT. The tail is visible at the splenic hilum on the highest slices and the uncinate process is the lowest part. Normal thickness of the head is 2 cm, the neck 0.5–1 cm and the body and tail 1–2 cm The height of the head is very variable and may measure up to 8 cm and the body and tail may measure 3–4 cm.

The normal pancreatic duct is visible in 60–70% of scans if slices are thin. The common bile duct is often visible in the pancreatic head. The formation of the portal vein is seen behind the neck and the mesenteric vessels are seen to pass anterior to the uncinate process.

Magnetic resonance imaging of the pancreas

Limited by respiratory movement, bowel peristalsis and the lack of oral contrast, nonetheless the gland and its vessels are well seen, with the anterior and posterior pancreaticoduodenal arcades visible in many cases. The intensity of the pancreatic gland is less than that of the liver on T1-weighted and greater on T2-weighted sequences. The nondilated common bile duct is visible within the pancreatic head but the normal pancreatic duct is seldom visible.

Endoscopic retrograde cholangiopancreatography (see Fig. 5.25)

ERCP visualizes the pancreatic duct by injection of contrast after cannulization via duodenal endoscopy. The main duct is cannulated in common with the bile duct when the anatomy of the bile duct is normal. The main duct is seen to begin by the union of small ducts in the tail. It passes obliquely downwards and to the right across the L1 vertebra and ends in a dilated ampulla before entering the duodenum. The duct is 16 cm long and up to 4 mm diameter in the head. The accessory duct may be filled via its communication with the main duct and is seen to pass anteriorly and superiorly to the main duct.

Branches join the main duct at right angles. A pancreatogram is obtained when enough contrast is injected to fill the acini. This is undesirable since it is associated with a higher incidence of post-ERCP complications.

The pancreatic duct is foreshortened in PA views on ERCP because of the posterior course of part of the gland between the head, which lies on the aorta, and IVC and the tail, which lies in the paravertebral gutter. Right posterior oblique views may be helpful.

Angiography of the pancreas

This technique shows the vessels as described. Coeliac and superior mesenteric arteries must be opacified.

Venography of the pancreas

This technique is sometimes undertaken for venous sampling to identify the site of a hormone-producing tumour. A transhepatic approach to the portal, splenic and superior mesenteric veins is used.

THE SPLEEN (Fig. 5.31)

The spleen is found in the left upper quadrant of the abdomen. It is the size of a fist, measuring up to 12 cm long, 7 cm wide and 7 cm in thickness. Its long axis is in the line of the tenth rib and its lower pole does not usually extend beyond the mid-axillary line.

The spleen has a smooth diaphragmatic surface related through the diaphragm to the costodiaphragmatic recess of the pleura and the ninth, tenth and eleventh ribs. The visceral surface of the spleen faces anteroinferiorly and to the right. Its contours correspond to its relationship to the stomach anteriorly, the splenic flexure of the colon inferiorly and the left kidney posteriorly. The splenic artery enters and the splenic vein leaves the spleen as four or five branches each at the hilum between the gastric and renal impressions. The tail of the pancreas also lies at the splenic hilum.

The spleen is covered with peritoneum on its visceral and diaphragmatic surfaces. At the hilum it is attached by peritoneum to the posterior abdominal wall — the phrenicosplenic and lienorenal ligaments — and to the greater curve of the stomach — the gastrosplenic ligament. The splenic vessels and the pancreatic tail pass towards the spleen in the former and the short gastric and left gastroepiploic vessels pass in the latter.

BLOOD SUPPLY OF THE SPLEEN

The splenic artery arises from the coeliac trunk. The splenic vein receives the inferior mesenteric vein and joins with the superior mesenteric vein to form the portal vein.

Fig. 5.31 Spleen: (a) visceral surface; (b) diaphragmatic surface and peritoneal attachments. (Courtesy of Prof. JB Coakley.)

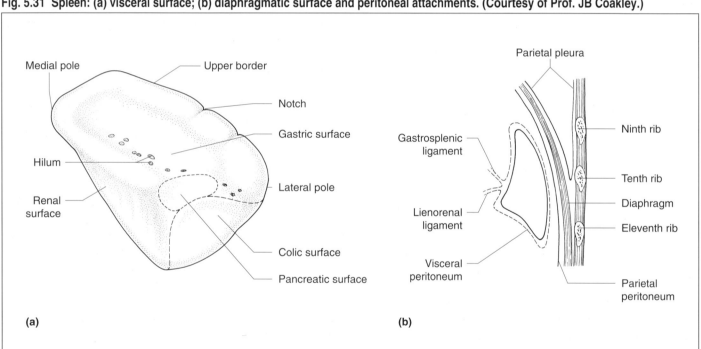

VARIANTS

The spleen develops in many parts in the dorsal mesentery of the stomach at 5–7 weeks of intrauterine life. These parts are represented in the adult by the segments supplied by each branch of the artery. The adult may, however, have *multiple spleens* or may retain some *fetal lobulation.* Up to 10% of normal adults have, in addition to a normal spleen, accessory spleens called *splenunculi.* These occur most commonly in the splenic hilum or near the pancreatic tail but may also be found in the small intestinal mesentery or in the greater omentum.

Anatomical asplenia and polysplenia (several small rudimentary splenic bodies) are associated with congenital heart disease and isomerism (bilateral right- or left-sided anatomy of the heart, bronchi and abdominal structures). This reflects the development of the spleen and the heart at the same period of intrauterine life. *Functional aspenia* occurs where, due to interruption of blood supply or diffuse disease, no spleen is seen in imaging such as scintigraphy, which depends on functioning splenic tissue.

A *'wandering spleen'* is a condition related to age, where lax suspensory ligaments allow great splenic mobility and the ectopic spleen may simulate a mass elsewhere.

RADIOLOGICAL FEATURES OF THE SPLEEN

Plain films of the abdomen

The spleen is often not visible but its lower pole may be outlined by fat. Its size and position may be deduced from the distance between air in the lung and its impression on the gastric or colonic gas shadows. Assessing its size by measurement of its width 2 cm above the splenic tip on plain films is less accurate than measurement of its length from the dome of the diaphragm to the tip. This is usually less than 14 cm.

The relationship of the spleen to the ninth, tenth and eleventh ribs is important in plain films of trauma cases where fracture of these ribs is associated with splenic rupture.

Ultrasound of the spleen

The spleen is less echogenic than the normal liver. Splenic length may be measured (normally less than 12 cm). The splenic vessels are best seen when enlarged.

The spleen enlarges anterior to the colon and becomes easier to see on ultrasound. Retroperitoneal masses, by comparison, may be masked by colonic gas.

Accessory spleens can be identified by ultrasound by demonstrating supply by the splenic artery and drainage by the splenic vein.

Computed tomography (see Figs 5.2, 5.3, 5.10 and 5.11)

On CT the spleen is seen as homogenously enhancing. Its relationship to the diaphragm, pleura and ribs and to the pancreas, stomach, colon and left kidney can be appreciated. Normal size is difficult to define because of respiratory movement between cuts but it is assessed by the number of cuts on which the spleen is visible. The spleen is enlarged if anterior to the aorta or extending below the ribs.

Portography

(See also the section on portal system.)
This may be performed by splenic puncture via the ninth or tenth interspace posteriorly, remembering that the costodiaphragmatic recess of the pleura always extends to the level of the lower pole of the spleen.

Magnetic resonance imaging

The spleen is visible on coronal or sagittal views on MRI and its relations to the kidney, adrenal gland and the diaphragm can be appreciated. Poor differentiation between the normal spleen and tumour may be improved by the use of reticuloendothelial contrast agents.

Scintigraphy

Activity may be seen in splenunculi in addition to the normal spleen.

THE PORTAL VENOUS SYSTEM (Fig. 5.32)

Blood from the gastrointestinal tract (not including the anus), the spleen, pancreas and the gall bladder drains to the liver via the portal venous system. This consists of the superior and inferior mesenteric and the splenic veins, which unite to form the portal vein. There are valves in this system in the fetus and young infant but not in the adult.

SUPERIOR MESENTERIC VEIN

This lies to the right of the superior mesenteric artery and drains the area supplied by this artery. Its branches are similar except proximally and are as follows:

- Right gastroepiploic and inferior pancreatico-duodenal proximally;
- Jejunal and ileal branches to its left side;
- Ileocolic, right colic and mid-colic branches to its right side.

INFERIOR MESENTERIC VEIN

This lies to the left of the inferior mesenteric artery and drains its area of supply in the colon via the:

- Left colic, sigmoid and superior rectal veins; and
- Some pancreatic branches.

THE SPLENIC VEIN

Four or five branches leave the splenic hilum and unite to form the splenic vein. Occasionally, a vein from the upper pole of the spleen joins the splenic more proximally (the superior polar vein). Proximally the splenic vein receives the short gastric veins and the gastroepiploic vein from the stomach. It receives multiple pancreatic branches and the inferior mesenteric vein as it passes posterior to the tail and body of the pancreas. The splenic vein then unites with the superior mesenteric vein to form the portal vein behind the neck of the pancreas.

THE PORTAL VEIN

The portal vein passes behind the neck of the pancreas and receives the superior pancreatico-duodenal vein. It then passes behind the first part of the duodenum and receives the right gastric and left gastric (also known as the coronary vein) veins. It passes in the free edge of the lesser omentum posterior to the common bile duct and the hepatic artery. Here it is separated from the IVC by

Fig. 5.32 Portal venous system. (Courtesy of Prof. JB Coakley.)

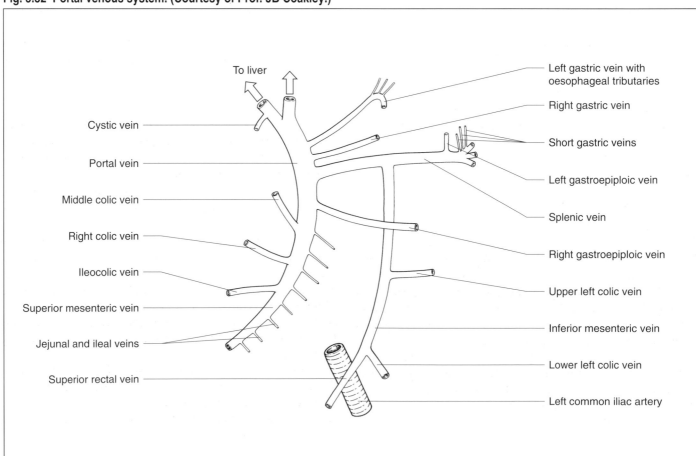

the epiploic foramen.

At the porta hepatis the portal vein divides into right and left branches. The right branch receives the cystic vein if one is formed and the left receives the paraumbilical veins. Attached to the left portal vein is the ligamentum teres and its continuation — the ligamentum venosum. Within the liver the portal vein is distributed with the branches of the hepatic artery.

PORTOSYSTEMIC ANASTOMOSES

Portal venous pressure is raised when there is obstruction to blood flow in the portal vein, the liver or the hepatic veins. Portosystemic collateral pathways then open where these two systems communicate (see **Table 5.3**).

RADIOLOGICAL FEATURES OF THE PORTAL VENOUS SYSTEM

Plain films of the abdomen

The normal portal veins are not visible. If there is gas in the portal veins in the liver it is distinguished from gas in the bile ducts by its peripheral position.

Ultrasound (see Figs 5.23 and 5.26)

The portal vein is visible on ultrasound as it passes towards the liver posterior to the common bile duct and hepatic artery (see **Fig. 5.26**). Its diameter is variable but always greater than the normal bile duct. Portal vein branches in the liver are seen as having more echogenic walls than the branches of the bile duct.

The splenic vein is an important landmark in ultrasound as it passes posterior to the pancreas (see **Fig. 5.23**). It helps identify this gland. An abnormality in its course around the vertebrae and prevertebral structures can be an indication of a mass here.

Computed tomography
(see Figs 5.2, 5.3, 5.10 and 5.11)

The portal vein can be seen in the porta hepatis and its branches are seen in the liver generally posterior to the bile duct and hepatic artery branches. The portal vein is seen posteriorly in the free edge of the lesser omentum. Here it is separated by the epiploic foramen from the IVC. This space, called the portocaval space, is the site of normal lymph nodes in the lesser omentum and of abnormal masses.

The splenic vein is seen posterior to the pancreas and unites with the inferior mesenteric vein laterally and the superior mesenteric vein behind the neck of the pancreas (see **Fig. 5.32**). It lies anterior to the left kidney and its hilum, the renal vein and IVC.

Table 5.3 Portosystemic anastomoses

Site	Portal system	Systemic veins
Gastro-oesophageal junction	Left gastric vein	Oesophageal veins
Rectum	Superior rectal veins	Inferior rectal veins
Retroperitoneum	Tributaries in mesentery	Retroperitoneal, renal, lumbar and phrenic veins
Umbilicus	Paraumbilical veins with ligamentum t eres	Veins of the abdominal wall

The superior mesenteric vein is seen to the right of the artery on lower slices and together these pass anterior to the uncinate process of the pancreas.

Portography

Direct

This includes *splenoportography,* where contrast is introduced directly into the spleen and outlines the splenic vein and the portal vein.

A *transhepatic* route can also be used to cannulate the portal vein and via this the splenic or other veins. This can be used to sclerose oesophageal varices or to do venous sampling to isolate a hormone-producing pancreatic tumour.

Transumbilical portography can be performed in the neonate by catheterizing the umbilical vein, which drains to the left portal vein.

Indirect

This is the most commonly used method today and *digital subtraction angiography (DSA)* makes visualization of the portal system by this method easier. Contrast is injected into the coeliac and superior mesenteric arteries (sequentially or together) and films are taken in the venous phase. To show the inferior mesenteric vein that artery must also be injected.

If the spleen is very large the splenic vein may be difficult to visualize because of pooling if contrast in the spleen.

Flow of blood is slow in the portal venous system and there is poor mixing of blood from the splenic and superior mesenteric veins with the former supplying principally the left lobe of the liver and the latter the right lobe. This should not be misinterpreted when only one artery is injected.

Contrast in the liver preferentially fills the right lobe of the liver in the supine patient because of the more posterior position of this lobe. To overcome this effect of gravity it may be necessary to rotate the patient.

THE KIDNEYS (Figs 5.33–5.35)

The kidneys lie retroperitoneally in the paravertebral gutters of the posterior abdominal wall. They lie obliquely with their upper poles more medial and more posterior than their lower. The kidneys measure approximately 12 cm long, are 6 cm wide and 3.5 cm thick. Their size is approximately that of three-and-one-half lumbar vertebrae and their associated discs on a radiograph.

On coronal section (see **Fig. 5.33**) each kidney is seen to have an outer cortex and an inner medulla. Extensions of cortex centrally as columns (of Bertin) separate the medulla into pyramids whose apices, jutting into the calyces, are called the papillae. Minor calyces combine to form two or three major calyces, which in turn unite to form the pelvis of the kidney. The pelvis may be entirely intrarenal or entirely extrarenal. The gap between the renal substance and the pelvis is called the renal sinus and is filled with fat.

The functional subunit of the kidney is called the **nephron** and consists of a glomerulus in the cortex and a tubule in the medulla. This drains to a collecting duct, which empties into the calyx at the tip of the medulla.

The **hilum** of the kidney lies medially; that of the right at L1 vertebral level and that of the left at L1/L2 level. At the hilum, the pelvis lies anteriorly and the renal vein posteriorly with the artery in between. Lymph vessels and nerves also enter at the hilum.

THE RELATIONS OF THE KIDNEYS

These are as follows:

■ Posteriorly:
— Upper third, diaphragm and twelfth rib and the costodiaphragmatic recess of the pleura
— Lower third, medial to lateral: psoas, quadratus lumborum and transverses abdominis muscles.
■ Superiorly: the adrenal gland — more medial on the right kidney; and
■ Anteriorly:
— Right kidney:
liver
second part of the duodenum
ascending colon
small intestinal loops
—Left kidney:
stomach
pancreas and its vessels
spleen
splenic flexure of the colon
jejunal loops.

Fig. 5.33 Internal structure of the kidney.

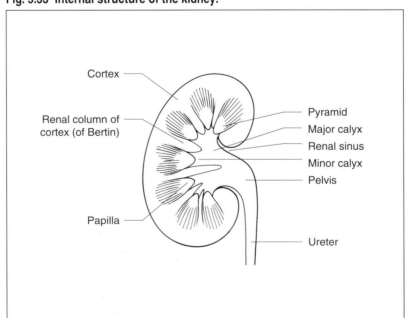

Cortex

Renal column of cortex (of Bertin)

Papilla

Pyramid
Major calyx
Renal sinus
Minor calyx
Pelvis

Ureter

Fig. 5.34 Kidneys: (a) posterior relations of right kidney; (b and c) anterior relations of kidneys.(Courtesy of Prof. JB Coakley.)

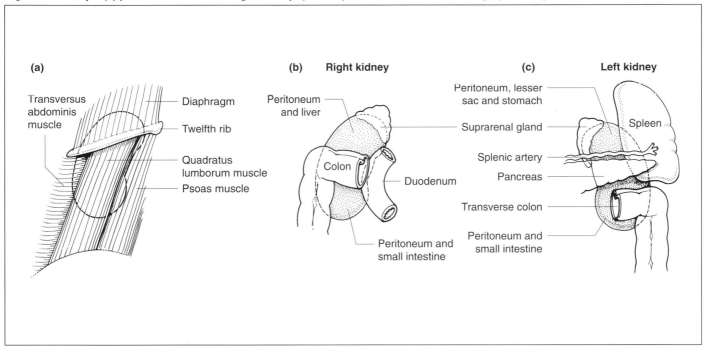

BLOOD SUPPLY OF THE KIDNEYS

The renal arteries arise from the aorta at L1/L2 level. The right renal artery is longer and lower than the left and passes posterior to the IVC. Each renal artery divides in three branches: one passes posterior to the renal pelvis and supplies the posterior upper part of the kidney; another anterior branch supplies the upper anterior kidney; and the third branch passes anterior to the renal pelvis and supplies the entire lower part of the kidney.

These arteries further subdivide into segmental, interlobar, arcuate (at the base of the pyramids) and interlobular arteries.

VENOUS DRAINAGE

The renal veins drain directly to the IVC. The left renal vein is longer and must pass anterior to the aorta to reach the IVC. It also receives the inferior phrenic, adrenal and gonadal veins of that side.

FASCIAL SPACES AROUND THE KIDNEYS (see **Fig. 5.35**)

A true *fibrous capsule* surrounds the kidney. This, in turn, is surrounded by perinephric fat, which separates the kidney from the surrounding organs including the adrenal gland. A condensation of fibroareolar tissue around this fat forms the *renal fascia*. This has an anterior lamella *(Gerota's fascia)* and a posterior lamella *(Zuckerkandl's fascia)*. These lamellae are fused laterally as the lateral conal fascia, which is continuous with the fascia on the deep surface of the tranversalis abdominis muscle. Above, the layers are also fused and blend with the diaphragmatic fascia. Medially, the anterior lamella fuses with the sheaths of the aorta and the IVC. The posterior lamella fuses with the psoas muscle.

The renal fascia encloses the *perirenal space*. The adrenal gland lies within the perirenal space separated from the kidney by fat. Below, this space is relatively open. The anterior layer merges with the areolar tissue that binds the peritoneum with the posterior abdominal wall and the posterior lamella becomes continuous with the fascia over the iliacus muscle. The fat within the perirenal space has septa that can lead to loculation of urine, blood or pus that escapes into this space.

The space between the anterior pararenal fascia and the posterior peritoneum is called the *anterior pararenal space*. It is continuous across the midline and contains the pancreas, duodenum and ascending and descending duodenum. Some writers describe this as a multilaminar rather than a single space.

Posterior to the renal fascia and anterior to the muscles of the posterior abdominal wall is the *posterior pararenal space*. This is limited medially by the attachment of the

Fig. 5.35 Fascial spaces of the retroperitoneum.

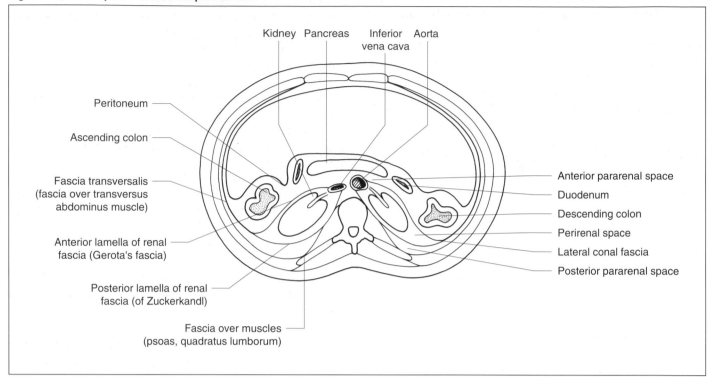

THE DEVELOPMENT OF THE KIDNEY

renal fascia to psoas muscle but is continuous laterally with the extraperitoneal fatty tissue deep to the transversalis muscle. It extends inferiorly to the fat anterior to the iliacus muscle.

THE DEVELOPMENT OF THE KIDNEY

The glomerulus and proximal ductal system of the definitive kidney are derived from the metanephros (the pronephros and mesonephros are transient in man). The collecting duct, calyces and ureter are derived from the metanephric duct.

The kidney is formed in the pelvis in twelve distinct lobules and assumes its adult position by the differential growth of the ureters relative to the trunk. It is supplied first by branches of the iliac artery and subsequently by series of vessels from the abdominal artery, each of which disappears as the kidney develops a new supply.

Developmental abnormalities and variants

The adult kidney may retain some degree of *fetal lobulation.* This may involve the entire kidney or just the middle and lower thirds. It is frequently bilateral. Fetal lobulation is distinguished from pathological scarring by the position of the surface notches — in fetal lobulation surface notches are between the calyces, while scarring occurs directly over the calyces.

One or both kidneys may stay in the pelvis as a *pelvic kidney* supplied by a branch of the internal iliac artery. Both kidneys are pelvic and fused in a *pancake kidney.* A very rare anomaly called *thoracic kidney* (although the diaphragm is usually intact) occurs when the kidney is found higher than its normal position; this may cause an opacity on a chest radiograph. The kidney may ascend to a normal position but retain a supply from an *accessory artery*, which usually enters the lower pole below the hilum. The lower poles of both kidneys may be fused forming a *horseshoe kidney,* or the lower pole of one kidney may be fused with the upper pole of the kidney from the other side — a condition known as *crossed fused ectopia.*

Rarely (in 1 in 1500 births) one kidney is congenitally absent.

RADIOLOGICAL FEATURES OF THE KIDNEY

Plain films of the abdomen

Perirenal fat often makes part or all of the renal outlines visible. Renal *size* is variable with a normal range of 11–15 cm on a radiograph or approximately three-and-one-half vertebral bodies in height. The left kidney is usually bigger but a difference in size of greater than 2 cm is abnormal. The kidneys are relatively bigger in the child (approx. four vertebral bodies in height) and normal limits of size have been plotted against height or age.

The kidneys are seen to move with changes from supine to erect positions and, because of their relationship with the diaphragm, to move with respiration. These moves may be greater than 5 cm and are generally greater in women than men. As the kidney moves inferiorly, its degree of tilt increases with its lower pole becoming more anterior. It may, as a result, appear foreshortened on a radiograph.

Since the colon is anterior to both kidneys and the stomach is anterior to the left kidney and the duodenum to the right, gas in these organs may overlie the renal outlines in a radiograph. Confusing gas and faecal shadows in the colon can be minimized by bowel preparation prior to radiography. Stomach rugal-fold patterns can also cause misleading shadows. The anterior relationship of the stomach is used to advantage in filling the stomach with gas, for example, by a carbonated drink in renal radiography, especially in children.

Intravenous urography (Fig. 5.36)

The renal outline can be seen in the nephrographic phase of intravenous urography (IVU) in most cases. *CT* can help eliminate overlying bowel gas and other shadows. Tomographic cuts for the upper pole are more posterior to those for the lower pole because of the slope of the kidney. Features of size and of renal movement are as for the plain film. Fetal lobulation and its relationship to the calyces can be appreciated. Prominence of the midportion of the lateral border of the left kidney is a normal variant called a *splenic hump* because of the proximity of the spleen.

In the urographic phase the calyceal system can be seen. Minor and major calyces are seen. These are connected to the pelvis of the kidney by infundibulae, which may be long or short. Occasionally a calyx is connected directly to the pelvis of the kidney. The papillae are conical and indent the calyces with surrounding sharp fornices. Contrast in the collecting tubules in the papilla is responsible for the papillary blush that is sometimes seen. Several papillae may indent a single calyx — known as a complex calyx — an arrangement that is more common in the upper pole.

Renal vessels passing close to the renal pelvis and calyces can cause filling defects. These *vascular impressions* are less obvious in well-filled collecting systems.

The renal pelvis is bifid in 10% of cases. This may be associated with complete or partial renal duplication. Partial renal duplication may lead to hypertrophy of septal cortex in the mid-portion of the kidney — known as hypertrophied column of Bertin — causing a pseudomass appearance.

If renal sinus fat is prominent this may cause thinning and elongation of the infundibulae on IVU.

Ultrasound examination of the kidneys

This is nearly always possible unless bowel gas obscures the view, which is more likely in the left side. The renal size is not magnified and so is smaller than on radiographs with normal upper limit of length at 12 cm.

The cortex is distinguishable from the less echogenic medulla — a difference that is more marked in the young infant.

Fat in the renal sinus is very echogenic and a lucent area within this due to the renal pelvis may be the first sign of hydronephrosis.

The aorta, IVC and renal artery and vein are visible on ultrasound. The structures at the hilum (i.e. the pelvis, artery and vein from anterior to posterior) can also be identified.

In addition, the relationship of the right kidney to the liver and the left to the spleen and pancreas can be appreciated. Gas in the stomach, duodenum, small intestine and colon, which are anterior to the kidneys, may obscure their view on ultrasound.

Computed tomography (see Figs 5.3 and 5.4)

The kidneys are seen on slices from T12 to L3 vertebral levels. At the hilum the kidney measures 5 cm transversely and 4 cm sagitally. The renal parenchyma is 1.5 cm thick. Its length is judged by the scanning distance from upper to lower pole.

Posterior relations (i.e. diaphragm, pleura and ribs, psoas, quadratus lumborum and transversus abdominis muscles) and anterior relations (i.e. liver, pancreas, spleen and gastrointestinal tract) can be seen on noncontrast studies.

The kidney is seen to be surrounded by perinephric fat. This is most abundant medial to the lower pole of the kidney and this is a favoured site of accumulation of blood or urine in the ruptured kidney and of pus in a perirenal abscess. The renal fascia is less than 1 mm thick in the normal subject and is only well seen, unless thickened by disease, if it is vertical through the CT slice in a subject with adequate fat.

The renal substance is homogenous on plain scans. After intravenous contrast the cortex is first opacified and then the medulla and pyramids making it possible to distinguish between them. The pyramids are only seen from base to tip at the hilum and are cut at various degrees of obliquity in other slices.

Intravenous contrast scans are best also to visualize the renal vessels.

Magnetic resonance imaging

This technique is not so good as ultrasound for masses less than 3 cm in diameter but is useful for imaging the renal vessels, including the assessment of these in tumour staging.

Fig. 5.36 Intravenous urogram. The right kidney has three major calyces. The left kidney has two major calyces, and a bifid pelvis. Note the course of the lower ureters. The distal part of the ureter passes behind the bladder.

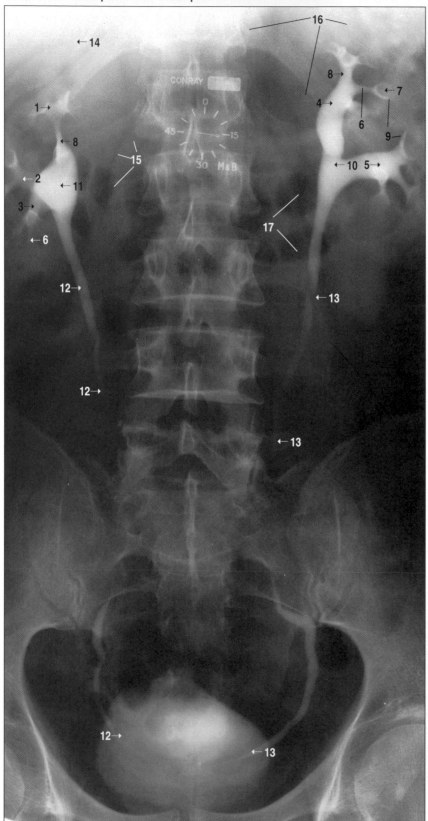

1. Right upper-pole (major) calyx
2. Right middle (major) calyx
3. Right lower-pole (major) calyx
4. Left upper-pole (major) calyx
5. Left lower-pole (major) calyx
6. Minor calyx (infundibulum of)
7. Papilla
8. Infundibulum
9. Fornix
10. Bifid left renal pelvis
11. Right renal pelvis
12. Right ureter
13. Left ureter: vascular impression
14. Upper pole right kidney
15. Right psoas outline
16. Gas in body of stomach
17. Gas in transverse colon

Renal cortex and medulla have different signal intensities resulting in good contrast between these, especially on short TR sequences. As with ultrasound, fat is visible in the renal sinus and the renal pelvis is not easily seen within this unless dilated. Renal vessels are well seen and MRI is useful for evaluation of renal artery stenosis and of tumour or thrombus within the renal vein.

As with CT, the renal capsule and the perinephric fascia are not always visible if normal but perinephric fat is seen surrounding the kidney and separating it from other retroperitoneal structures.

Arteriography of the kidneys

Although needed less often now with the use of ultrasound and CT, this still has a role in assessment of vascular and other lesions of the kidneys. Aortography is performed prior to selective studies and identifies accessory renal arteries if present. These are found in >20% of arteriograms and are even commoner in horseshoe and ectopic kidneys. Aortography also establishes the presence and gross function of both kidneys.

In selective studies, the upper pole is seen to be supplied by anterior and posterior branches of the renal artery, and the lower pole by an anterior branch. Owing to the posterior angulation of the renal artery from the aorta, it is best seen by oblique views with the side of interest uppermost in the supine patient.

Renal venography

This is performed via the inferior vena cava. Venography of the left adrenal and of the left gonad is also performed via left renal venography because of the common drainage of veins from these organs on this side.

The renal veins are seen to have valves. These are commoner on the left side.

The right renal vein is multiple in 10% of venograms and receives the right gonadal vein in 6% of cases.

The left renal vein is more than twice as long as the right. It is multiple in 14% of venograms, splits to surround the aorta in 7% and is retroaortic in 3.5%.

Interventional procedures in the kidney

Performed via fluoroscopy, ultrasound, CT and angiography. Points of anatomical interest in these procedures include:

- The posterior relationship of the diaphragm causes the kidney to move with respiration and most punctures must be performed in suspended respiration;
- The posterior relationship of the pleura makes an approach to the lower pole safer than to an upper pole; and
- A puncture of the kidney in its mid-lateral border is relatively bloodless because of the branching of the renal artery into three branches with separate areas of supply.

Scintigraphy of the kidney

This method is used primarily in the study of the physiology of the kidney. Technetium-labelled dimercaptosuccinic acid (Tc^{99m} DMSA) static scans have some anatomical uses. These are used to establish how much of the fused part of horseshoe kidneys is made of functional renal tissue. Static scans are also useful in the evaluation of pseudotumours of the kidney due to hypertrophy of a column of Bertin.

THE URETER (see Fig. 5.36)

The ureters convey urine from the kidneys to the bladder. Each is 25–30 cm long and is described as having a pelvis and abdominal, pelvic and intravesical parts.

The pelvis has been described with the kidney. The remainder of the ureter has a diameter of about 3 mm but is narrower at the following three sites:

- The junction of the pelvis and ureter;
- The pelvic brim; and
- Where it enters the bladder — this is narrowest of all.

The abdominal ureter passes on the medial edge of the psoas muscle, which separates it from the tips of the transverse processes. On the right side, it is related to the second part of the duodenum, it is crossed by the gonadal, the right colic and the ileocolic vessels and lies lateral to the IVC. On the left side, it is crossed by the gonadal and left colic vessels and has jejunal loops anterior to it, and is crossed at the pelvic brim on the left side by the mesentery of the sigmoid colon and is posterior to this part of the colon.

The ureter enters the pelvis at the bifurcation of the common iliac artery anterior to the sacroiliac joint. It then lies on the lateral wall of the pelvis in front of the iliac artery to a point just anterior to the ischial spine where it turns forwards and medially to enter the bladder.

Close to the bladder in the male, the ureter passes above the seminal vesicle and is crossed by the vas deferens. In the female this part of the ureter is close to the lateral fornix of the vagina and 2.5 cm lateral to the cervix. It passes under the uterine artery in the base of the broad ligament.

The intravesical portion of the ureter has an oblique course of 2 cm through the bladder wall. The vesical muscle has a sphincteric action and the obliquity has a valve-like action.

BLOOD SUPPLY OF THE URETER

The ureter is supplied by branches of nearby arteries and drains to corresponding veins, that is the aorta and IVC and renal, gonadal, internal iliac and inferior vesical vessels.

THE DEVELOPMENT OF THE URETER

The ureter develops as a blind diverticulum from the metanephric duct and grows first posteriorly and then cranially to unite with the developing kidney.

Developmental abnormalities and variants

Duplication of part or all of the ureter occurs in about 4% of subjects. It is the commonest significant congenital anomaly of the urinary tract. Duplication is two to three times commoner in females. When complete duplication occurs, the ureter serving the upper renal moiety drains fewer calyces and is inserted lower into the bladder than that draining the lower moiety — known as the *Weigert-Meyer law*. The low insertion may extend to the bladder neck or the urethra or, in females, the vestibule or vagina.

Ureteric *ectopy* is most common in association with duplication but may occur alone.

Ureterocoele is a dilation of the intramural portion of the ureter due to narrowing of its orifice. This is most common in a duplicated system when it occurs in the ureter draining the upper renal moiety and is usually ectopic.

RADIOLOGICAL FEATURES OF THE URETER

Plain films of the abdomen

The ureter is not visible but a knowledge of its course in relation to the skeleton is necessary when looking for radio-opaque calculi. The ureters pass anterior to the tips of the transverse processes of L2 to L5 lumbar vertebrae and anterior to the sacroiliac joint. They then pass laterally to the ischial spines and medially again to the bladder (see also the course visible on IVU in **Fig. 5.36**).

Intravenous pyelography (see Fig. 5.36)

The ureters are visible completely or in part when filled with contrast. Their course is as above. The ureter passes anteriorly from the kidney to its position near the psoas muscle. Prone views aid ureteric filling. The ureter enters the posterior part of the bladder and oblique views are therefore helpful in imaging the ureterovesical junction.

Varying degrees of ureteric duplication may be seen with the ureters uniting at any point of their course. Other variants already discussed may also be identified.

Ultrasound

Only the proximal and distal ureters are visible on ultrasound and these only when dilated. Intestinal gas obscures the remainder.

Computed tomography

Ureteric calculi not visible on radiographs may be visible on CT scans The ureter itself is easier to identify if it contains contrast medium (see **Fig. 6.7**). It is visible medial to the lower pole of the kidney, anterior to psoas. More distally the ureter remains anterior to the psoas muscle and is lateral to the great vessels. Having crossed the bifurcation of the common iliac artery, the ureter in the pelvis is medial to the iliac arteries and veins. It enters the bladder posterolaterally. Variants such as duplication are easily identified.

THE ADRENAL GLANDS (Fig. 5.37)

The adrenal glands lie retroperitoneally above each kidney. The renal surface is moulded to the kidney and is separated from it by the perirenal fat. The adrenal gland is enclosed within the perirenal fascia but is in a separate compartment from the kidney. The posterior surface of each adrenal gland lies on the crus of the diaphragm. Anteriorly the right gland is related to the liver and the IVC and the left gland is related to the stomach and the pancreas.

The right adrenal gland is lower and more medial in relation to the spine than the left. On cross-section it is linear or 'V'-shaped with a larger medial limb and a smaller lateral limb.

The left adrenal gland is more semilunar and it extends down the superomedial border of the kidney towards the hilum. On cross-section it is triangular or 'Y'-shaped.

At birth the adrenal glands are relatively much bigger than in the adult — one third the size of the kidney at birth and one thirtieth in the adult. The adult gland measures approximately 4 cm high, is 3 cm wide and 1 cm thick.

The adrenal glands have an outer cortex derived from mesoderm and an inner medulla (10% of weight of the gland), which is derived from the neural crest and is related to the sympathetic nervous system.

ARTERIAL SUPPLY

Three arteries supply these glands on each side, namely:

- The superior adrenal artery from the inferior phrenic artery;
- The middle adrenal artery from the aorta; and
- The inferior adrenal artery from the renal artery.

VENOUS DRAINAGE

One vein drains the adrenal gland on each side. The right adrenal vein drains to the IVC and the left adrenal vein drains to the left renal vein.

VARIANTS

Small masses of adrenal cortical tissue called *'cortical bodies'* are often found near the adrenal glands. These may become attached to other organs early in embryology and migrate with these organs to be found in such places as the broad ligament of the uterus, the spermatic cord and even the epididymis.

RADIOLOGICAL FEATURES OF THE ADRENAL GLANDS

Plain films of the abdomen

The adrenal glands are visible only if calcified and are then seen to be lateral to the spine at the level of the upper pole of the kidneys.

Computed tomography (see Fig. 5.11)

The adrenal glands can be identified in more than 95% of subjects if a narrow slice technique is used. The shape of the adrenal gland on CT cuts is variable with a linear, 'V'-shaped one being commonest on the right and triangular or 'Y'-shaped on the left. Its craniocaudal extent is less than 4 cm and limb thickness is usually less than 1 cm.

The right adrenal gland is seen posterior to the IVC. More laterally it lies between the liver and the crura of the diaphragm. The left adrenal extends more laterally anterior to the kidney from which it is separated by perirenal fat. Contrast medium may be necessary to distinguish it from the adjacent splenic vessels.

Fig. 5.37 Adrenal glands: (a) right adrenal; (b) left adrenal. (Courtesy of Prof. JB Coakley.)

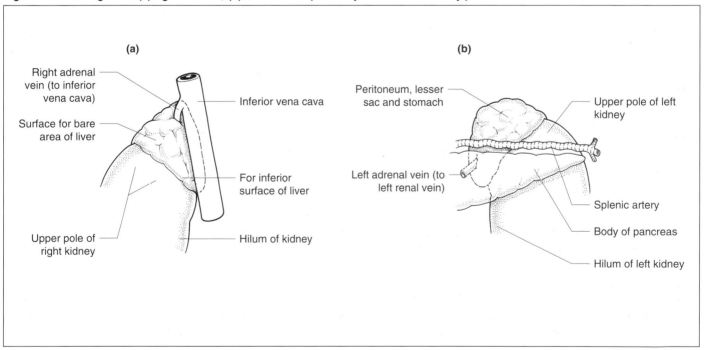

Ultrasound

The adrenal glands can be seen between the kidney and liver on the right and between the kidney and pancreatic tail on the left. Gas in the stomach may make visualization of the left adrenal difficult.

Adrenal venography

This may be performed for venous sampling in addition to imaging the veins. The right adrenal vein enters the IVC 3 cm above the renal vein near the neck of the twelfth rib close to the entry of the hepatic veins. The left adrenal vein is easier to cannulate than the right. It enters the left renal vein near the lateral border of the vertebral body and receives the inferior phrenic vein.

Arteriography of the adrenal gland

All three supplying arteries must be visualized on each side to be studied as follows:

- The *superior adrenal artery* usually consists of several branches from the inferior phrenic artery. It may arise separately from the aorta usually above the coeliac artery but may arise below this or from the renal artery;
- The *middle adrenal artery* arises from the aorta and is multiple in more than 30% of studies; and
- The *inferior adrenal artery* may arise from the renal artery directly or with the superior capsular artery.

Other arteries to the adrenal gland may arise from the gonadal arteries.

Magnetic resonance imaging

The adrenal glands are well seen with anatomical features similar to CT. Owing to greater contrast than CT, MRI can distinguish between the adrenal gland and nearby vessels and diaphragmatic crura without intravascular contrast.

THE ABDOMINAL AORTA
(Fig. 5.38; see Fig. 6.10)

The aorta enters the abdomen through the aortic hiatus of the diaphragm between the crura at T12 vertebral level. It lies anterior to L1–L4 vertebral bodies close to the left psoas muscle. The left lumbar veins pass behind it. Anteriorly it is related to the pancreas, which separates it from the stomach, to the third part of the duodenum and to the coils of small intestine.

The abdominal aorta is 12 cm long and ends by dividing into the right and left common iliac arteries at L4 vertebral level.

BRANCHES OF THE ABDOMINAL AORTA

These are as follows:

- Three unpaired anterior branches:
  — Coeliac trunk at T12/L1 (**Fig. 5.39**; see **Fig. 5.12**)
  — Superior mesenteric artery at L1 (**Fig. 5.40**; see **Fig. 5.19**)
  — Inferior mesenteric artery at L3 (**Fig. 5.41**; see **Fig. 5.20**)
- Three lateral paired visceral arteries:
  — Adrenal arteries at L1
  — Renal arteries at L1-L2
  — Gonadal arteries at L3
- Five lateral paired parietal branches:
  — Inferior phrenic arteries at T12
  — Four pairs of lumbar arteries; and
- Terminal arteries:
  — The common iliac arteries
  — Median sacral artery.

RADIOLOGICAL FEATURES OF THE AORTA

Plain films of the abdomen

The aorta is visible only if calcified. It is then seen as linear calcification vertically in the midline and to the left of this. Tortuosity of the aorta in the elderly may cause considerable variation in the site of this calcification.

Proximity of the vertebral bodies may lead to bony erosion by aneurysms of the aorta, which may be detectable on radiographs.

Ultrasound

This is a useful means of studying the aorta particularly for aneurysm formation. It can be visualized posterior to the pancreas where its coeliac and superior mesenteric branches can be easily seen. Where it passes posterior to loops of small intestine it is often obscured by gas.

The aortic diameter is 2–3 cm depending on age; the diameter diminishes as the aorta progresses caudally. The aorta can be distinguished from the IVC on ultrasound of the upper abdomen by its course near the diaphragm. The aorta remains posteriorly placed to reach the aortic hiatus posterior to the crura of the diaphragm. The IVC, on the other hand, passes ventrally to pierce the central tendon of the diaphragm.

Computed tomography

The aorta can be seen throughout its course, as can its terminal division into right and left common iliac arteries. Its coeliac trunk can be identified above the pancreas. The

Fig. 5.38 Major blood vessels: (a) abdominal aorta; (b) inferior vena cava.

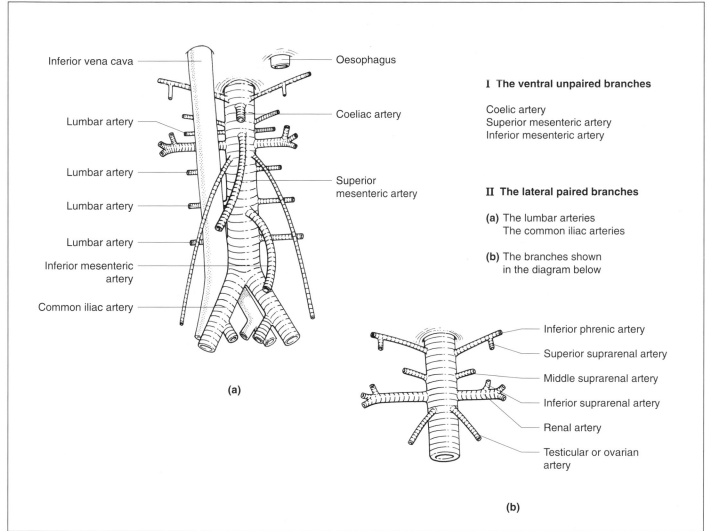

Inferior vena cava

Lumbar artery

Lumbar artery

Lumbar artery

Lumbar artery

Inferior mesenteric artery

Common iliac artery

Oesophagus

Coeliac artery

Superior mesenteric artery

(a)

I The ventral unpaired branches

Coelic artery
Superior mesenteric artery
Inferior mesenteric artery

II The lateral paired branches

(a) The lumbar arteries
The common iliac arteries

(b) The branches shown
in the diagram below

Inferior phrenic artery

Superior suprarenal artery

Middle suprarenal artery

Inferior suprarenal artery

Renal artery

Testicular or ovarian artery

(b)

common hepatic artery can often be identified so far as its gastroduodenal branch. The obliquity of this branch in relation to axial CT cuts makes it difficult to see. The left gastric artery can be traced to the stomach but the splenic artery is very tortuous and can only be seen in sections.

The superior mesenteric artery is usually surrounded in fat even in the cachectic subject, aiding its CT visualization. The inferior mesenteric artery, on the other hand, is not always seen even with intravenous contrast. The renal arteries are seen and the left renal vein is seen passing anterior to the aorta. The lumbar arteries are sometimes visible.

Magnetic resonance imaging

This technique is useful for visualization of the aorta without contrast medium. Anterior branches are visible on sagittal views and lateral branches are best seen in planes parallel to their course.

Angiography (see Figs 5.12, 5.19, 5.20 and 6.10)

The anatomy as described above is best imaged by aortography or selective arteriography of its branches.

Fig. 5.39 Branches of the coeliac artery. (Courtesy of Prof. JB Coakley.)

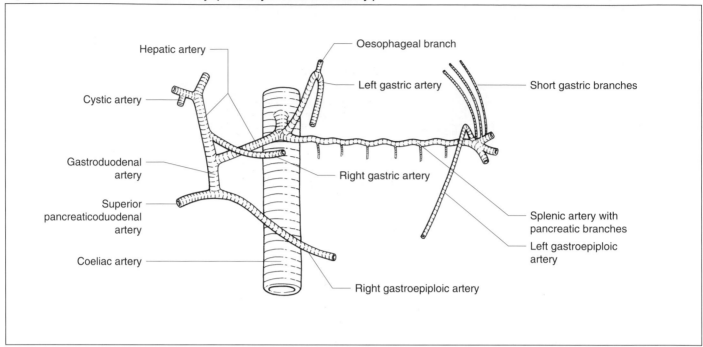

Fig. 5.40 Branches of the superior mesenteric artery. (Courtesy of Prof. JB Coakley.)

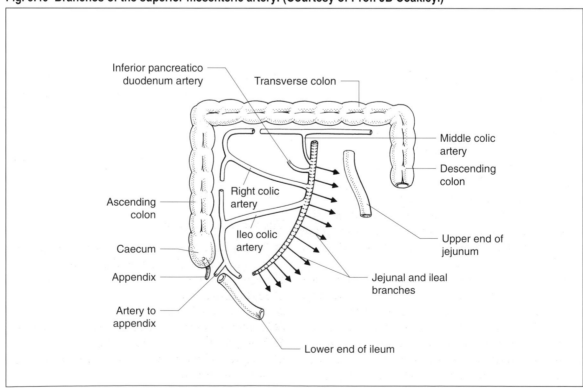

Fig. 5.41 Branches of the inferior mesenteric artery. (Courtesy of Prof. JB Coakley.)

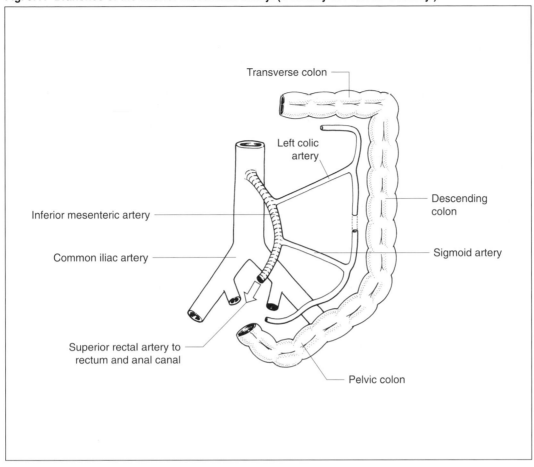

THE INFERIOR VENA CAVA (see Fig. 5.38)

The inferior vena cava (IVC) is formed by the union of the right and left common iliac veins at L5 vertebral level behind the right common iliac artery. It passes to the right of the aorta so far as T12 level, where it is separated from it by the right crus of the diaphragm. The IVC pierces the diaphragm at T8 level, passes through the pericardium and enters the right atrium. An incomplete semilunar valve is found at its entry to the atrium. Otherwise the IVC has no valves.

The IVC lies on the bodies of the lumbar vertebrae. Part of the right adrenal gland and the right inferior phrenic, right adrenal, right renal and right lumbar arteries pass posterior to it. It is related anteriorly from below upwards, to coils of small intestine and the root of the mesentery, the third part of the duodenum, the head of the pancreas and the common bile duct, the first part of the duodenum and the epiploic foramen, with the portal vein anterior to it. It then passes in a deep groove in the liver (sometimes a tunnel) before piercing the diaphragm and entering the heart.

TRIBUTARIES OF THE INFERIOR VENA CAVA

These are as follows:

- Third and fourth lumbar veins (upper two to the azygous vein, the fifth to the ileolumbar vein);
- Right gonadal vein;
- Right renal vein;
- Right adrenal vein;
- Small veins from right and caudate lobes of liver;
- Right, middle and left hepatic veins; and
- Right inferior phrenic vein (left drains to left suprarenal vein.

EMBRYOLOGY AND VARIANTS

The IVC arises embryologically by a complex series of fusion of primitive veins. As a result of this its lower tributaries lie posterior to the aorta, while its upper tributaries lie anterior to the aorta. *Variation* in this development can give rise to several congenital abnormalities of the IVC. It may, for example be double below the renal veins due to persistence of a primitive vein on the left side. This may be associated with a failure of union of the common iliac veins. Occasionally, the IVC is continuous with a much enlarged azygous vein, which carries all of its blood to the superior vena cava (SVC). The IVC may be left-sided so far as the renal veins and then cross over (retroaortically) and continue as a right-sided IVC through the liver to the heart.

RADIOLOGY OF THE INFERIOR VENA CAVA

Chest radiography

The inferior vena cava can be identified as it pierces the right hemidiaphragm and enters the heart. On a lateral chest radiograph it identifies a hemidiaphragm as right.

Cavography

The IVC can be opacified by contrast medium that is introduced either simultaneously into the dorsal pedal veins of both feet or via both femoral veins or by a catheter that is introduced into the vessel itself. Some contrast may be introduced into its tributaries by the performance of a Valsalva manoeuvre.

Ultrasound

The IVC can be identified where it is not obscured by intestinal gas. Its hepatic and proximal course are best seen using ultrasound. It can be seen posterior to the portal vein at the epiploic foramen. The hepatic veins can be seen draining to the IVC before it enters the right atrium. The IVC curves ventrally just before piercing the diaphragm, unlike the aorta, which passes posterior to the diaphragm, thus distinguishing these vessels.

Computed tomography

The IVC is seen on the right of the aorta. It is a transverse oval in cross-section but its shape varies from slit-like on inspiration to circular on expiration. The right adrenal gland is seen to be partly posterior to the IVC. Some liver tissue may also be found posterior to it in its upper course. The right aortic branches that pass behind the IVC may or may not be visible.

The union of the common iliac veins to form the IVC can be identified, and the right common iliac vein is seen to be posterior to the left common iliac artery. In fact, all the pelvic veins are dorsal to the corresponding arteries.

Magnetic resonance imaging

The IVC can be noninvasively visualized by a few coronal sections.

VEINS OF THE POSTERIOR ABDOMINAL WALL (Fig. 5.42)

The internal and external vertebral venous plexuses drain via segmental lumbar veins. The lumbar veins are joined on each side by an ascending lumbar vein, which also connects the lateral sacral and iliolumbar vein (which drains into the common iliac vein). The lumbar vein ascends on the vertebral bodies at the root of the transverse processes deep to the psoas muscle.

The azygous vein may arise in one of three ways. It may be simply the continuation of ascending lumbar vein on the right side entering the thorax with the aorta or by piercing the right crus of the diaphragm; it may arise from the back of the IVC at the level of the renal veins; or it may begin as the continuation of the subcostal vein.

Similarly, the hemiazygous vein may be the continuation of the left ascending lumbar vein and enter the thorax by piercing the left crus. It may arise from the posterior aspect of the left renal vein or it may be the continuation of the left subcostal vein.

In the event of congenital absence of, or obstruction of, the IVC, the ascending lumbar and azygous system of veins convey blood to the SVC. The role of this system in the spread of malignant and other disease is controversial.

RADIOLOGICAL FEATURES OF THE VEINS OF THE POSTERIOR ABDOMINAL WALL

Azygous and ascending lumbar venography

These veins are filled with contrast by one of several routes to identify pathology in the spinal canal. Both femoral veins may be injected while the IVC is obstructed by external compression, or one or both ascending lumbar veins may be selectively cathetherized via the femoral and iliac veins. Intraosseus phlebography by injection of a spinous process of a lumbar vertebra is theoretically possible. With the advance of CT and MRI, these techniques are now seldom used.

Contrast-enhanced computed tomography

The ascending lumbar veins, the azygous and hemiazygous veins, may be visible deep to psoas distally or close

Fig. 5.42 Veins of the posterior abdominal wall.

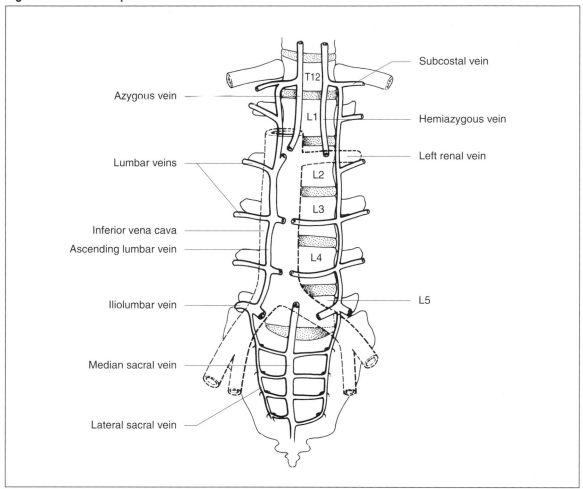

to the aorta proximally as it passes between the crura of the diaphragm. These veins are much more easily seen if enlarged, as occurs in obstruction of the IVC or SVC.

LYMPHATIC DRAINAGE OF THE ABDOMEN

Lymph channels in the abdomen travel with the arteries. Most lymph drains nodes around the abdominal aorta. These are arranged into four groups:

■ Preaortic;
■ Right para-aortic;
■ Left para-aortic; and
■ Retroaortic.

All of these drain to the cisterna chyli, which is an elongated lymph channel that continues in the thorax as the thoracic duct.

PREAORTIC NODES

These are arranged around the coeliac trunk and the superior and inferior mesenteric arteries. They drain lymph in the areas supplied by these arteries, that is, the gastrointestinal tract, the liver, gall bladder, pancreas and spleen. Lymph from these viscera pass through visceral nodes such as the nodes in the porta hepatis and nodes near the intestinal wall and along the course of the arteries before reaching the para-aortic nodes. Lymph from the preaortic nodes passes in the *intestinal trunk* to the cisterna chyli.

PARA-AORTIC NODES

These nodes lie on either side of the aorta in relation to its lateral paired branches. They lie anterior to the lateral margin of psoas and the crura of the diaphragm. They receive lymph from the structures supplied by these branches including the posterior abdominal wall, the diaphragm, the kidneys and adrenals and the gonads.

Lymph from the legs drains via the deep inguinal and external and common iliac nodes to the para-aortic nodes. Lymph from the pelvis drains via internal and common iliac nodes to the para-aortic nodes.

Efferent vessels from these nodes unite to form the *right and left lumbar trunks.*

RETROAORTIC NODES

These nodes drain no area in particular and are really only posteriorly placed nodes of the lateral group. They are worthy of mention only because very little else lies between the aorta and the vertebral bodies and a mass posterior to the aorta is therefore likely to have arisen in lymph nodes.

CISTERNA CHYLI

This thin-walled sac, 6 mm wide and 6 cm long, is really the dilated proximal end of the thoracic duct before it passes through the aortic hiatus of the diaphragm. It lies in front of the bodies of L1 and L2 to the right crus of the aorta. The cisterna chyli receives the intestinal trunk, the right and left lumbar trunks and paired descending intercostal trunks.

RADIOLOGICAL FEATURES OF THE ABDOMINAL LYMPHATICS

Computed tomography

Lymph nodes with normal lengths of 0.5–1 cm are within the resolution of CT; however, internal architecture is not visible. Thus nodes are designated abnormal only if enlarged. CT cannot detect abnormalities in nodes less than 1 cm in diameter.

Nodes may be visualized in any of the sites mentioned above but are best seen around the aorta. Unlike lymphography, CT may visualize hepatic, visceral and preaortic nodes, especially if these are enlarged.

Lymphography

Contrast is introduced into lymph vessels of the feet to visualize the lymph channels and nodes of the posterior abdominal wall. Lymph channels are visible within hours and should clear in less than 24 hours. Lymph nodes are best seen after 24 hours when contrast has accumulated within them and the channels are clear.

Normal lymph nodes have a fine reticular appearance on lymphography. Vessels pass directly through any fatty filling defect but are deflected by more significant pathology. Normal lymph nodes are no longer than 3.5 cm long with their long axis in the line of the lymph vessels; however, some abnormal lymph nodes may measure less than this.

Lymphography by this method shows the deep inguinal nodes, the external iliac nodes and the common iliac nodes. The para-aortic nodes are seen as right and left lumbar chains of nodes along the tip of the transverse processes of the lumbar vertebrae to L2 level where they drain to the cisterna chyli. In about 60% of cases, a middle chain arises from the right chain. Fine, tortuous, transverse vessels link the chains. Gaps in the right chain are frequent and associated with bypass vessels but there are no gaps in the left chain. The upper left lumbar nodes are particularly numerous and are called the 'upper lumbar clump'.

On an AP view, the distance between the lateral border of a vertebral body and the most lateral lymph node should not be greater than 2 cm. On a lateral view the distance between the anterior border of T12–L2 vertebrae and the lymph nodes or cisterna chyli should be less than 3 cm.

Lymphography is associated with a risk of respiratory compromise due to pulmonary contrast emboli. This procedure is contraindicated in patients with poor respiratory reserve but can be undertaken in patients with moderate dyspnoea if less contrast is used. In these cases only the right foot is cannulated because of the greater incidence, as described above, of right to left crossover of lymphatics.

Magnetic resonance imaging

As with CT, abnormal lymph nodes are defined in terms of size rather than internal architecture. Spatial resolution is less than CT but greater contrast resolution allows differentiation from nearby vessels, bowel loops and other retroperitoneal structures.

THE PERITONEAL SPACES OF THE ABDOMEN (Figs 5.43 and 5.44)

The normal peritoneum cannot be seen by any imaging modality. It is important, however, because its anatomy determines the pathways and sites of collections of intraperitoneal fluid, blood and pus.

The peritoneal cavity is described as having a greater sac, the main cavity of the abdomen, and a lesser sac (or omental bursa), a diverticulum of this behind the stomach. The posterior wall of the *lesser sac* is formed by the peritoneum over the pancreas and the left adrenal and upper pole of the left kidney; whereas its anterior wall is formed by the peritoneum over the posterior wall of the stomach and the lesser omentum. It is limited laterally by the spleen and its attached gastrosplenic and lienorenal ligaments. The lesser sac is partially divided by the fold of peritoneum over the left gastric artery, the pancreato-gastric fold.

Medially the lesser sac communicates with the general cavity of the peritoneum via the *epiploic foramen (of Winslow)*. The boundaries of the epiploic foramen are:

Fig. 5.43 Peritoneal attachments to the posterior abdominal wall showing the peritoneal spaces.

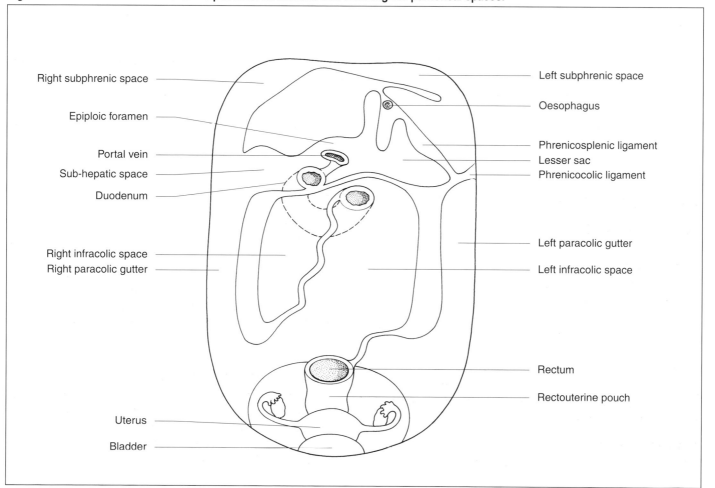

Right subphrenic space

Epiploic foramen

Portal vein

Sub-hepatic space

Duodenum

Right infracolic space

Right paracolic gutter

Uterus

Bladder

Left subphrenic space

Oesophagus

Phrenicosplenic ligament

Lesser sac

Phrenicocolic ligament

Left paracolic gutter

Left infracolic space

Rectum

Rectouterine pouch

Fig. 5.44 Sagittal view of the peritoneal spaces.

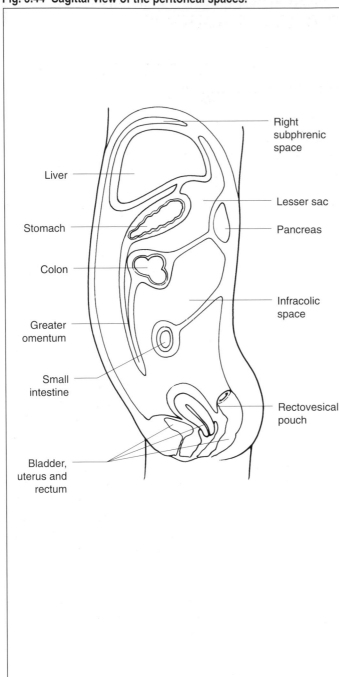

- Posteriorly: the IVC;
- Anteriorly: the free edge of the lesser omentum containing;
  — The portal vein
  — The hepatic artery and the common bile duct;
- Superiorly: the caudate process of the liver; and
- Inferiorly: the first part of the duodenum.

The *peritoneum over the liver* (see **Fig. 5.21b**) is continuous with that on the abdominal surface of the diaphragm except for a bare area posterosuperiorly. The peritoneal reflections that form the boundaries of the bare area are called ligaments:

- The left triangular ligament on the left; and
- The superior and inferior coronary ligaments on the right, with the right triangular ligament where these meet laterally.

These peritoneal reflections form the boundaries of the subphrenic and subhepatic spaces that are common sites of intraperitoneal collections.

The *subphrenic space* lies anterosuperiorly between the diaphragm and the liver. It is incompletely divided by the falciform ligament. The *subhepatic space* lies posteroinferiorly between the liver and the abdominal viscera. It communicates anteriorly (see **Fig. 5.44**) and laterally with the subphrenic space, and laterally with the right paracolic gutter. The posterior part of the subhepatic space between the liver and the kidney is called the hepatorenal pouch (Morrison's pouch). This is the deepest point of the abdominal cavity in a supine patient and is therefore a common site of collection of pus.

On the *left side,* the subphrenic space lies between the left lobe of the liver and the fundus of the stomach and the spleen. It is partially separated from the left paracolic gutter by a fold of peritoneum called the phrenicocolic ligament.

The stomach is suspended from the liver by two layers of peritoneum called the lesser omentum, which separate to enclose the stomach and are continued at the greater curve as the greater omentum. This turns back on itself to the transverse colon and its layers are fused to form an apron, which hangs from the stomach and the transverse colon over the loops of small intestine.

Below the mesocolon (the mesentery of the transverse colon) the *infracolic space* is divided into right and left parts by the root of the mesentery. *Right and left paracolic spaces (gutters)* are found lateral to the ascending and descending colon. The infracolic and paracolic spaces are continuous with the rectovesical and rectouterine pouches of the pelvis.

RADIOLOGICAL FEATURES OF THE PERITONEAL SPACES

Plain films of the abdomen
The peritoneum is not visible in the normal abdomen but in pneumoperitoneum gas may outline the subphrenic space, the falciform ligament, the umbilical ligaments (see section on the abdominal wall) or the lesser sac.

Ultrasound
This is a good method of visualization of fluid collections in the right subphrenic and subhepatic spaces. The left subphrenic space between the left lobe of the liver or the spleen and the diaphragm can also be visualized. Gas in the stomach may obscure part of this space. Pelvic ultrasound or transrectal or transvaginal ultrasound may show fluid collections in the pelvic part of the peritoneal cavity.

Gas in the stomach may obscure the lesser sac. Bowel gas obscures the remainder of the peritoneal cavity.

Computed tomography
The subphrenic and subhepatic spaces are well seen if they contain fluid or gas. Collections in the hepatorenal space can be distinguished from other peri- and pararenal collections. The lesser sac and its limits can also be seen. The inframesocolic spaces are difficult to evaluate, especially if the contrast filling of bowel loops is less than optimal because of the variable nature of intestinal loops on serial scanning.

CROSS-SECTIONAL ANATOMY OF THE UPPER ABDOMEN

AXIAL SECTION AT LEVEL OF T10 (Fig. 5.45; see Fig. 5. 10)

Body wall
The ribs and intercostal muscles are sectioned obliquely around most of the perimeter of the section. Anteriorly the costal cartilages forming the costal margin are separated by the two rectus abdominus muscles and the midline linea alba between. Superficial to the ribs and intercostal muscles lie the serratus anterior muscles laterally and the latissimus dorsi muscles postero-laterally. The erector spinae muscles lie posterior to the vertebra on each side.

The diaphragm
The domes of the diaphragm can be distinguished from the liver and other intra-abdominal viscera only where these are separated by fat. The crura are visible anterior to the vertebral bodies. With the adjoining diaphragm these form linear structures extending from the posterior aspect of the liver and spleen to the anterior surface of the abdominal aorta. The *retrocrural space* so formed is the lowest recess of the mediastinum. In addition to the aorta it contains the azygous vein on the right side and the hemiazygous vein on the left side, the thoracic duct on the right posterior to the aorta (not usually visible on CT scans unless dilated), lymph nodes and fat. The IVC remains on the abdominal side, that is, lateral to the crura below T8 level, where it pierces the diaphragm.

Liver
The liver occupies most of the right half of this section. Its anatomical right and left lobes are separated by the attachment of the falciform ligament on the anterior surface and by the fissure for the ligamentum venosum on

the visceral surface. Although above the porta hepatis, some branches of the portal veins and bile ducts may be seen at this level.

Spleen

Lying posteriorly on the left, close to the diaphragm and the ribs, the spleen has a smooth diaphragmatic surface and a concave visceral surface in axial section.

Other viscera

The antrum of the stomach lies deep to the left lobe of the liver. The hepatic flexure of the colon lies between these. The splenic flexure is found anterior to the spleen. Jejunal loops, variable in size and position, occupy most of the remaining cross-sectional area at this level.

AXIAL SECTION AT THE LEVEL OF T11 (see **Fig. 5.11**)

Body wall

This is as for the T10 level. The gap between the costal margins becomes progressively wider in lower cuts.

Diaphragm

As for T10 level. Usually only the crura and adjacent diaphragm are visible.

Liver

Anatomical right and left lobes are distinguished on the visceral surface by the fissure for the ligamentum teres between the inferior border of the liver and the porta hepatis and by the fissure for the ligamentum venosum between this and the IVC at the diaphragm.

On this section, a line dividing the liver that passes through the gall bladder and the IVC defines the morphological right and left lobes. That part of the anatomical right lobe left of this line and anterior to the porta is the quadrate lobe and that part posterior to the porta is the caudate lobe.

At the porta hepatis, the portal veins lie posteriorly with the branches of the hepatic artery and of the bile ducts anteriorly.

Adrenal glands

The right adrenal gland is a linear structure directly behind the IVC between the crura and the liver. The left adrenal gland extends deeper in front of the left kidney than does the right. Nearby splenic vessels may be confused with an adrenal abnormality.

Spleen

This section may pass through the splenic hilum. Vessels are seen dividing into branches just medial to the spleen. The splenic vein passes from the spleen posterior to the pancreas and is often visible throughout its length on one or two sections. The splenic artery has a tortuous course and only short segments are visible on axial sections.

Fig. 5.45 Axial section at level T10.

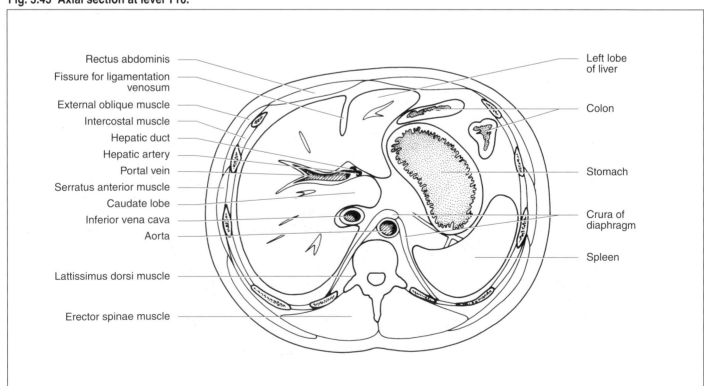

Other viscera

The aorta lies in the retrocrural space and its coeliac branch may be seen at this level. The IVC lies close to the liver as above.

The gastric antrum, jejunum and colon are seen as on the higher section.

AXIAL SECTION AT THE LEVEL OF T12 (see **Fig. 5.2**)

Body wall

The ribs and intercostal muscles are seen as before. The latissimus dorsi is more lateral in position than before and the serratus anterior muscle is seen interdigitating with the external oblique muscle. The internal oblique muscle is seen arising from the deep aspect of the ribs.

Liver

The left lobe of the liver is smaller or not seen at this level. The gall bladder is still visible below the porta hepatis.

Pancreas

The tail and body lie higher than the head of the pancreas. The tail of the gland is related to the splenic hilum.

The body of the pancreas is seen anterior to the splenic vein and the aorta.

Other viscera

The adrenal glands are still visible on this section. The upper pole of the left kidney (higher than that of the right) is visible.

The first part of the duodenum lies superior to the pancreatic head. The ascending and descending colon are seen, as are the jejunal loops.

The lower pole of the spleen lies behind the colon and the left kidney.

AXIAL SECTION AT THE LEVEL OF L1 (**Fig. 5.46**; see **Fig. 5.3**)

Body wall

The abdominal wall proper is now visible with the recti on each side of the linea alba and the three muscle layers of the abdominal wall — the internal and external oblique and transversus abdominis muscles — between the recti and the lower ribs.

Liver

The lowermost part of the right lobe lies posteriorly on this section

Fig. 5.46 Axial section at level L1.

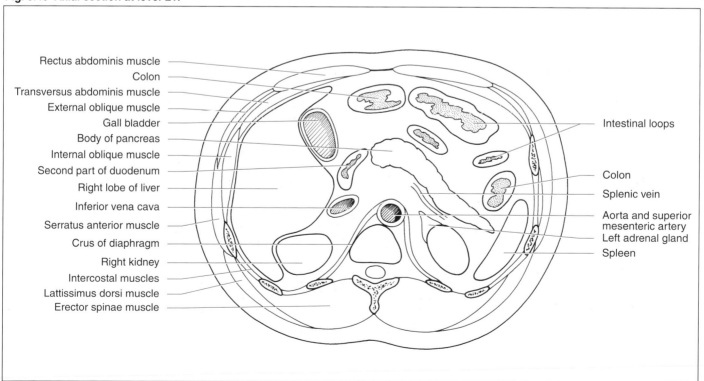

Rectus abdominis muscle
Colon
Transversus abdominis muscle
External oblique muscle
Gall bladder
Body of pancreas
Internal oblique muscle
Second part of duodenum
Right lobe of liver
Inferior vena cava
Serratus anterior muscle
Crus of diaphragm
Right kidney
Intercostal muscles
Lattissimus dorsi muscle
Erector spinae muscle

Intestinal loops

Colon
Splenic vein

Aorta and superior mesenteric artery
Left adrenal gland
Spleen

The aorta and the inferior vena cava

The aorta remains between the crura. Its superior mesenteric branch is visible at this level. The IVC is separated from the aorta by the crura and, at this level, is free from the liver.

Pancreas

The body of the pancreas lies anterior to the splenic vein at this level. In lower sections the head of the pancreas is seen to be separated from the uncinate process by the superior mesenteric vessels (the vein lies left of the artery).

Kidneys

Both kidneys are visible at this level.

Other viscera

The second part of the duodenum lies lateral to the pancreatic head. The loops of small intestine lie anterior to the pancreas. Vessels and fat are seen in its mesentery. Ascending and descending colon lie laterally on each side.

AXIAL SECTION AT THE LEVEL OF L2 (Fig. 5.47; see Fig. 5.4)

Body wall

The crura of the diaphragm are seen as muscular columns that are not connected to one another. The right crus is often bigger than the left (and extends further caudally).

The psoas muscle lies along the lateral aspect of the vertebral bodies and, although thin here, it increases in bulk in lower cuts. Other muscles are as described in previous sections.

Liver and spleen

The lowermost part of the right lobe of the liver is seen in this section; usually the spleen does not extend to this level.

Kidneys and renal vessels

This section includes one or both renal hila (the left hilum is slightly higher than the right). The left renal vein is seen passing to the IVC from the left hilum anterior to the aorta. The renal arteries pass between the veins and the renal pelvices, which are most posterior of all.

Renal medullary pyramids can be demonstrated in their full length at the level of the hilum, whereas they are intersected at various planes to their long axis above and below this because of their orientation towards the hilum.

The duodenum

The third part of the duodenum is seen passing between the aorta and the superior mesenteric artery.

The colon and jejunum

The transverse colon is seen close to the anterior abdominal wall with the ascending and descending colon laterally. Loops of jejunum and their mesentery occupy most of the anterior part of this section.

Fig. 5.47 Axial section at level of L2.

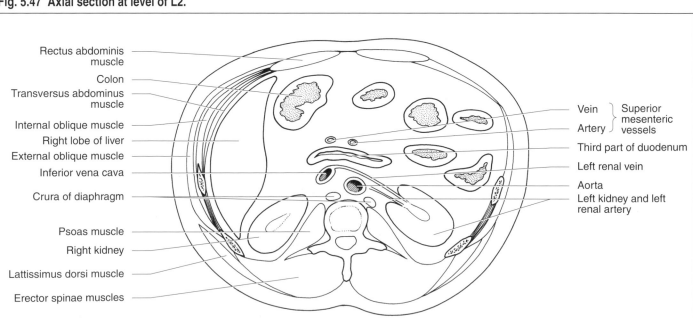

CHAPTER 6 *THE PELVIS*

The bony pelvis, muscles and ligaments

The pelvic floor

The sigmoid colon, rectum and anal canal

The blood vessels, lymphatics and nerves

The lower urinary tract

The male reproductive organs

The female reproductive organs

Cross-sectional anatomy

THE BONY PELVIS, MUSCLES AND LIGAMENTS (Figs 6.1–6.6)

The pelvis (**Fig. 6.1**) is a bony ring comprised of paired *innominate bones*, the *sacrum* and *coccyx*. The innominate bones articulate with each other anteriorly and with the sacrum posteriorly. Each innominate bone is composed of three parts, which fuse at the acetabulum.

The *ilium* is a flat curved bone and bears the *iliac crest* superiorly. The *anterior* and *posterior superior iliac spines* are on either end of the iliac crest, with the anterior and posterior inferior iliac spines below these. The inner surface of the bone is smooth and has the *iliopectineal line* running from front to back, demarcating the true from the false pelvis.

The *pubic bone* consists of a *body*, and *inferior and superior rami*. The body of the pubic bone articulates with its fellow at the *symphysis pubis*. It bears a tubercle on its superolateral aspect. The articular surfaces of the symphysis pubis are covered in hyaline cartilage with a fibrocartilaginous disc between them. The pubic bone is strengthened on all sides by dense ligaments.

The *ischium* is composed of a body and an inferior ramus, which joins the inferior pubic ramus. The body bears a tuberosity inferiorly and a spine posteriorly. The *ischial spine* defines the greater and lesser sciatic notches above and below.

The *obturator foramen* is bounded by the body and rami of the pubic bone and the body and ramus of the ischial bone.

The sacrum

Five fused vertebrae comprise this triangular bone, which is curved posteriorly. The anterior part of its upper end is termed the sacral promontary. It articulates with the lumbar spine superiorly and with the coccyx inferiorly. Anteriorly the sacrum has four pairs of sacral foramina, which transmit nerves from the sacral canal. Lateral to these are the lateral masses or alae of the sacrum. The sacrum also bears four pairs of posterior sacral foramina and the canal ends posteriorly in the sacral hiatus — a midline opening that transmits the fifth sacral nerve.

The coccyx

This is composed of three to five fused vertebrae. The first segment is often separate. It articulates at an acute angle with the sacrum.

The sacroiliac joints

The sacroiliac joints are covered with cartilage and lined

Fig. 6.1 Bony pelvis.

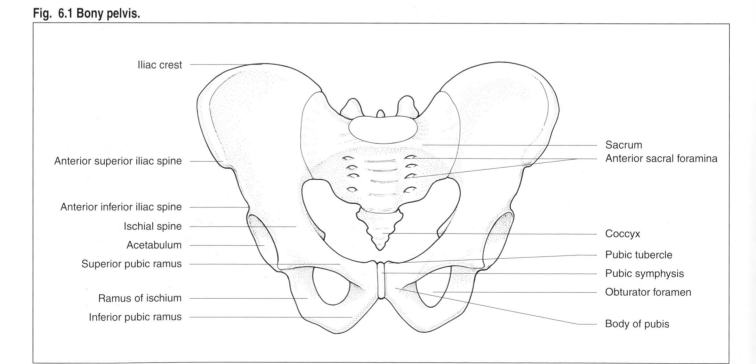

Iliac crest

Anterior superior iliac spine

Anterior inferior iliac spine

Ischial spine

Acetabulum

Superior pubic ramus

Ramus of ischium

Inferior pubic ramus

Sacrum
Anterior sacral foramina

Coccyx

Pubic tubercle

Pubic symphysis

Obturator foramen

Body of pubis

with synovium. The joint surface is flat and uneven and this irregularity helps lock the sacrum into the iliac bones. Ligaments support the front and back of the joint. The dense interosseous *sacroiliac ligaments* unite the bones above and behind the joint.

The *sacrotuberous ligament* runs from the ischial tuberosity to the sides of the sacrum and coccyx. It defines the posterior limit of the *lesser sciatic foramen.*

The *sacrospinous ligament* runs from the ischial spine to the sides of the sacrum and coccyx. It defines the posterior limit of the *greater sciatic foramen.*

The *iliolumbar ligament* runs from the transverse process of L5 to the posterior part of the iliac crest, further stabilizing the joint.

The pelvic muscles are shown in **Fig. 6.2.** At the level of the iliac crest the paired *psoas muscles* lie on either side of the spine. They descend anteriorly, fusing with the *iliacus muscle,* which arises from the inner surface of the ilium. The fused *iliopsoas muscle* passes anteriorly under the inguinal ligament to insert into the lesser trochanter of the femur.

The *piriformis muscles* pass obliquely from the anterior aspect of the sacrum through the greater sciatic foramen behind the acetabulum to insert into the greater trochanter of the femur.

The *obturator membrane* closes the obturator foramen. The *obturator internus muscle* arises from the anterior and lateral walls of the pelvis covering the obturator foramen. Its fibres converge towards the lesser sciatic foramen as it hooks around the posterior part of the ischium between its tuberosity and spine. It passes through the lesser sciatic foramen to insert into the greater trochanter of the femur.

The aponeurosis of the abdominal wall muscles inserts into the superior surface of the pubic bone. A thickening of the aponeurosis is the *inguinal ligament,* which runs from the pubic tubercle to the anterior superior iliac spine. All the muscles of the anterior, lateral and posterior abdominal walls insert, to some degree, into the iliac crest, inguinal ligament and pubic bone.

The gluteal muscles arise from the external surface of the iliac bone and the iliac crest and insert into the upper femur. *Gluteus maximus* is the largest, the most superficial and the most posterior gluteal muscle, covering the posterior part of the ilium and the sacroiliac joints. *Gluteus medius* and *minimus* are more anteriorly placed, gluteus minimus being the smallest and the most deeply placed.

Fig.6.2 Pelvic muscles: (a) coronal section; (b) viewed from inside the pelvis.

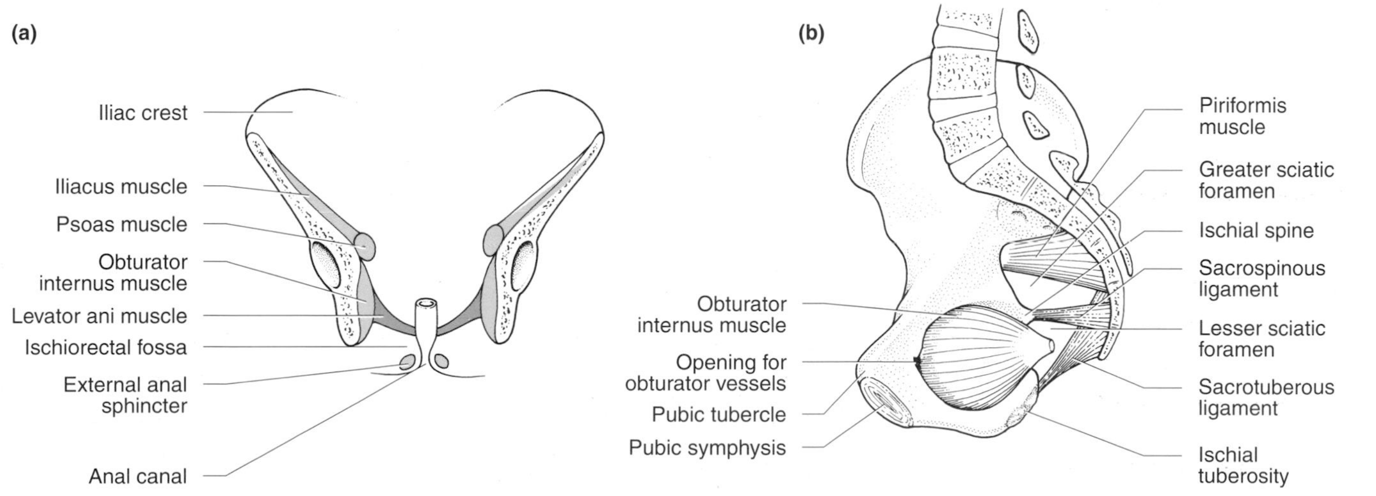

RADIOLOGY OF THE PELVIC RING

Plain films

The bony landmarks may be identified on the plain radiograph (**Fig. 6.3**). The sacral promontary and superior part of the pubic bone define the pelvic inlet and separate the true pelvis below from the false pelvis above. The sacroiliac joints are not optimally seen on the frontal view due to their obliquity. Special views may be performed so that the X-ray beam passes through the joint to demonstrate it clearly.

Some variations of the lower lumbar spine and sacrum occur. The first sacral segment may be partially or completely separate — so-called lumbarization of the sacrum.

Fig. 6.3 AP radiograph of male pelvis.

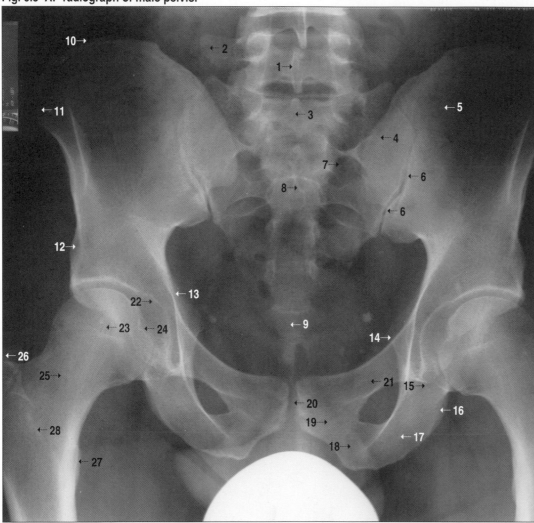

1. Spinous process of L5 vertebra
2. Transverse process of L5 vertebra
3. Spinous process of first sacral segment
4. Lateral sacral mass
5. Ilium
6. Sacroiliac joint
7. Sacral foramen of S2 vertebra
8. Spinous process of S3 vertebra
9. Coccyx: first segment of three
10. Iliac crest
11. Anterior superior iliac spine
12. Anterior inferior iliac spine
13. Pelvic brim
14. Ischial spine
15. Body of ischium
16. Ischial tuberosity
17. Ramus of ischium
18. Inferior pubic ramus
19. Body of pubic bone
20. Pubic symphysis
21. Superior pubic ramus
22. Acetabulum
23. Head of femur
24. Fovea
25. Neck of femur
26. Greater trochanter of femur
27. Lesser trochanter of femur
28. Intertrochanteric femur

Similarly, the lowest lumber vertebra may be partially or completely fused to the sacrum — known as sacralization of the lumbar spine. The posterior elements of the lower lumbar vertebra or the sacral vertebrae may not be fused in some people, with no apparent sequelae.

The male and female pelvises have several differences. The muscle attachments are more prominent in the male. The pelvic inlet is heart-shaped in the male and oval in the female. The angle between the inferior pubic rami is narrow in the male and wide in the female.

Cross-sectional imaging

The muscles of the pelvis may be seen on CT and MR images (**Fig. 6.4**; see **Figs 6.2** and **6.7**). The ability of MRI to yield sagittal and coronal views of the pelvis gives a

Fig. 6.4 CT scan of pelvis: axial section through male bladder. Rectal and intravenous contrast have been given. The full bladder displaces small bowel loops superiorly.

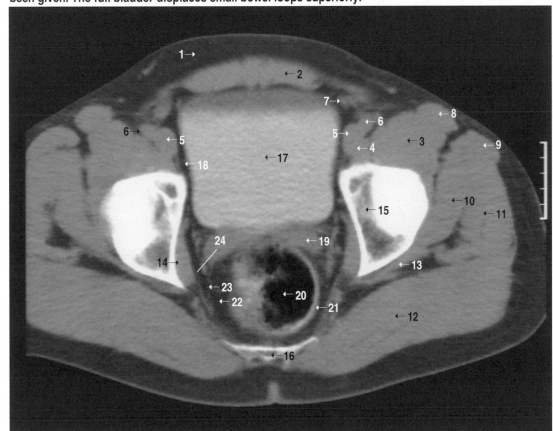

1. Subcutaneous fat
2. Rectus abdominis muscle
3. Iliacus muscle
4. Psoas muscle and tendon
5. External iliac vein
6. External iliac artery
7. Inferior epigastric vessels
8. Sartorius muscle
9. Tensor fascia lata muscle
10. Gluteus minimus muscle
11. Gluteus medius muscle
12. Gluteus maximus muscle
13. Piriformis muscle
14. Obturator internus muscle
15. Acetabulum
16. Lower sacral segment: S4 vertebra
17. Bladder: full of layering urine and contrast
18. Perivesical fat
19. Seminal vesicle
20. Rectum containing air, faeces and contrast medium
21. Wall of rectum
22. Perirectal (mesorectal) fat
23. Perirectal fascia (known as Denonvillier's fascia anteriorly)
24. Pararectal fat

clear appreciation of the anatomy of the pelvic floor. CT is an excellent way to image the sacroiliac joints. High-resolution scans taking narrow slices parallel to the long axis of the joint, or axially, give very good bony detail.

THE PELVIC FLOOR (Figs 6.5–6.7)

A sling of muscles closes the floor of the pelvis. The urethra and rectum and the vagina in the female pierce the pelvic floor. The floor is composed of two muscular layers — the levator ani/coccygeus complex and the perineum.

The *levator ani* muscle is the principal support of the pelvic floor. It arises from the posterior aspect of the pubis, the fascia covering the obturator internus muscle on the inner wall of the ilium and the ischial spine. Its fibres sweep posteriorly, inserting into the *perineal body* (a fibromuscular node behind the urethra in males or urethra and vagina in females), the *anococcygeal body* (a fibromuscular node between the anus and coccyx) and the coccyx. The fibres of levator ani sling around the prostate gland or vagina and rectum, blending with the *external anal sphincter*. The components of levator ani are named according to their attachments — *puborectalis, pubococcygeus* and *iliococcygeus*. Levator

Fig. 6.5 MR scan of pelvis: coronal section. This coronal scan is taken through the posterior part of the prostate gland and seminal vesicles. The anterior part of rectum, bulging forward over the prostate gland between the seminal vesicles, is also included.

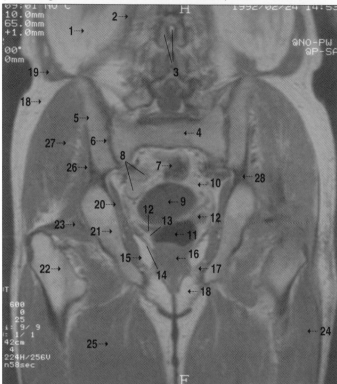

ani provides muscular support for the pelvic organs and reinforces the urethral and rectal sphincters. The coccygeus muscle is in the same tissue plane as levator ani. It arises from the ischial spine and sacrotuberous ligament and inserts into the side of the coccyx and lower sacrum. It aids levator ani in supporting the pelvic organs.

The perineum is the diamond-shaped space between the pubis, ischial tuberosities and coccyx. It is divided into two compartments by the transverse perineal muscles, which arise from the ischial tuberosity and run medially to insert into the perineal body.

The anterior compartment is the *anterior urogenital triangle.* The anterior urogenital triangle contains a tough

1. Perirenal fat cone, below lower pole of kidney
2. Medial aspect of psoas muscle
3. Posterior elements of L3 vertebra
4. Body of sacrum
5. Ilium
6. Sacroiliac joint
7. Sigmoid colon
8. Small bowel loops
9. Bladder
10. Perivesical fat
11. Anterior part of rectum
12. Seminal vesicle
13. Fat above levator ani muscle
14. Levator ani muscle
15. Fat in ischiorectal fossa
16. Posterior part of prostate gland
17. Perineum (urogenital diaphragm)
18. Subcutaneous fat
19. Muscles of abdominal wall
20. Obturator internus muscle
21. Ischium
22. Intertrochanteric part of femur
23. Piriformis muscle
24. Vastus muscles
25. 'Hamstring' (posterior femoral) muscles
26. Gluteus minimis muscle
27. Gluteus medius muscle
28. Upper part of greater sciatic foramen

Fig. 6.6 CT scan of pelvis: axial section through male perineum.

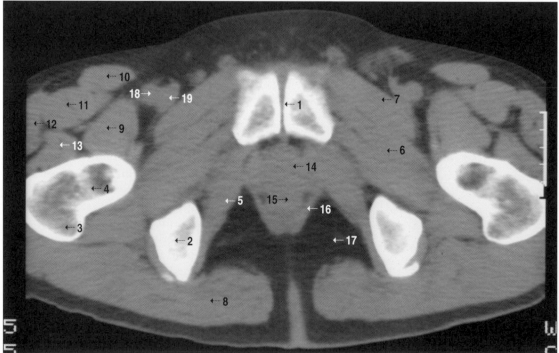

1. Symphysis pubis
2. Ischium
3. Femur: greater tuberosity
4. Femur: neck
5. Obturator internus
6. Obturator externus
7. Pectineus muscle
8. Gluteus maximus muscle
9. Iliacus muscle
10. Sartorius muscle
11. Retus femoris muscle
12. Tensor fascia lata muscle
13. Vastus lateralis muscle
14. Prostate gland
15. Anorectal junction
16. Levator ani muscle (lowermost fibres: pubococcygeus)
17. Fat in ischiorectal fossa
18. Common femoral artery
19. Common femoral vein

sheet of fascia — the perineal membrane — which is pierced by the urethra and also the vagina in females. The external urethral sphincter is reinforced by this layer. Its *inferior surface* gives attachment to the bulb and crura of the penis or clitoris (*bulbocavernosus* and *ischiocavernosus*).

The posterior compartment is the *anal triangle*. It contains the anus and its sphincters with the *ischiorectal fossa* on either side. The ischiorectal fossa is the space below and lateral to the posterior part of levator ani and medial to the inner wall of the pelvis (**Fig. 6.2a**). It is bounded posteriorly by sacrotuberous ligaments and the gluteus maximus muscle, laterally by the fascia of the obturator internus muscle and anteriorly by the perineal body. It is largely full of fat. It is of importance in pathological conditions of the rectum. The anococcygeal body extends from the anus to the coccyx posteriorly. It receives fibres from the anal sphincter and levator ani muscles.

RADIOLOGY OF THE PELVIC FLOOR
Magnetic resonance imaging
The muscles of the pelvic floor are elegantly demonstrated by sagittal and coronal sections using MRI (see **Figs 6.5, 6.15** and **6.20**). The low-signal intensity of the muscles contrasts with the high-signal intensity of the pelvic fat. No other imaging modality approaches MRI for demonstration of the pelvic floor anatomy. The bones have a low-intensity cortex with a high-intensity marrow cavity. The pubic symphysis is of intermediate signal intensity.

Computed tomography
Axial CT scanning may also demonstrate the muscles of the pelvic floor (see **Fig. 6.6**).

Fig. 6.7 Male pelvis: (a) sagittal section showing pelvic floor and urethra; (b) coronal section showing the pelvic floor (courtesy of Prof. JB Coakley).

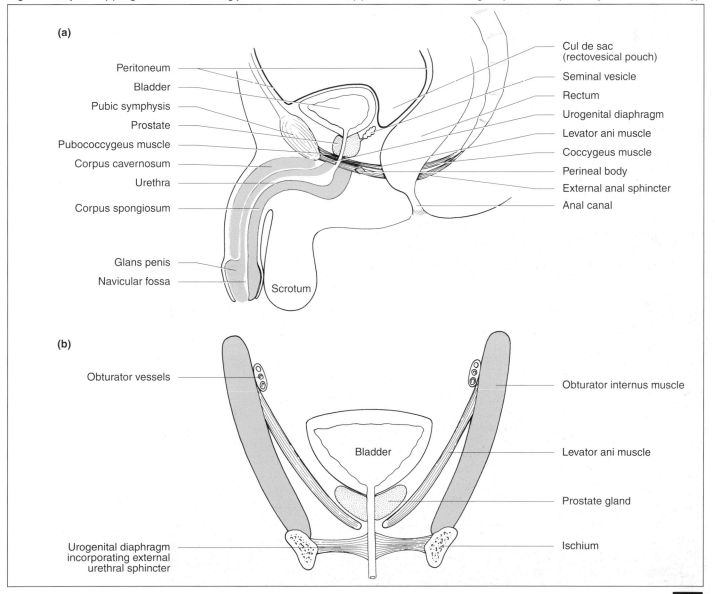

THE SIGMOID COLON, RECTUM AND ANAL CANAL (Fig. 6.8; see Fig. 5.20)

THE SIGMOID COLON

The sigmoid colon is variable in length (12–75 cm, average 40 cm). It is covered by a double layer of peritoneum, supported on its own mesentery, which is attached to the posterior and left lateral pelvic wall. It has the same sacculated pattern as the rest of the colon in young people. It may appear featureless in older subjects. The redundant sigmoid lies on the other pelvic structures.

Blood supply (see Fig. 5.20)

The arterial supply is from the inferior mesenteric artery via the sigmoid arteries, which join in the arterial cascade of the large bowel. Venous drainage is to the portal system via the inferior mesenteric vein.

.Fig. 6.8 Rectum: (a) anterior view and blood supply; (b) lateral view showing peritoneal reflections. (Courtesy of Prof. JB Coakley.)

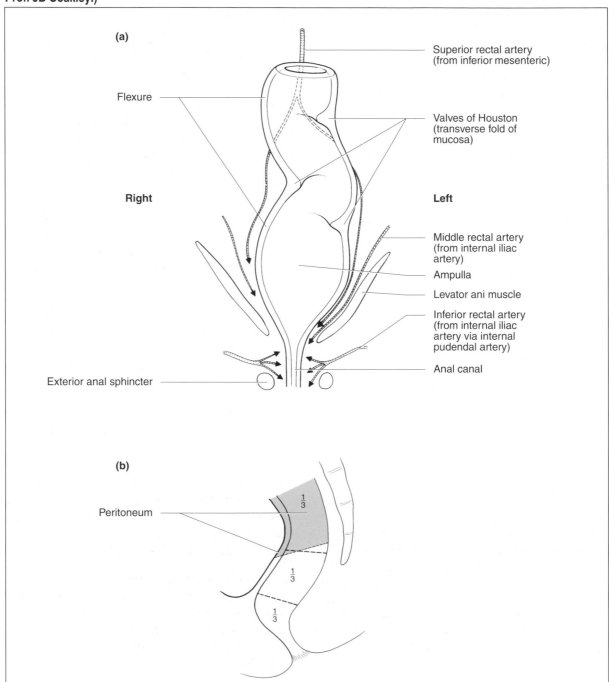

Lymph drainage

This is via the blood supply to preaortic nodes around the origin of the inferior mesenteric artery.

THE RECTUM

This is about 12 cm long. It commences anterior to S3 and ends in the anal canal 2–3 cm in front of the tip of the coccyx. It forms an anteroposterior curve in the hollow of the sacrum. The rectum has no sacculations or mesentery. Its upper third is covered by peritoneum on its front and sides; its middle third has peritoneum on its anterior surface only, while its lower third has no peritoneum. The lower part of the rectum is dilated into the rectal ampulla. The mucosa of the rectum has three to four longitudinal mucosal folds in the resting state — known as the *columns of Morgagni*. The taenia coli fuse in the rectum. Some longitudinal shortening of the rectum occurs, giving the rectum a slight 'S' shape. This creates three lateral mucosal folds — left, right and left from above downward. These are known as the *valves of Houston.*

Posteriorly are the sacrum and coccyx. Anteriorly, loops of small bowel and sigmoid colon lie in the peritoneal cul-de-sac between upper two-thirds of rectum and bladder or uterus. The lower third is related to the vagina in the female and to the seminal vesicles, prostate and bladder base in the male.

The rectum is surrounded by *perirectal fat*. Fascia known as the *perirectal fascia* surrounds the perirectal fat, and lateral to the perirectal fascia is the *pararectal fat*. The perirectal fascia separates the seminal vesicles and prostate from the rectum anteriorly.

THE ANAL CANAL

This is directed posteriorly almost at right angles to the rectum. It is a narrow, muscular canal. It has an internal sphincter of involuntary muscle and an outer external sphincter of voluntary muscle, which blends with levator ani. Anteriorly, the perineal body separates it from the vagina in the female and the bulb of the urethra in the male. Posteriorly, the anococcygeal body is between it and the coccyx, and laterally is the ischiorectal fossa.

Blood supply (see Fig. 5.20)

The superior, middle and inferior rectal (haemorrhoidal) arteries form a rich submucous plexus supplying the rectum and anal canal. The superior rectal artery is a branch of the inferior mesenteric artery. The middle and inferior arteries arise from the internal iliac artery. The plexus drains via a superior rectal vein to the inferior mesenteric vein and via middle and inferior veins to the internal iliac vein. This represents a communication between systemic and portal systems.

Lymph drainage

The rectum and upper anal canal drain to pararectal nodes, and from here to preaortic nodes around the inferior mesenteric artery and to internal iliac nodes. The lower anal canal drains to superficial inguinal nodes.

RADIOLOGY OF THE SIGMOID AND RECTUM

Plain films (see Fig. 5.1)

The sigmoid colon and rectum may be identified on plain radiographs outlined by air, faeces, or both. The sigmoid colon has a characteristic 'S'-shaped curve as it joins the descending colon to the rectum, which lies anterior to the sacrum.

Barium enema (see Fig. 5.18)

This is the main radiological examination used to assess these structures. The best detail is attained by the double-contrast technique, that is, the use of a small amount of barium to coat the mucosa and sufficient air or gas to distend the bowel. The valves of Houston are the lateral mucosal folds of the rectum and are usually less than 5 mm thick. The longitudinal columns of Morgagni are best identified after evacuation of barium when the rectum is not distended. These measure 3 mm in width. On the lateral view, the postrectal space is measured between the posterior wall of the rectum and the anterior part of the sacrum at the level of S4. This measurement should not exceed 1 cm. The posterior impression of the pubococcygeal fibres of levator ani may be identified at the lower limit of the rectum. The anal canal may be identified if outlined with barium paste; it makes an acute, posteriorly directed, angle with the rectum.

Computed tomography

The rectum and perirectal tissues are readily assessed by CT. Visualization of the rectum on CT may be improved by the administration of dilute rectal contrast (see **Figs 6.4** and **6.23**). CT is usually performed to assess the rectum in neoplastic or inflammatory processes, where it also important to image the surrounding soft tissues and bone. The rectal wall, perirectal fat and fascia and pararectal fat may be identified.

Magnetic resonance imaging

More recently, MRI is being used to image the sigmoid colon and rectum. The ability to obtain coronal and sagittal images in addition to axial scans is a great advantage, particularly to assess tumour spread (see **Figs 6.5, 6.15** and **6.20**).

BLOOD VESSELS, LYMPHATICS AND NERVES OF THE PELVIS

OVERVIEW OF THE ARTERIES AND VEINS

The aorta bifurcates at the level of L4/L5 slightly to the left of midline. At the level of the iliac crest, the common iliac arteries are slightly anterior to the common iliac veins. Both vessels are located on the medial border of the psoas muscle as this passes anteriorly into the pelvis. The vessels pass behind the distal ureters. At the level of the pelvic inlet, the internal iliac vessels run medially and posteriorly towards the sciatic notch, while the external iliac vessels continue down on the medial aspect of iliopsoas muscle, passing under the inguinal ligament to enter the thigh.

INTERNAL ILIAC ARTERY (Fig. 6.9; see Fig. 6.10)

This artery arises in front of the sacroiliac joint at the level of L5/S1 or the pelvic inlet. It descends to the sciatic foramen and divides into an anterior trunk, which continues down towards the ischial spine and a posterior trunk, which passes back towards the foramen. Anterior to the internal iliac artery are the distal ureters and the ovary and fallopian tube in the female. The internal iliac vein is posterior and the external iliac vein and psoas muscle are lateral. Peritoneum separates its medial aspect from loops of bowel.

Branches of the anterior trunk

These are as follows:

- Superior vesical artery — this runs medially to supply the upper part of bladder;
- Inferior vesical artery — this supplies lower bladder and ureter, prostate and seminal vesicles;
- Middle rectal artery — this usually arises with the inferior vesical artery and it supplies the rectum with branches to prostate and seminal vesicles;
- Uterine artery — this runs medially and ascends tortuously in the broad ligament. It supplies the uterus, cervix, and tubes with branches to the ovary and vagina;
- Vaginal artery — this corresponds to the inferior vesicle in the male and anastomoses with the uterine artery;
- Obturator artery — this passes anteriorly through the obturator foramen and gives branches to muscle and bone;
- Internal pudendal artery — this curves around the ischial spine to pass through the lesser sciatic foramen. It supplies the external genitalia and gives off the inferior rectal artery; and
- Inferior gluteal artery — this passes through the greater sciatic foramen to supply the muscles of the buttock and thigh.

Fig. 6.9 Internal iliac artery and branches (diagrammatic view).

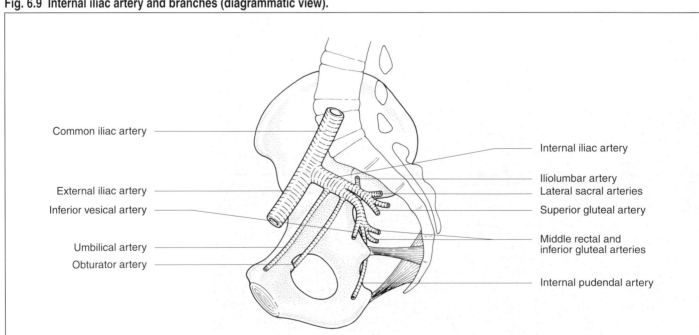

Common iliac artery

External iliac artery

Inferior vesical artery

Umbilical artery

Obturator artery

Internal iliac artery

Iliolumbar artery
Lateral sacral arteries

Superior gluteal artery

Middle rectal and inferior gluteal arteries

Internal pudendal artery

Branches of the posterior trunk

These are as follows:

- Iliolumbar artery — this ascends in front of the SI joint. It supplies psoas and iliacus muscles and gives a branch to the cauda equina;
- Lateral sacral arteries — usually two. These pass through anterior sacral foramina and exit through the posterior sacral foramina. They supply the contents of sacral canal and muscle and skin of the lower back; and
- Superior gluteal artery — a continuation of the posterior trunk. This passes through the greater sciatic foramen to supply the muscles of the pelvic wall and gluteal region.

Radiological point of interest

The umbilical artery is the first branch of the internal iliac artery in the fetus. It ascends on the inner surface of the anterior abdominal wall to the umbilicus and into the cord. It persists as a fibrous cord after birth — called the *medial umbilical ligament*. It may be identified if outlined by air on the plain radiograph as in pneumoperitoneum (see also Chapter 5).

EXTERNAL ILIAC ARTERY (Fig. 6.10)

This runs downwards and laterally on the medial border of the psoas muscle to a point midway between the ante-

Fig. 6.10 Aortogram: external and internal iliac arteries.

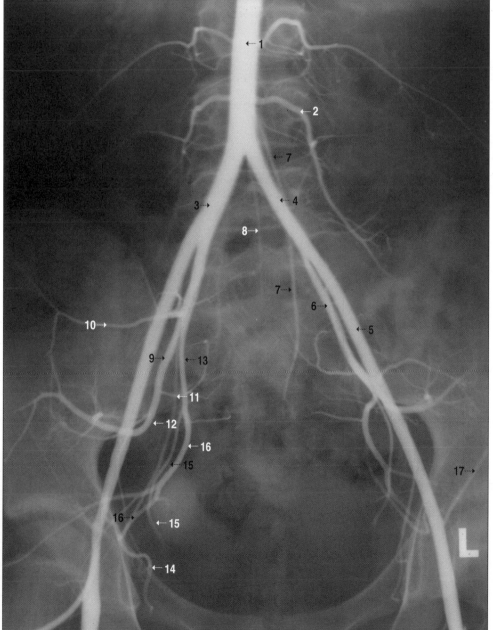

1. Abdominal aorta
2. Lumbar artery
3. Right common iliac artery
4. Left common iliac artery
5. Left external iliac artery
6. Left internal iliac artery
7. Inferior mesenteric artery
8. Median sacral artery
9. Posterior trunk of right internal iliac artery
10. Iliolumbar artery (branch of **9**)
11. Lateral sacral artery (branch of **9**)
12. Superior gluteal artery (branch of **9**)
13. Anterior trunk of right internal iliac artery
14. Obturator artery (branch of **13**)
15. Vesical artery (branch of **13**)
16. Inferior gluteal artery (branch of **13**)
17. Deep circumflex iliac artery

rior superior iliac spine and the pubic symphysis. At this point, it passes under the inguinal ligament to become the common femoral artery. In front of and medial to the vessel, peritoneum separates it from loops of bowel. Its origin may be crossed by the ureter. In the female it is crossed by the ovarian vessels. In the male it is crossed by the testicular vessels and the ductus deferens. The external iliac vein is posterior to its upper part and medial to its lower part.

Branches

Both branches arise just above the inguinal ligament and are as follows:

- Inferior epigastric artery — this runs superiorly on the posterior surface of anterior abdominal wall to enter the rectus sheath; and
- Deep circumflex iliac artery — this ascends laterally to the anterior superior iliac spine behind the inguinal ligament and passes back on the inner surface of the iliac crest, supplying the abdominal wall muscles.

THE ILIAC VEINS (see **Figs 6.4** and **6.23**)

The external and internal iliac veins accompany the arteries. They run medial to the arteries lower down. As the veins ascend, they become posterior to the arteries. The upper part of the left common iliac vein then passes to the right behind its artery to form the inferior vena cava by joining with its fellow behind and to the right of the aortic bifurcation. The tributaries of the iliac veins match the arterial branches.

RADIOLOGY OF THE ILIAC VESSELS (see **Fig. 6.10**)

Angiography

The iliac arteries are demonstrated by angiography. In most cases this is performed by injecting contrast medium under high pressure into the distal aorta via a pigtail catheter, which is inserted retrogradely through a common femoral artery. Images may be acquired using plain radiographs or using digital-subtraction angiography where information is acquired on an image intensifier and processed by computer. Digital-subtraction techniques may also demonstrate the arteries after a large dose of *intravenous* contrast, but detail is inferior.

Venography

The external iliac veins may be demonstrated by injection of intravenous contrast into leg veins. Contrast opacification of the internal iliac veins requires intraosseous injection of contrast, often into the bodies of the pubic bones.

This technique is rarely performed now since cross-sectional imaging may be used to assess the pelvic veins.

Computed tomography

CT during the administration of intravenous contrast gives excellent cross-sectional information about the vessels in the pelvis and their relationship to surrounding structures. The arteries have a round, even calibre, while the veins are relatively collapsed and more oval-shaped in the supine position.

Magnetic resonance imaging

MRI has some advantages over CT. Contrast is not required as flowing blood shows as a black signal void. The vessels may be imaged along in their own plane giving an equivalent image to an angiographic study.

Ultrasound

This may also identify the common and external iliac vessels, although visualization is somewhat dependent on unpredictable factors such as bowel gas and body habitus of the subject. The vessels are seen as anechoic linear structures. Colour doppler techniques demonstrate direction of blood flow and facilitate identification.

THE LYMPHATICS

Lymph drainage runs in lymphatic channels related to the blood vessels. Three chains accompany the external iliac vessels — one (antero)lateral to the artery, one (postero)medial to the vein and a variable middle chain anteriorly between the vessels. The obturator node is part of the middle chain. These chains drain to the common iliac and para-aortic nodes. The internal iliac lymph vessels and nodes drain to nodes around the common iliac and from here superiorly to para-aortic nodes. Sacral nodes drain to the internal chain.

RADIOLOGY OF THE LYMPHATICS

Lymphangiography

Although performed less often in recent times with the increasing use of CT, lymphangiography is the only radiological method available for direct demonstration of the lymphatics. A lipid-based contrast agent is injected slowly into a lymphatic vessel in either foot. The external iliac, obturator, common iliac and para-aortic nodes are demonstrated. The internal iliac nodes are not visualized using this method.

Cross-sectional imaging

CT and MRI may demonstrate the lymph nodes, particularly if enlarged.

IMPORTANT NERVES OF THE PELVIS

The *femoral*, *sciatic* and *obturator* nerves pass through the pelvis to supply the lower limb. They are formed by the union of various branches of the *lumbosacral plexus* of nerves. The obturator nerve descends medial to the psoas muscle, runs along the lateral pelvic wall and through the upper part of the obturator foramen into the thigh. It is posteromedial to the common iliac vein in the pelvis. The femoral nerve, surrounded by fat, descends between the psoas and iliacus muscles, passing under the inguinal ligament into the thigh. The sciatic nerve is the largest in the body. It is formed from the lumbosacral plexus on the anterior surface of the sacrum and piriformis. It passes through the greater sciatic foramen into the gluteal region. Nerves to the organs of the pelvis are derived from the lumbosacral plexus, which lies on the sacrum and piriformis muscle.

Fig. 6.11 Bladder: (a) lateral view (undistended); (b) posterior surface in male (the prostate gland has been removed). (Courtesy of Prof. JB Coakley.)

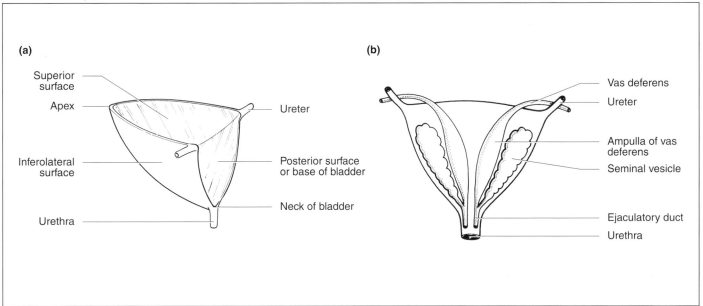

THE LOWER URINARY TRACT (Fig. 6.11; see Fig. 6.7)

THE PELVIC URETERS

The distal ureters enter the pelvis anterior to the psoas muscle. They pass anterior to the bifurcation of the iliac vessels and run on the lateral wall of the pelvis. Just in front of the ischial spine, they turn medially to enter the posterolateral aspect of the bladder. The distal ureter lies above the seminal vesicles in the male and is crossed by the vas deferens. The distal ureter passes above the lateral vaginal fornix in the female, lateral to the cervix and under the uterine vessels in the broad ligament. The intravesical ureter tunnels obliquely through the bladder wall. The bladder muscle exerts a sphincter-like action on the lower ureter.

THE BLADDER (see Fig. 6.11)

This is a pyramidal muscular organ when empty. It has a base posteriorly and an apex behind the pubic symphysis. It has one superior and two inferolateral walls. The ureters enter the posterolateral angles and the urethra leaves inferiorly at the narrow neck, which is surrounded by the (involuntary) internal urethral sphincter.

The urethra is separated from the pubic symphysis by the fatty space of Retzius, which contains a venous plexus as well as nerves and lymphatics. Perivesical fat surrounds the bladder. The obturator internus muscle is anterolateral and the levator ani muscle inferolateral to this. Superiorly it is loosely covered by peritoneum, which separates it from loops of small bowel and sigmoid colon.

In the female, the body of the uterus rests on its posterosuperior surface and the cervix and vagina are posterior, with the rectum behind. In the male, the termination of the vasa and seminal vesicles are between the posterior bladder and the rectum. In the female, the bladder neck rests on the pelvic fascia. In the male, it is fused with the prostate. The trigone is the triangular inner wall of the bladder between the ureteric and urethral orifices. This part of the wall is smooth, the remainder of the bladder wall is coarsely trabeculated by criss-cross muscle fibres.

The bladder is an extraperitoneal structure. As it fills it becomes ovoid and rises into the abdomen, stripping the loose peritoneum off the anterior abdominal wall. The peritoneum is loose over the bladder, except posteriorly. The bladder is relatively fixed inferiorly via condensations of pelvic fascia, which attach it to the back of the pubis, the lateral walls of the pelvis and the rectum. Its continuity with the prostate in the male makes it even more immobile at this point due to the strong pubo-prostatic ligaments.

Peritoneal reflections

In the female, the peritoneum is reflected from the superior surface of the bladder to the anterior surface of the uterus. This peritoneal fold is known as the 'pouch of Douglas'. The peritoneum is further reflected from the posterior part of the uterus to the rectum and this fold is known as the cul-de-sac. In the male, the peritoneum is reflected off the bladder to the rectum, forming the rectovesical pouch or cul-de-sac. These peritoneal pouches usually contain loops of bowel.

Blood supply of the bladder

The bladder is supplied via the internal iliac artery via superior and inferior vesical arteries. Venous drainage is via a venous plexus to the internal iliac vein.

Lymph drainage

This is along the blood vessels to internal iliac and thence to para-aortic nodes.

Applied anatomy

Bladder rupture may occur with fractures of the pelvis due to the rigid fixture of the bladder neck to the pelvis. Ruptures are usually extraperitoneal; however, intraperitoneal rupture may occur in blunt trauma to the abdomen when the bladder is full. The point of tear is usually at the junction of the loose and the fixed peritoneum at the posterior part of the bladder.

RADIOLOGY OF THE BLADDER

Plain films

The bladder may be identified on plain films, especially when full. It is seen as a round soft-tissue density surrounded by a lucent line of the perivesical fat. It should be smooth and symmetrical. The median umbilical ligament is a fibrous remnant of the urachus, which runs from the apex of the bladder to the umbilicus in the fetus. This may be seen outlined by air in pneumoperitoneum.

Contrast studies

The bladder may be filled with contrast either after intravenous injection in the intravenous urogram or retrogradely via the urethra. The corrugations of the bladder wall are seen. The smooth impression of the uterus may be seen posterosuperiorly. The prostatic impression is seen inferiorly in the male. Irregular collections of contrast may be trapped between muscle fibres after micturition.

Cross-sectional imaging

The bladder is readily identified by ultrasound, CT and MR — especially when distended. Ultrasound is best for assessing its internal anatomy. CT and MR imaging have the advantage of also being able to assess the surrounding structures.

THE MALE URETHRA (Fig. 6.12; see Fig. 6.13)

The male urethra may be divided into posterior and anterior parts. The posterior urethra comprises the prostatic and membranous urethra and the anterior part comprises the bulbous and penile urethra.

The prostatic urethra traverses the ventral part of the prostate and is the widest part. It is about 3 cm long. It has a longitudinal midline ridge known as the prostatic crest. Several prostatic ducts open into the prostatic sinus — a shallow longitudinal depression on either side of the prostatic crest. The prostatic crest bears a prominence called the verumontanum. A small blindly ending sinus opens onto this — the prostatic utricle. (This is thought to be the developmental male equivalent of the vagina). On either side of the prostatic utricle the ejaculatory ducts open. These are the common termination of the seminal vesicles and the vasa. The lower part of the prostatic urethra is immobile as it is fixed by the puboprostatic ligaments.

The membranous urethra is so called as it traverses the membranous urogenital diaphragm, which forms the (voluntary) external urethral sphincter. It is the narrowest part of the urethra and is about 2 cm long. The urethra is relatively immobile at this point.

The bulbous urethra lies in the bulb of the penis. It has a localized dilatation called the infrabulbar fossa. It is sur-rounded by the corpus spongiosum.

The penile urethra is long and narrow, except for a localized dilatation at its termination — the navicular fossa. It is surrounded by the corpus spongiosum of the penis.

Applied anatomy

Proximal urethral injuries are common with pelvic fractures owing to the fixed attachment of the distal prostatic and membranous urethra to the pelvic bones.

Fig. 6.12 Male bladder and urethra: (a) sagittal section; (b) diagram of prostatic urethra to show ducts.

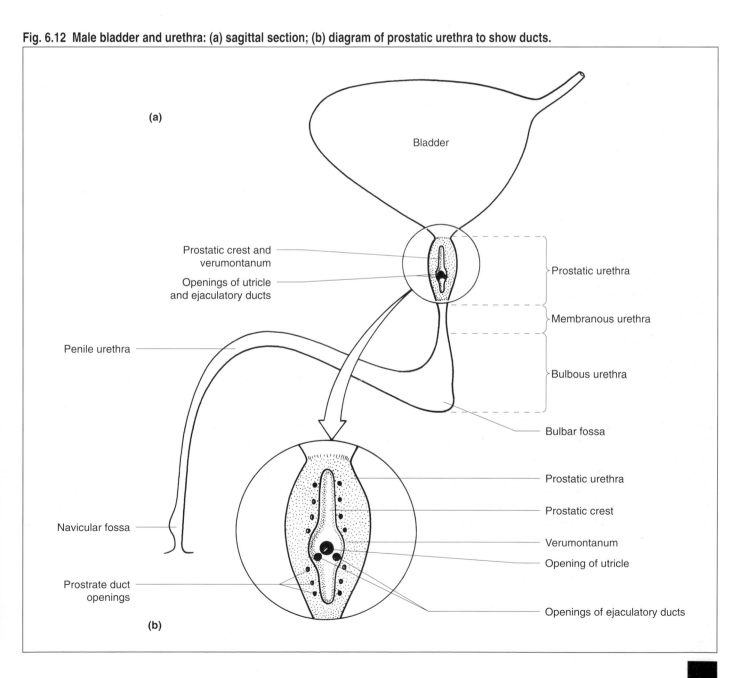

RADIOLOGY OF THE MALE URETHRA (Fig. 6.13)

The male urethra may be outlined by contrast, which is usually introduced retrogradely via a soft catheter in the navicular fossa. The infrabulbar fossa is seen and the various parts of the urethra are recognized by position and calibre. The verumontanum appears as a posterior filling defect in the prostatic urethra, and the utricle may fill.

THE FEMALE URETHRA

This is 4 cm long and traverses the urogenital diaphragm anterior to the bladder. The external urethral sphincter is at the urogenital diaphragm but is less well developed than that in the male. The involuntary internal urethral sphincter at the bladder neck appears to be more important in females.

Fig. 6.13 Retrograde urethrogram in the male: oblique view.

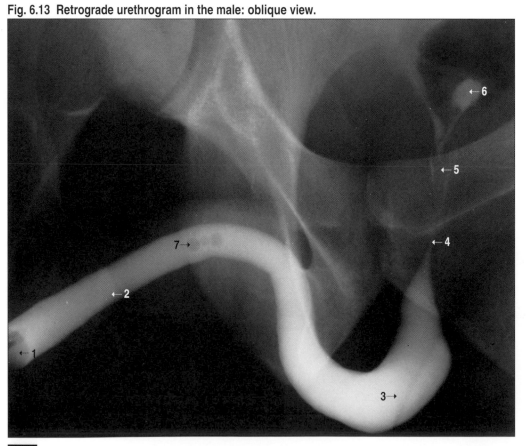

1. Balloon of catheter in navicular fossa
2. Penile urethra
3. Bulbous urethra
4. Membranous urethra
5. Impression of verumontanum in prostatic urethra
6. Filling of utricle (not usually seen)
7. Air bubbles in contrast

THE MALE REPRODUCTIVE ORGANS
(see Figs 6.7, 6.11, 6.12, 6.15 and 6.16)

THE PROSTATE GLAND (Fig. 6.14)

This gland is shaped like a truncated cone and surrounds the base of the bladder and the proximal (prostatic) urethra, extending inferiorly to the urogenital diaphragm and external sphincter. It has a base superiorly, an apex inferiorly, and an anterior wall, a posterior wall and two lateral walls. Anteriorly is the fatty space of Retzius and pubic bone. Laterally are the muscles of the pelvic wall. Posteriorly are the seminal vesicles. Fascia known as Denonvillier's fascia separates the prostate and seminal vesicles from the rectum. The puboprostatic ligament runs from the front of the gland to the pubic bone and provides support.

The structure of the gland is arranged into three lobes — a right and a left lobe posteriorly and a median lobe anteriorly. The right and left lobes are continuous anteriorly but are separated posteriorly by a median sulcus (which is palpable on rectal examination). The median lobe projects anteriorly between the openings of the ejaculatory ducts, which traverse the upper part of the gland to open into the prostatic urethra. A narrow isthmus of prostate encircles the anterior part of the urethra.

The internal architecture of the gland is described as having three zones, which may be distinguished by some imaging techniques. There is a central zone, which surrounds the urethra, a narrow transitional zone and an outer peripheral zone. With ageing, the peripheral zone hypertrophies — a condition known as benign prostatic hyperplasia.

THE SEMINAL VESICLES
(see **Figs 6.4** and **6.11**)

These are paired sacculated diverticula that lie transversely behind the prostate and store seminal fluid. These convoluted tubes narrow at their lower end to fuse with the vasa to become the ejaculatory ducts.

Blood supply of prostate gland and seminal vesicles

Blood supply is via the inferior vesical artery. Venous drainage is via the prostatic venous plexus to the internal iliac vein. Blood also drains from the prostate gland to a vertebral venous plexus, providing a route for the spread of prostatic cancers.

Lymph drainage

This is via lymphatic channels that accompany blood vessels to internal iliac nodes.

Fig. 6.14 Prostate gland: diagram of axial section showing lobar anatomy and prostatic urethra.

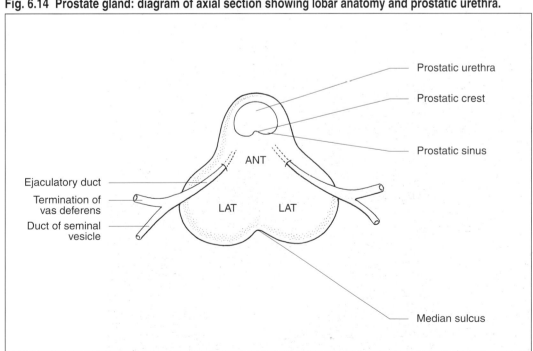

RADIOLOGY OF THE PROSTATE GLAND AND SEMINAL VESICLES

Ultrasound

The prostate gland may be imaged by ultrasound. The best visualization is achieved with an ultrasound probe in the rectum. In this situation, the prostate gland is imaged directly. In-built linear and sector scanners allow longitudinal and transverse images. The prostate gland yields uniform, low-level echoes. The right and left lobes are identified adjacent to the transducer, with the median lobe and urethra anterior to them. The seminal vesicles can be identified as sacculated structures posterolateral to the gland.

Cross-sectional imaging

MRI is an excellent method of imaging the prostate. The zonal anatomy is seen on the T2-weighted image. The peripheral zone is of uniformly high intensity and contrasts with the intermediate signal intensity of the transitional and central zones. The urethra is of relatively high signal intensity on T2-weighted images. The periprostatic venous plexus is of high signal intensity on T2 images as is the fat in the retropubic space of Retzius, contrasting with the low-intensity puboprostatic ligament and pubococcygeus muscle. Denonvillier's fascia may be identified as a low-intensity line between the posterior aspect of the prostate and the rectum. On T1-weighted images, the prostate and the venous plexus are of relatively low signal intensity and the zonal anatomy cannot be identified. The zonal anatomy is not seen on CT.

The seminal vesicles are seen posterior to the prostate and bladder on axial CT, and on axial or sagittal MR images (**Fig. 6.15**).

Fig. 6.15 MRI scan of male pelvis: sagittal T1-weighted image.

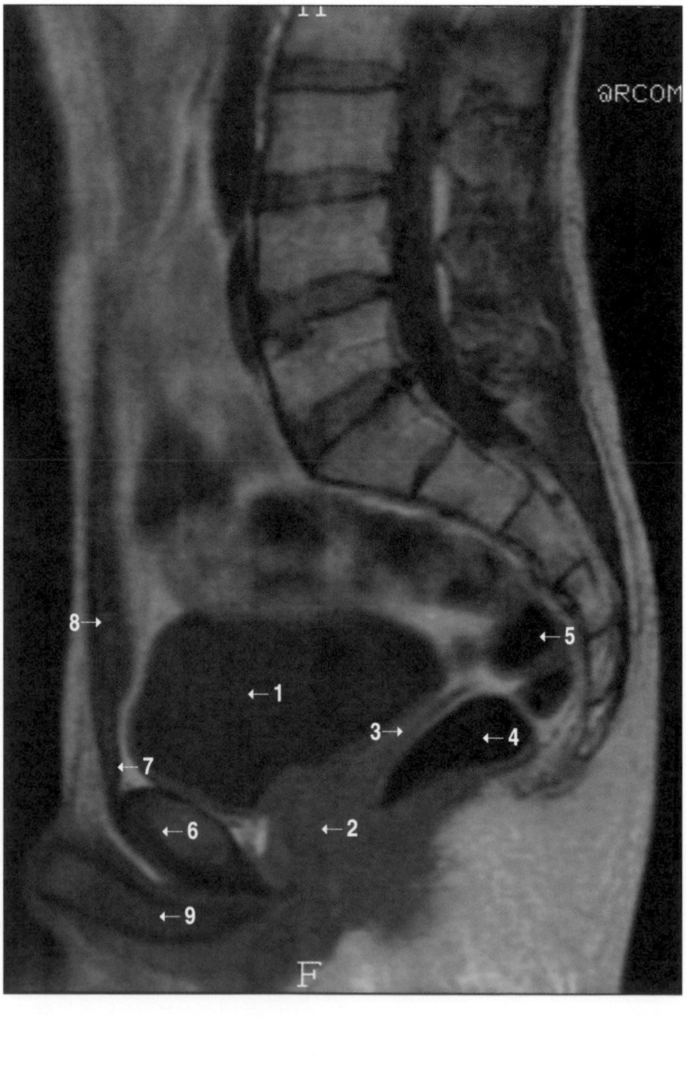

1. Bladder
2. Prostate gland
3. Seminal vesicle
4. Rectum
5. Sigmoid colon
6. Pubic bone
7. Aponeurosis of rectus sheath
8. Rectus muscle
9. Corpus cavernosum

THE TESTIS, EPIDIDYMIS AND SPERMATIC CORD
(Fig. 6.16; see Fig. 6.17)

The testis

This as an oval sperm-producing gland that is described as having upper and lower poles. It is suspended by the spermatic cord in the scrotal sac and is covered by a fibrous capsule called the tunica albuginea, which is thickened posteriorly to form an incomplete fibrous septum known as the *mediastinum* of the testis. Fibrous septa arise from the mediastinum, dividing the testis into lobules of sperm-producing cells. These are drained by *seminiferous tubules* to the *rete testis* in the mediastinum. From here, ductules pierce the tunica near the upper pole to convey sperm to the head of the epididymis.

The testis is invaginated anteriorly into a double serous covering — the *tunica vaginalis* (analogous to the invagination of bowel into the peritoneum). The tunica vaginalis is continuous with the peritoneum during development via the *processus vaginalis.* This is normally obliterated at birth.

The testis is separated from its fellow by an incomplete midline scrotal septum. The upper pole has a small sessile projection called the *appendix* of the testis, which is situated just below the head of the epididymis.

Fig. 6.16 Male reproductive organs: (a) testis and epididymis; (b) scrotum — transverse section.

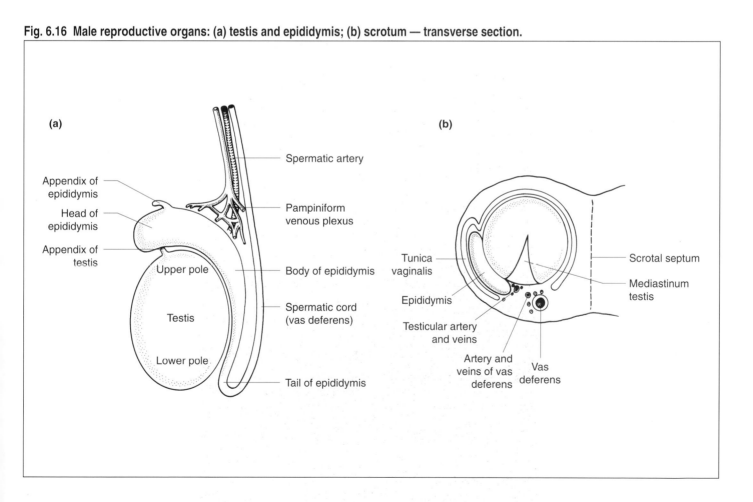

The epididymis

This is a convoluted duct that measures about 6 m when unravelled. It is intimately applied to the testis with its *head* lying on the upper pole, its *body* along the posterolateral aspect of the testis and its *tail* lying inferiorly. From here it continues superiorly as the spermatic cord. The head of the epididymis has a small sessile projection superiorly known as the *appendix* of the epididymis.

The spermatic cord

This extends from the tail of the epididymis through the scrotum, inguinal canal and pelvis to fuse with the seminal vesicle just above the prostate.

Fluid collections in the scrotum

Fluid may be present in the sac of the tunica vaginalis in a condition known as *hydrocoele*. If the tunica communicates with the peritoneal cavity via an open processus vaginalis, the fluid collection is called a *congenital* hydrocoele. Cysts related to the spermatic cord are seen when isolated areas of the processus vaginalis have failed to obliterate.

Cysts of the epididymis arise from the efferent spermatic ducts in the head of the epididymis. They are found above and behind the testis and are known as *spermatocoeles.*

Blood supply

The testis is supplied by the *testicular artery,* which arises directly from the aorta at the level of the renal arteries. Venous drainage is via a plexus of veins called the *pampiniform venous plexus.* This is above and behind the testis and becomes one vein at the upper end of the inguinal canal. The right vein drains into the inferior vena cava and the left into the left renal vein.

The spermatic cord and epididymis are supplied by the internal iliac artery via a branch of the inferior vesical artery.

The scrotum is supplied by the external pudendal branches of the femoral artery.

Lymph drainage

The testis drains to para-aortic nodes via the testicular vessels.

The scrotum drains to superficial inguinal nodes.

RADIOLOGY OF THE TESTIS

Ultrasound (Fig. 6 17)

The testes may be imaged by ultrasound as oval structures of uniform low-level echoes. On longitudinal scans, the upper and lower poles are identified. The head of the epididymis is seen to rest on the upper pole posteriorly.

Fig. 6.17 Ultrasound of testis: (a) longitudinal scan; (b) transverse scan.

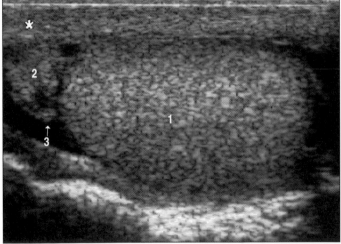

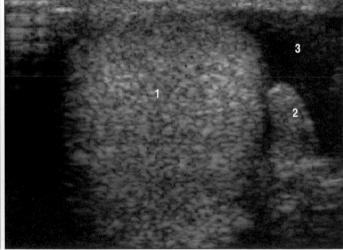

(a)
1. Testis
2. Head of epididymis
3. Fluid around testis

(b)
1. Testis
2. Epididymis
3. Fluid around testis

The appendices may be identified on high-resolution images. The mediastinum is seen as an echogenic line posteriorly. The epididymis is seen posterolateral to the testis and the spermatic cord is posteromedial to it. The scrotal septum is seen between the testes. A small amount of anechoic fluid may surround the normal testis. Coronal scans show the mediastinum as a line of high echogenicity in the posterior part of the testis.

The tortuous veins of the pampiniform plexus may be seen related to the cord above the upper pole. Slow venous flow may be demonstrated by colour doppler techniques.

Magnetic resonance imaging

Use of a surface coil improves resolution. The tunica albuginea and mediastinum testis are of low signal intensity compared with the high signal intensity of normal testicular tissue. The epididymis is of variable intensity.

THE PENIS

The penis comprises three cylinders of erectile tissue, which arise from the perineum: a ventral *corpus spongiosus*, which surrounds the urethra, and paired dorsal *corpora cavernosa*. The corpus cavernosum is expanded to form the *glans penis* inferiorly and the *bulb* superiorly. The corpora are surrounded by a common fibrous envelope in the penis and diverge posterosuperiorly to form the *crura.*

RADIOLOGY OF THE PENIS

Ultrasound

The corpora and urethra may be identified by ultrasound. The corpora yield low-level echoes and the urethra is seen as a circular anechoic structure. The penile artery may be imaged using the colour flow Doppler technique.

Magnetic resonance imaging

This will also show the corpora, which are of high signal intensity on T2-weighted images.

Cavernosography

This entails the injection of contrast into the corpora. This examination is performed for the investigation of erectile dysfunction.

THE FEMALE REPRODUCTIVE TRACT

THE VAGINA (Figs 6.18–6.20)

This muscular canal extends from the uterus to the vestibule, opening between the labia minora behind the urethra and clitoris. It has a rectangular shape, being flattened from front to back. Superiorly the cervix of the

Fig. 6.18 Female pelvis: sagittal section showing pelvic floor.

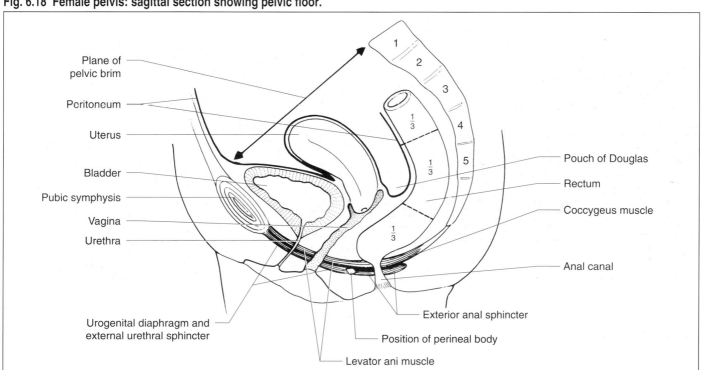

uterus projects into its anterior wall at an acute angle. The cervix invaginates the upper vagina and arbitrarily divides it into a shallow anterior and deep posterior and lateral recesses or *fornices*. In front is the base of the bladder and the urethra. Behind the upper vagina is the *pouch of Douglas,* containing loops of bowel. Below this is the rectum, and the anococcygeal body separates the lower vagina from the anal canal. On either side are the levator ani muscles and the pelvic fascia. The ureters pass medially above the lateral fornices. The vagina traverses levator ani and the urogenital diaphragm, which have a sphincter-like action.

Blood supply

Vaginal branches of the internal iliac and the uterine arteries supply the vagina. Venous drainage is via a plexus on its lateral walls to the internal iliac vein.

Lymph drainage

The upper two-thirds drains to internal and external iliac nodes. The lower third drains to superficial inguinal nodes.

THE UTERUS (Figs 6.18–6.22)

This is a pear-shaped muscular organ lying between the bladder and rectum. It has a *fundus*, a *body* and a *cervix*. It lies on the posterosuperior surface of the bladder with its cervix projecting into the anterior wall of the upper vagina, forming an acute angle. The cavity of the uterus is triangular in coronal section, but its anterior and posterior wall are apposed, giving it a slit-like appearance in the sagittal plane. The fallopian tubes open into the cornua of the uterus superolaterally. The uterus leads to the vagina via the *cervical canal*. Just above the cervical canal the uterus narrows to an isthmus. The *internal os* is at the upper end of the cervical canal and the *external os* at its lower end.

The inner lining of the uterus is the *endometrium,* which undergoes cyclical changes of proliferation and desquammation in the premenopausal female.

Peritoneum covers the fundus, body, cervix and upper part of the vagina posteriorly. From here it is reflected onto the anterior surface of the rectum, forming the pouch of Douglas. Anteriorly, the peritoneum is reflected

Fig. 6.19 Uterus and fallopian tubes: coronal section showing blood supply and ureter relative to uterine artery, cervix and vagina.

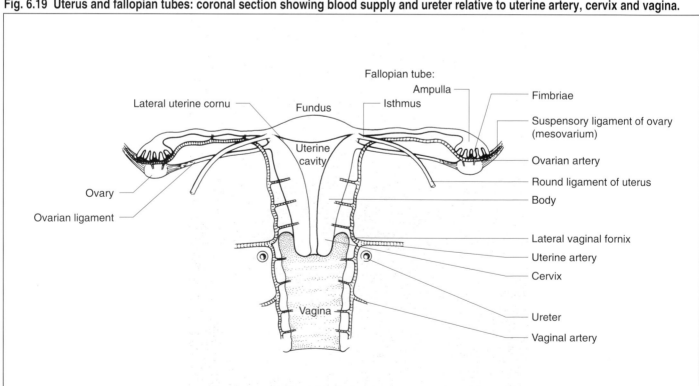

from the upper part of the body to the superior surface of the bladder forming the *uterovesical pouch.*

On either side of the uterus, the peritoneum is reflected to the lateral pelvic walls covering the fallopian tubes. The fold of peritoneum so formed is called the *broad ligament.* Several important structures run in this fold.

Ligamentous support of the uterus

The major support is by the *parametrial ligaments* anchoring the cervix to the walls of the pelvis. These are condensations of the fibrous tissue, which surrounds the cervix to form *pubocervical, lateral cervical* and *uterosacral ligaments* on the upper surface of the levator ani muscle.

The *round ligament* is a fibromuscular band that passes from the upper lateral part of the uterus to the inguinal canal, ending in the labium majus.

Normal variants of the uterus

The uterus may be retroverted, that is, lie in a posterior plane with the axis of the cervix directed upwards and backwards. It may also be retroflexed. Here the cervix bears the usual relationship with the vagina but the uterus is bent backwards on the cervix. These positions are not of clinical importance but make visualization of the uterus by ultrasound difficult.

In children the cervix is twice the size of the uterus. The uterus grows disproportionately until they are of equal size at puberty. In adulthood the converse is true.

Fig. 6.20 MRI scan of female pelvis: sagittal T1-weighted image.

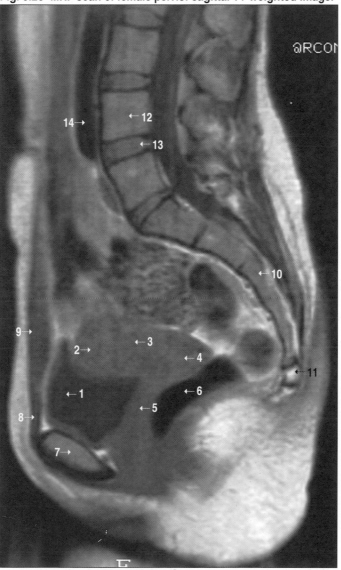

1. Bladder
2. Uterus: fundus
3. Uterus: body
4. Uterus: cervix
5. Vagina
6. Rectum
7. Pubic bone
8. Aponeurosis of rectal sheath
9. Rectus abdominis muscle
10. Sacrum
11. Coccyx
12. L4 vertebral body
13. L4/L5 disc space
14. Abdominal aorta

THE FALLOPIAN TUBES

The fallopian (uterine) tubes lie in the 'free edge' of the broad ligament and convey ova from the ovaries to the uterus. They open into the uterine *cornua*. They are described as having four parts as follows:

- The uterine part — this is the part within the wall of the uterus;
- The isthmus — this is long and narrow and leads to the ampulla;
- The ampulla — this is a wide, dilated, tortuous part at the outer end; and
- The infundibulum — this is the outer extremity of the tube. It is funnel-shaped and its rim is fimbriated. It extends out beyond the broad ligament and opens into the peritoneal cavity. It embraces the upper surface of the ovary. One of the fimbriae is longer than the rest. This is called the ovarian fimbria as it is closely applied to the ovary.

Blood supply of the uterus and fallopian tubes

The uterine artery, a branch of the internal iliac, runs medially in the base of the broad ligament to reach the lower lateral wall of the uterus. It ascends tortuously within the broad ligament to supply the uterus and tubes and anastomoses with the ovarian artery.

Venous drainage is via a venous plexus in the base of the broad ligament to the internal iliac vein.

Lymph drainage

The fundus drains along ovarian vessels to para-aortic nodes.

The body drains via the broad ligament to nodes around the external iliac vessels and occasionally via the round ligament to inguinal nodes. The cervix drains to external and internal iliac nodes and posteriorly to sacral nodes.

Fig. 6.21 Ultrasound of uterus and vagina: longitudinal image.

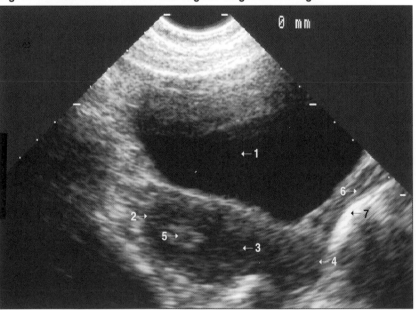

1. Urine-filled bladder
2. Fundus of uterus
3. Body of uterus
4. Cervix uteri
5. Endometrium
6. Vaginal stripe
7. Gas in rectum

THE BROAD LIGAMENT

This fold of peritoneum encloses the fallopian tubes superiorly. The uterine artery runs medially in its base. The ureter loops under the uterine artery within the ligament, passing just lateral to the cervix above the lateral vaginal fornix to enter the bladder. The uterine plexus of veins in the base of the broad ligament communicates with the veins of the vagina and bladder via the pelvic plexus of veins.

THE OVARIES (Fig. 6.22)

These are paired oval organs measuring approximately 3 cm × 2 cm × 2 cm. They lie on the posterior surface of the broad ligament in close contact with the infundibulum of the fallopian tube and attached to its ovarian *fimbria*. A fold of peritoneum, the *suspensory ligament of the ovary*, runs from the side wall of the pelvis to the ovary. The ovarian vessels run in this, crossing over the external iliac vessels. Each ovary is attached to the back of the broad ligament by the *meso-ovarium*, which is continuous with its outer coat. A fourth attachment, the *ovarian ligament* attaches the ovary to the side of the uterus. Despite all its attachments, the ovary is very mobile, especially in women who have had children. It is frequently found behind the uterus in the pouch of Douglas.

Blood supply

Arterial supply is via the ovarian artery, which arises directly from the aorta at the level of the renal arteries.

Venous drainage is via the right ovarian vein into the inferior vena cava, and via the left ovarian vein into the left renal vein.

Lymph drainage

Along the ovarian vessels to preaortic nodes.

RADIOLOGY OF THE FEMALE PELVIS

Ultrasound (Figs 6.21 and 6.22)

Ultrasound is probably the commonest radiological method of imaging the female reproductive tract. The urine-filled bladder lifts gassy loops of bowel out of the way and provides an acoustic window through which the pelvic organs may be visualized.

The uterine myometrial wall yields uniform low-level echoes. The endometrium yields a high-level echo that is seen as a long white stripe on longitudinal images and a central echo on transverse images. This is thicker and more obvious perimenstrually. The vagina is also seen as a white stripe of increased echogenicity on longitudinal images. The vaginal stripe makes an acute angle with the

Fig. 6.22 Ultrasound of uterus and ovaries: transverse image.

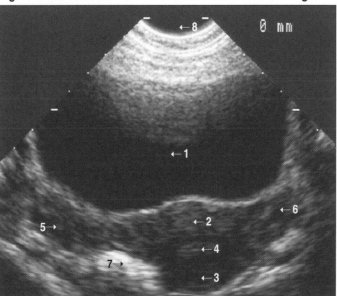

1. Bladder
2. Body of uterus: anterior aspect
3. Body of uterus: posterior aspect
4. Endometrial stripe
5. Right ovary
6. Left ovary
7. Acoustic shadowing from bowel gas in cul-de-sac
8. Skin surface: anterior abdominal wall

Fig. 6.23 CT scan of pelvis: axial section though female bladder and uterus. The full bladder has pushed small bowel loops superiorly out of the plane of scanning. Intravenous and rectal contrast have been adminstered.

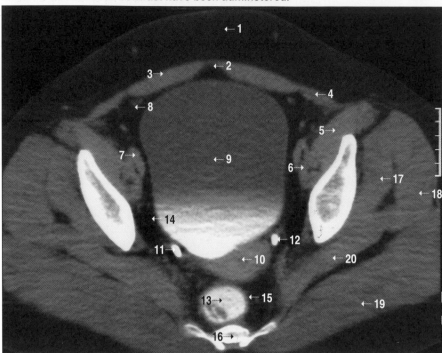

1. Subcutaneous fat
2. Rectus sheath aponeurosis (linea alba)
3. Rectus abdominis muscle
4. Transversus abdominis muscle with fused aponeurosis of external oblique and internal oblique muscles superficially
5. Iliacus muscle
6. Psoas muscle
7. External iliac artery and vein
8. Inferior epigastric vessels
9. Bladder with layering contrast
10. Uterus
11. Right ureter
12. Left ureter
13. Contrast in rectum
14. Perivesical fat
15. Perirectal fat
16. Lower sacrum
17. Gluteus minimus muscle
18. Gluteus medius muscle
19. Gluteus maximus muscle
20. Piriformis muscle

body of the uterus. Owing to the rectangular shape of the vagina, it is seen as a transverse line on transverse images. The ovaries are normally identified on either side of the uterus on transverse images. They may, however, lie in the pouch of Douglas or even fail to be identified in normal women. The normal ovary may contain small anechoic *follicles* in premenopausal women. In the late phase of the menstrual cycle, a small amount of fluid may be seen in the pouch of Douglas.

Endovaginal ultrasound is performed with an ultrasound transducer in the vagina. The basic ultrasound features are the same, but the resolution is better. There is improved visualization of the adnexal area and the internal architecture of the ovary as well the uterus and uterine cavity.

Computed tomography and magnetic resonance imaging (Fig. 6.23; see Fig. 6.20)

MRI is better than CT at imaging the uterus because it can image in various planes as well as having superior soft-tissue contrast. On T2-weighted images, the endometrium, endocervical canal and vaginal canal are all of high signal intensity. The inner zone of myometrium is of low signal intensity and is continuous with the fibrous stroma of the cervix. The outer myometrium is of moderate signal intensity. The ovaries are isointense with fat on T2-weighted images and the follicles stand out as hyperintense spots. They are of intermediate intensity on T1 images. The broad ligament is frequently seen as a low-intensity structure running posterolaterally from the uterus to the pelvic side wall. The round ligaments are also of low intensity, seen coursing anteriorly from the upper lateral part of the uterus to the inguinal canal.

On CT the uterus is seen as a round structure of soft-tissue density lying on the bladder. Oral contrast helps to differentiate loops of bowel, which lie on and around it. A tampon in the vagina may also aid interpretation, showing as a rounded air-density below the uterus on cross-sectional images.

Hysterosalpingography (Fig. 6.24)

This technique outlines the cavity of the uterus and tubes by injection of water-soluble contrast via the cervical canal. The cervical canal is approximately one-third the length of the entire uterine long axis. *Longitudinal ridges* are seen on the anterior and posterior walls of the cervical canal. These may have branches running laterally — the *plicae palmate* — in nulliparous women. *Cervical glands* may be outlined by contrast as outpouchings from the cervical canal. The isthmus is seen as a narrow area above the cervix, and the internal os may sometimes be identified as a constriction of the lumen of the isthmus. The uterine cavity is seen to be triangular on the frontal view. It is usually smooth-walled. The triangular cornua lead to the fallopian tubes, which are 5–6 cm long. The isthmus of the tube is uniformly narrow and opens into the wide ampulla. Contrast spills freely into the peritoneal cavity.

The walls of the uterus may demonstrate longitudinal folds. Polypoid filling defects may be seen in the secretory phase in normal women. Filling of endometrial glands may also be seen in normal women in the secretory phase.

Vaginography

This technique outlines the vagina with contrast. The characteristic rectangular shape of the vagina is demonstrated. It is of utmost importance to recognize this shape in the case of inadvertent filling of the vagina during a barium examination.

Fig. 6.24 Hysterosalpingogram.

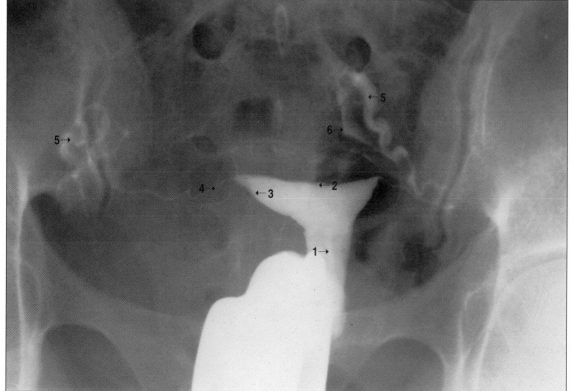

1. Body of uterus
2. Fundus of uterus
3. Uterine cornu
4. Isthmus of fallopian tube
5. Ampulla of fallopian tube
6. Peritoneal spill of contrast

CROSS-SECTIONAL ANATOMY (Figs 6.25–6.27; see Figs 6.4, 6.6 and 6.23)

The anatomy described can be identified on both CT and MRI images.

MID-SACRAL LEVEL — MALE OR FEMALE (Fig. 6.25)

This level is above the bladder. The sigmoid colon may be seen close to its junction with the rectum. Loops of small bowel lie in the pelvis, on top of the pelvic organs. Pelvic and mesenteric fat separate the various bowel loops. The sacrum is posterior, with the piriformis muscle arising from its anterior surface. The piriformis muscle passes anteriorly, inferiorly and laterally to insert into the greater tuberosity of the femur. The sciatic nerve lies on the piriformis. The gluteus muscles are posterior; gluteus maximus is the largest, most posterior and most superficial. Gluteus minimus is the smallest, most anterior and deepest gluteal muscle. The psoas and iliacus muscles are relatively anterior at this level, with the external iliac vessels lying on them, the vein being slightly anterior and lateral to the artery.

The ureters are lateral on the side wall of the pelvis and are extraperitoneal in location. At first they lie anterior to the bifurcation of the iliac artery. At a lower level they are more anteriorly located. In the male, the vasa deferentia pass over the ureters and may be identified by CT or MRI, running posteriorly from the inguinal canal around the side of the bladder to join with the ducts of the seminal vesicles at a lower level.

Fig. 6.25 Cross-section of male/female pelvis: mid-sacral level.

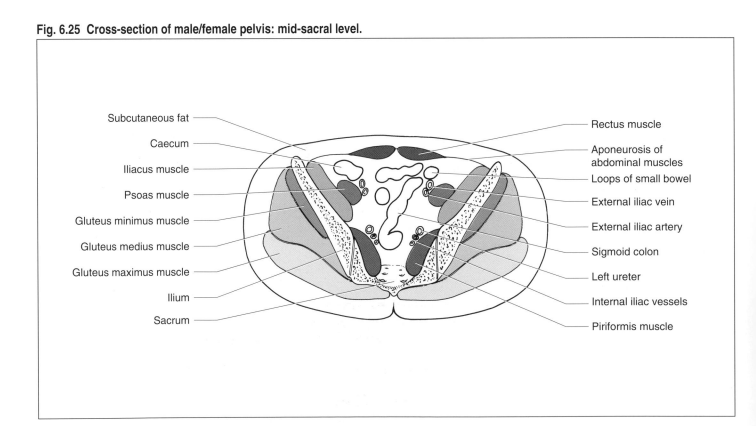

Subcutaneous fat

Caecum

Iliacus muscle

Psoas muscle

Gluteus minimus muscle

Gluteus medius muscle

Gluteus maximus muscle

Ilium

Sacrum

Rectus muscle

Aponeurosis of abdominal muscles

Loops of small bowel

External iliac vein

External iliac artery

Sigmoid colon

Left ureter

Internal iliac vessels

Piriformis muscle

LOWER SACRAL LEVEL — MALE (Fig. 6.26)

The bladder has a rather square shape when it contains urine. It extends anteriorly to the anterior abdominal wall. Posteriorly are the seminal vesicles. The rectum is just behind the seminal vesicles, separated from them by the perirectal fascia and is surrounded by perirectal fat.

Outside the perirectal fascia is the pararectal fat. This is continuous with the fat lining the pelvis above the levator ani muscle. The obturator internus muscle is deep to the lateral pelvic wall. It can be seen hooking around the posterior part of the ischium to insert into the greater trochanter of the femur. The ureters insert into the posterolateral aspect of the bladder. They are not be seen at the level of the seminal vesicles as they pass over these.

Fig. 6.26 Cross-section of male pelvis: lower sacral level.

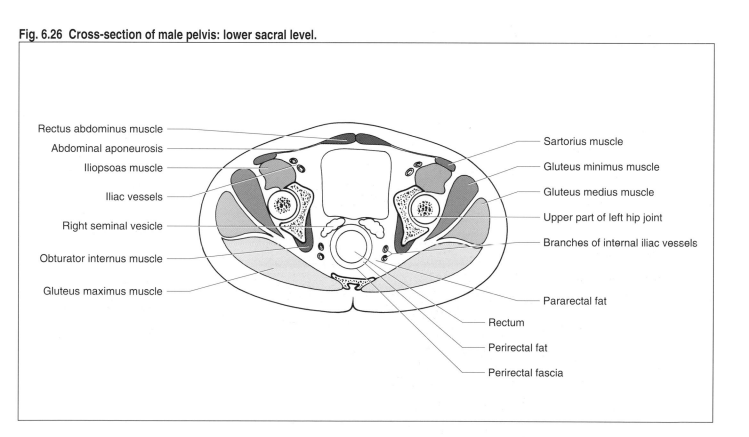

Rectus abdominus muscle
Abdominal aponeurosis
Iliopsoas muscle
Iliac vessels
Right seminal vesicle
Obturator internus muscle
Gluteus maximus muscle

Sartorius muscle
Gluteus minimus muscle
Gluteus medius muscle
Upper part of left hip joint
Branches of internal iliac vessels
Pararectal fat
Rectum
Perirectal fat
Perirectal fascia

LOWER SACRAL LEVEL — FEMALE (Fig. 6.27)

The uterus is seen closely applied to the posterior surface of the bladder. The position of the ovaries is variable and they may be found lateral to the uterus or behind it. The ureters are close to the posterolateral aspect of the bladder at this level. They hook medially in the broad ligament of the uterus (which cannot be identified as a separate structure), passing under the uterine artery and above the lateral vaginal fornix before entering the bladder.

SECTION THROUGH THE PERINEUM — MALE (see Fig. 6.6)

The anterior compartment (urogenital triangle) is immediately deep to the lower part of the symphysis pubis. It consists of the prostate gland and prostatic urethra.

Immediately behind is the anorectal junction in the posterior (anal) triangle. The ischiorectal fossa is seen on either side of and behind the anal canal (see earlier discussion for boundaries.) Note how far anterior the upper part of the anal canal is. The puborectalis fibres of levator ani surround the external anal sphincter. Laterally are the obturator internus muscle and the ischial tuberosity. The sacrotuberous ligament can usually be identified running laterally from the coccyx and sacrum to the ischial tuberosity. Posteriorly is the gluteus maximus muscle and the coccyx.

SECTION THROUGH THE PERINEUM — FEMALE

The posterior compartment is the same as that for the male. The anterior compartment has the urethra just behind the pubis, with the vagina immediately behind. These structures are seen more clearly with MRI than CT.

Fig. 6.27 Cross-section of female pelvis: lower sacral level.

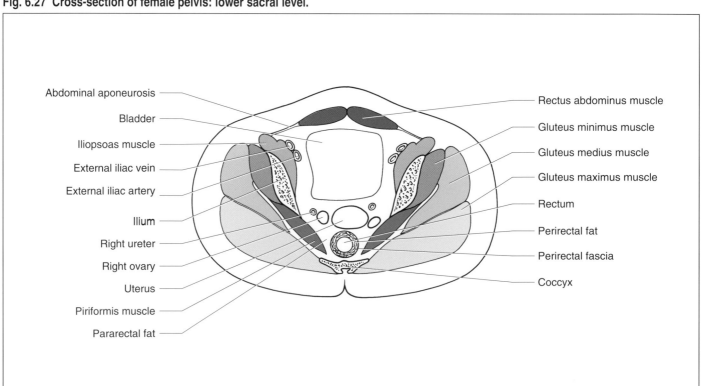

Labels (left): Abdominal aponeurosis, Bladder, Iliopsoas muscle, External iliac vein, External iliac artery, Ilium, Right ureter, Right ovary, Uterus, Piriformis muscle, Pararectal fat

Labels (right): Rectus abdominus muscle, Gluteus minimus muscle, Gluteus medius muscle, Gluteus maximus muscle, Rectum, Perirectal fat, Perirectal fascia, Coccyx

CHAPTER 7 *THE UPPER LIMB*

The bones

The joints

The muscles

The arteries

The veins

THE BONES OF THE UPPER LIMB

THE SCAPULA (Figs 7.1 and 7.2)

This flat triangular bone has three processes:

■ The *glenoid process*, which is separated from the remainder by the neck of the scapula. The glenoid cavity forms part of the shoulder joint;
■ The *spine*, which arises from the posterior surface of the scapula and separates the supraspinous and infraspinous fossae. The spine extends laterally over the shoulder joint as the *acromium* (see **Fig. 7.2**); and
■ The *coracoid process*, which projects anteriorly from the upper border of the neck of the scapula.

RADIOLOGICAL FEATURES OF THE SCAPULA

Plain radiographs

The *inferior angle* of the scapula lies over the seventh rib or interspace — this is a useful guideline in identifying ribs or thoracic vertebral levels.

The scapula lies over the ribs and obscures some of the lung fields in PA *chest radiographs* unless the shoulders are rotated forwards. In AP views it is not usually possible to rotate the scapulae off the lung fields. Similarly, in *AP views of the scapula* the beam is centred over the head of the humerus to project the thoracic cage away from the scapula.

Fig. 7.1 The scapula: (a) anterior view; (b) posterior view; (c) lateral view.

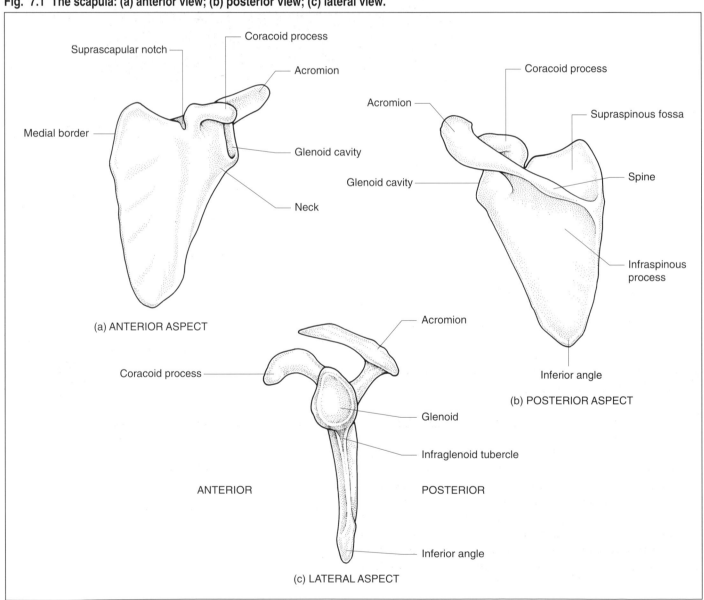

(a) ANTERIOR ASPECT

(b) POSTERIOR ASPECT

(c) LATERAL ASPECT

Fig. 7.2 Axial radiograph of the shoulder.

1. Medullary cavity of humeral shaft
2. Cortex
3. Head of humerus
4. Lesser tuberosity
5. Tip of acromion process
6. Lateral end of clavicle
7. Acromioclavicular joint
8. Clavicle
9. Glenoid fossa of scapula
10. Coracoid process of scapula
11. Acromion process of scapula

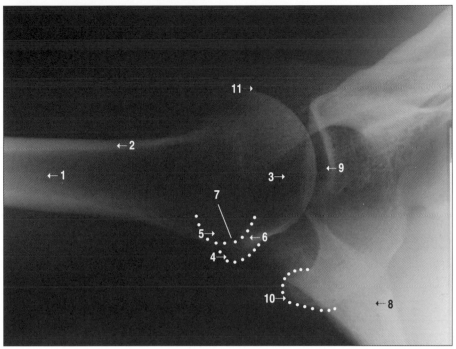

In *lateral chest radiographs*, the lateral border of the scapula may be confused with an oblique fissure. The inferior angle of the scapula may be slightly bulbous and simulate a mass on this view.

Isotope bone scan

The inferior angle of the scapula overlying the seventh rib may appear like a 'hot spot'.

Ossification

The scapula ossifies in the eighth week of fetal life. An ossification centre appears in the middle of the coracoid process in the first year of life and fuses at 15 years of age. Secondary centres appear in the root of the coracoid process, the medial border and the inferior angle of the scapula between 14 and 20 years and fuse between 22 and 25 years of age.

THE CLAVICLE (**Fig. 7.3**; see **Fig. 7.2**)

The clavicle lies almost horizontally between the sternoclavicular and the acromioclavicular joints. It is also attached to the first costal cartilage by the costoclavicular ligament, which arises from the rhomboid fossa on its inferomedial surface. It is connected to the coracoid process by the coracoclavicular ligament at the conoid tubercle and the trapezoid line on its inferolateral surface. The subclavian vessels and the trunks of the brachial plexus pass behind its medial third.

Fig. 7.3 The clavicle: (a) superior view; (b) inferior view.

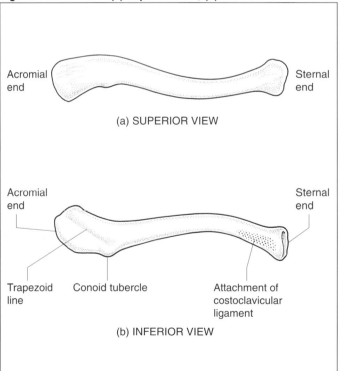

Acromial end — Sternal end

(a) SUPERIOR VIEW

Acromial end — Sternal end

Trapezoid line   Conoid tubercle   Attachment of costoclavicular ligament

(b) INFERIOR VIEW

RADIOLOGICAL FEATURES OF THE CLAVICLE

Chest radiograph

The clavicle overlies the apices of the lungs in chest radiographs. Apical or lordotic views are used to project the clavicles above the lungs to evaluate this area further. In portable AP chest radiography, if the patient is inclined backwards from a true vertical position, the horizontal beam projects the clavicles above the lungs.

On a chest radiograph, the distance between the medial end of the clavicle and the spine of the vertebrae is equal on both sides unless the patient is rotated.

Ossification

The clavicle begins to ossify before any other bone in body. It ossifies in membrane from two centres that appear at the fifth and sixth fetal weeks and fuses in the seventh week. A secondary centre appears at the sternal end at 15 years in females and 17 years in males and fuses at 25 years of age.

THE HUMERUS
(Figs 7.4 and 7.5; see Fig. 7.2)

The hemispherical head of the humerus is separated from the greater and lesser tubercle by the anatomical neck. Between the tubercles is the bicipital groove for the long head of the biceps. The shaft just below the tubercles is narrow and is called the surgical neck of the humerus.

The shaft is marked by a spiral groove where the radial nerve and the profunda vessels run. The deltoid tuberosity on the lateral aspect of the mid-shaft is the site of insertion of the deltoid muscle.

The lower end of the humerus is expanded and has medial and lateral epicondyles. The articular surface for the elbow joint has a capitellum for articulation with the radial head and a trochlea for the olecranon fossa of the ulna. Above the trochlea are fossae, the coranoid anteriorly and the deeper olecranon fossa posteriorly.

Fig. 7.4 The humerus: anterior and posterior views.

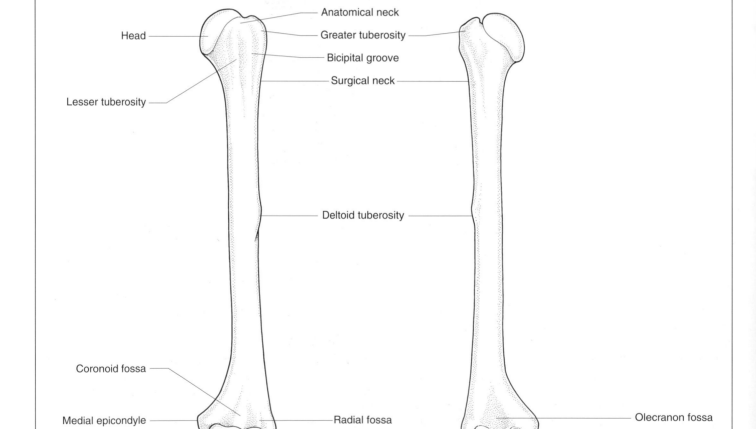

Fig. 7.5 AP radiograph of the elbow.

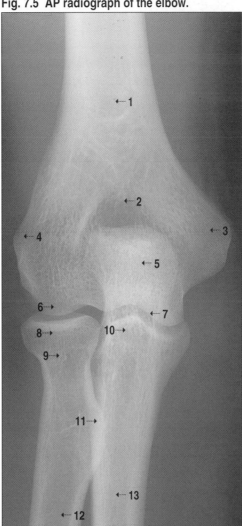

1. Shaft of humerus
2. Olecranon fossa
3. Medial epicondyle
4. Lateral epicondyle
5. Olecranon process
6. Capitulum
7. Trochlea
8. Head of radius
9. Neck of radius
10. Coronoid process of ulna
11. Radial tuberosity
12. Shaft of radius
13. Shaft of ulna

RADIOLOGICAL FEATURES OF THE HUMERUS

Plain radiographs

The lower epiphysis of the humerus lies at a 25° angle to the shaft so that a vertical line down the front of the shaft on a lateral radiograph, the *anterior humeral line,* bisects the capitellum.

An *olecranon foramen* may replace the olecranon fossa.

A hook-shaped projection of bone — termed the *supracondylar process* — occasionally occurs about 5 cm above the medial epicondyle. It varies in length between 2 and 20 mm and may be continuous with a fibrous band attached above the epicondyle to form a foramen that transmits the median nerve and the brachial artery.

Avulsion of the medial epicondyle

The flexor muscles of the forearm arise from the medial epicondyle of the humerus. Repeated contractions or a single violent contraction of these muscles in a child can result in avulsion of the apophysis (a secondary ossification centre occurring outside a joint) of the medial epicondyle.

Ossification

The primary centre for the humerus appears at the eighth week of fetal life. Secondary centres appear in the head of the humerus at 1 year, the greater tuberosity at 3 years and the lesser tuberosity at 5 years of age. These fuse with one another at 6 years and with the shaft at 20 years of age. Secondary centres appear in the capitellum at 1 year, the medial epicondyle at 5 years, the lateral epicondyle at 10 years and the trochlea at 11 years of age. These fuse at 17–18 years of age.

THE RADIUS AND ULNA (Figs 7.6 and 7.7; see Fig. 7.5)

The radius has a cylindrical head that is separated from the radial tubercle and the remainder of the shaft by the neck. Its lower end is expanded and its most distal part is the radial styloid. The radius is connected by the interosseus membrane to the ulna.

The upper part of the ulna — the olecranon — is hook-shaped, with the concavity of the hook — the trochlear fossa — anteriorly. A fossa found laterally at the base of the olecranon is for articulation with the radial head. The shaft of the ulna is narrow. The styloid process at the distal end is narrower and more proximal than that of the radius.

Fig. 7.6 The radius and ulna: anterior and posterior views.

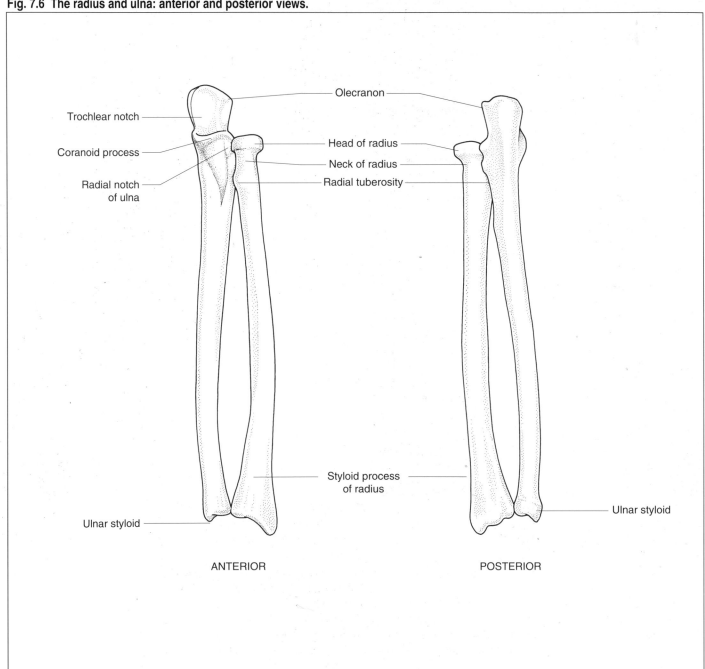

Trochlear notch

Coranoid process

Radial notch of ulna

Olecranon

Head of radius

Neck of radius

Radial tuberosity

Styloid process of radius

Ulnar styloid

Ulnar styloid

ANTERIOR

POSTERIOR

Fig. 7.7 AP radiograph of the wrist and hand.

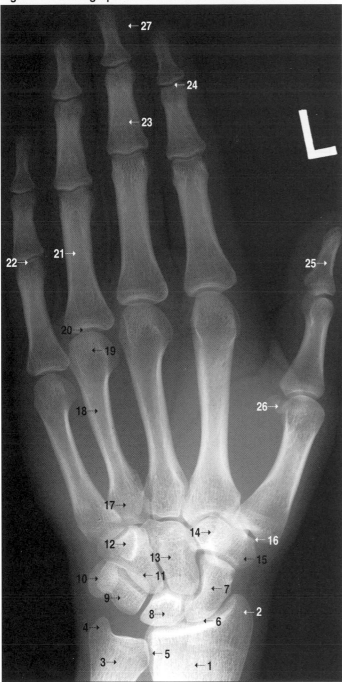

RADIOLOGICAL FEATURES OF THE RADIUS AND ULNA

Plain radiographs

The *head of the radius* has a single cortical line on its upper surface and is perpendicular to the neck in the normal radiograph (see **Fig. 7.5**). Angulation of the head or a double cortical line are signs of fracture of the radial head.

The triceps muscle is inserted into the tip of the *olecranon.* Fracture of the olecranon is therefore associated with proximal displacement by the action of this muscle.

The *ulnar styloid is proximal to the radial styloid,* with a line joining these on an AP radiograph lying at an angle of 110° with the long axis of the radius (see **Fig. 7.7**). In a lateral radiograph, the *articulating surface of the distal radius* is angled 20° to a line through the shaft of the radius. Recognition of these normal angles is important in reduction of fractures of the wrist.

The *pronator quadratus muscle* is a square, flat muscle that arises on the distal ulna and passes to the distal radius. A thin, fat pad overlying this muscle is visible as a linear lucency on a lateral radiograph of the wrist. Thickening of the muscle, such as by haematoma in fracture of the underlying bone, can be detected on a radiograph by bowing of the *pronator quadratus fat pad.*

Ossification of the radius

The primary ossification centre of the radius appears at the eighth week of fetal life. Secondary centres appear distally in the first year and proximally at 5 years of age. These fuse at 20 years and 17 years respectively.

Ossification of the ulna

The shaft of the ulna ossifies at the eighth week of fetal life. Secondary centres appear in the distal ulna at 5 years and in the olecranon at 10 years of age. These fuse at 20 and 17 years respectively.

1. Distal radius
2. Styloid process of radius
3. Distal ulna
4. Styloid process of ulna
5. Distal radioulnar joint
6. Radiocarpal joint
7. Scaphoid
8. Lunate
9. Triquetral
10. Pisiform
11. Hamate
12. Hook of hamate
13. Capitate
14. Trapezoid
15. Trapezium
16. First metacarpophalangeal joint
17. Base of fourth metacarpal
18. Shaft of fourth metacarpal
19. Head of fourth metacarpal
20. Fourth metacarpophalangeal joint
21. Shaft of proximal phalanx, ring finger
22. Proximal interphalangeal joint, little finger
23. Middle phalanx, middle finger
24. Distal interphalangeal joint, index finger
25. Distal phalanx, thumb
26. Sesamoid bone
27. Soft tissues overlying distal phalanx of middle finger

THE CARPAL BONES
(Fig. 7.8; see Fig. 7.7)

The carpal bones are arranged in two rows of four bones each. In the proximal row from lateral to medial are the scaphoid, lunate bone and triquetral bones, with the pisiform on the anterior surface of the triquetral. The trapezium, trapezoid, capitate and hamate make up the distal row.

Together the carpal bones form an arch, with its concavity situated anteriorly. The flexor retinaculum is attached laterally to the scaphoid and the ridge of the trapezium, and medially to the pisiform and the hook of the hamate. It converts the arch of bones into a tunnel, the carpal tunnel, which conveys the superficial and deep flexor tendons of the fingers and the thumb and the median nerve.

RADIOLOGICAL FEATURES OF THE CARPAL BONES

Radiography
These are radiographed in the anteroposterior, lateral and oblique positions (see **Fig. 7.7**). Carpal tunnel views are obtained by extending the wrist and taking an inferosuperior view that is centred over the anterior part of the wrist.

Supernumerary bones
These may be found in the wrist and include the *os centrale* found between the scaphoid, trapezoid and capitate, which may represent the tubercle of the scaphoid that has not fused with its upper pole, and the *os radiale externum,* which is found on the lateral side of the scaphoid distal to the radial styloid.

Nutrient arteries of the scaphoid
In 13% of subjects these enter the scaphoid exclusively in its distal half. If such a bone fractures across its midportion, the blood supply to the proximal portion is cut off and ischaemic necrosis is inevitable.

Ossification of the carpal bones
These ossify from a single centre each. The capitate ossifies first and the pisiform last but the order and timing of the ossification of the other bones is variable. Excluding the pisiform, they ossify in a clockwise direction from the capitate to trapezoid as follows: the capitate at 4 months; the hamate at 4 months; the triquetral at 3 years, the lunate bone at 5 years; and the scaphoid, trapezium and trapezoid at 6 years. The pisiform ossifies at 11 years of age.

Fig. 7.8 Bones of the hand.

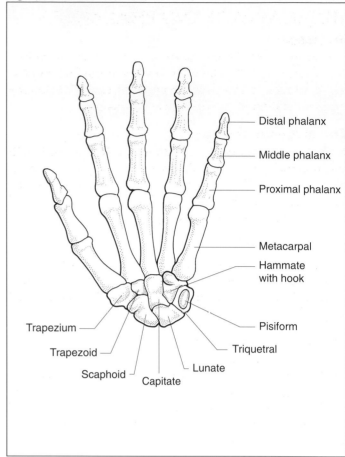

THE METACARPALS AND PHALANGES

The five metacarpals are numbered from the lateral to the medial side. Each has a base proximally that articulates with that of the other metacarpals, except in the case of the first metacarpal, which is as a result more mobile and less likely to fracture. The third metacarpal has a styloid process extending from its base on the dorsal aspect. Each metacarpal has a rounded head distally, which articulates with the proximal phalanx.

The phalanges are fourteen in number, three for each finger and two for the thumb. Like the metacarpals, each has a head, a shaft and a base. The distal part of the distal phalynx is expanded as the tuft of the distal phalynx.

RADIOLOGICAL FEATURES OF THE METACARPALS AND PHALANGES

Bone age

A radiograph of the left hand is used in the determination of bone age. Standards of age determined by epiphyseal appearance and fusion have been compiled for the left hand and wrist by Greulich and Pyle.

The metacarpal sign

A line tangential to the heads of the fourth and fifth metacarpals does not cross the head of the third metacarpal in 90% of normal hands — this is called the metacarpal sign. This line does, however, cross the third metacarpal head in gonadal dysgenesis.

The carpal angle

This is formed by lines tangential to the proximal ends of the scaphoid and lunate bone. The average angle in normal hands is 138°. It is reduced to an average 108° in gonadal dysgenesis.

The metacarpal index

This is calculated by measuring the lengths of the second, third, fourth and fifth metacarpals and dividing by their breadths taken at their exact mid-point. The sum of these divided by four is the metacarpal index and has a normal range of 5.4–7.9. An index greater than 8.4 suggests the diagnosis of arachnodactyly.

Sesamoid bones

Two sesamoid bones are found related to the anterior surface of the metacarpophalangeal joint of the thumb in the normal radiograph. A single sesamoid bone in relation to this joint in the little finger is seen in 83% of radiographs and at the interphalangeal joint of the thumb in 73%. These are occasionally found at other metacarpal and distal interphalangeal joints. The incidence of sesamoid bones is increased in acromegaly.

Tendons of the extensors of the fingers

These are inserted into the base of the dorsum of the phalanges. *Avulsion fractures* of this part of the phalanx are associated with proximal displacement of the fragment if the extensor tendon is attached to it and may need internal fixation. Small fractures of the base of the distal phalynx without displacement do not need fixation.

Ossification of the metacarpals and phalanges

These ossify between the ninth and twelfth fetal week. Secondary ossification centres appear in the distal end of the metacarpals of the fingers at 2 years and fuse at 20 years of age. Secondary centres for the thumb metacarpal and for the phalanges are at their proximal end and appear between 2 and 3 years and fuse between 18 and 20 years of age.

THE JOINTS OF THE UPPER LIMB

THE STERNOCLAVICULAR JOINT

Type

The sternoclavicular joint is a synovial joint divided into two parts by an articular disc.

Articular surfaces

The sternal end of the clavicle; the clavicular notch of the manubrium and the upper surface of the first costal cartilage.

Ligaments

These are the anterior and posterior sternoclavicular ligaments, costoclavicular ligament and the interclavicular ligament.

THE ACROMIOCLAVICULAR JOINT

Type

The acromioclavicular joint is a synovial joint.

Articular surfaces

These are the outer end of the clavicle and the acromium.

Ligaments

These are as follows:

- Acromioclavicular ligament, which is a thickening of the fibrous capsule superiorly; and
- Coracoclavicular ligament, which has conoid and trapezoid parts.

THE SHOULDER (GLENOHUMERAL) JOINT (Fig. 7.9)

Type

The glenohumeral joint is a ball-and-socket synovial joint.

Articular surfaces

These are as follows:

- Head of the humerus; and
- The glenoid cavity of the scapula, which is made deeper by a fibrocartilaginous ring — the labrum glenoidale.

Fig. 7.9 Coronal section through the shoulder joint as seen on coronal MRI scan.

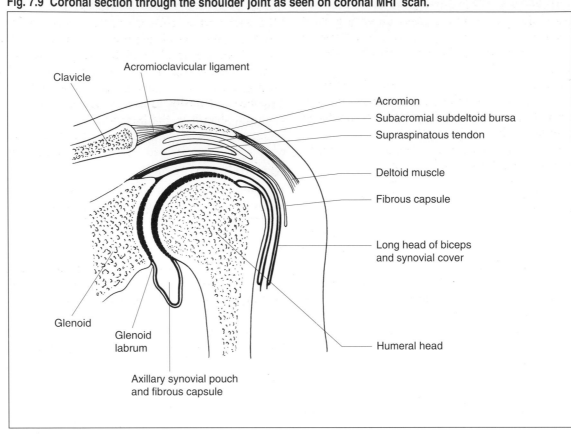

Capsule

This is attached to epiphyseal line of glenoid and humerus, except inferiorly where it extends downwards on the medial aspect of the neck of the humerus as the axillary pouch.

Synovium

In addition to lining the capsule of the joint, the synovium extends along the tendon of the long head of the biceps and beneath the tendon of subscapularis muscle as the subscapular bursa.

Ligaments

These are as follows:

- Three glenohumeral ligaments: anterior thickenings of the capsule passing from the upper part of the glenoid to the lesser tuberosity and the inferior part of the head of the humerus;
- The coracohumeral ligament; and
- The transverse humeral ligament between the greater and the lesser tuberosities of the humerus.

Stability

In addition to ligaments, the stability of the shoulder joint depends upon the surrounding muscles. These are:

- The short muscles known as the *rotator cuff muscles* (i.e. subscapularis, infraspinatus and teres minor muscles); and
- The longer muscles including the long head of biceps, pectoralis major, latissimus dorsi, teres major and deltoid muscles.

The inferior part of the joint is least well protected by either ligaments or muscles.

RADIOLOGICAL FEATURES OF THE SHOULDER JOINT

Plain radiographs

The *supraspinatus muscle* passes on the superior aspect of the shoulder joint to the greater tuberosity of the humerus. Calcification occurs in this muscle due to degenerative change and may be visible on radiographs.

The supraspinatus muscle is separated from the acromium by the subacromial-subdeltoid bursa, the largest bursa in the body. This bursa does not communicate with the shoulder joint unless supraspinatus is ruptured by trauma or degeneration. This communication is then visible on *arthrography*. *MRI* can also be used to detect this rupture.

The capsule of the shoulder joint is lax and relatively unprotected by ligaments or muscles inferiorly. This is the site of accumulation of fluid in effusion or haematoma of the joint. Similarly, dislocation of the joint occurs most often inferiorly with the head of the humerus coming to lie inferior to the coracoid process.

Arthrography with or without computed tomography

In the shoulder joint, arthrography is achieved by injection of contrast into the joint below and lateral to the coracoid process. It shows the features of the joint as outlined above. In particular, the axillary pouch can be seen inferior to the humeral head on external rotation of the arm and the subscapular (subcoracoid) bursa can be seen on internal rotation of the arm. The subacromial (subdeltoid) bursa is not filled unless the supraspinatus tendon is completely ruptured.

The tendon of the long head of biceps is seen as a filling defect within the joint and its synovial sheath is opacified outside the joint along the bicipital groove of the humerus.

Magnetic resonance imaging

MRI with surface coils is used increasingly to image the shoulder joint. Axial imaging demonstrates the relationship of the humeral head to the glenoid. The glenoid labrum has low-signal intensity and is triangular on axial section anteriorly and more rounded posteriorly. The long head of biceps muscle is visible, surrounded by its synovial sheath in the bicipital groove. Coronal oblique images are taken parallel to the supraspinatous muscle, which is seen separated from the acromium by fat within the subacromial bursa.

THE ELBOW JOINT (Fig. 7.10)

Type

The elbow joint is a synovial hinge joint, which incorporates the humeroulnar, the humeroradial and superior radioulnar joints as one cavity.

Articular surfaces

These are the trochlea and capitellum of the humerus; the head and ulnar notch of the radius and the trochlear fossa and radial notch of the ulna.

Capsule

This is attached to the margins of the articular surfaces of

Fig. 7.10 Humeroulnar component of the elbow joint: (a) sagittal section; (b) coronal section.

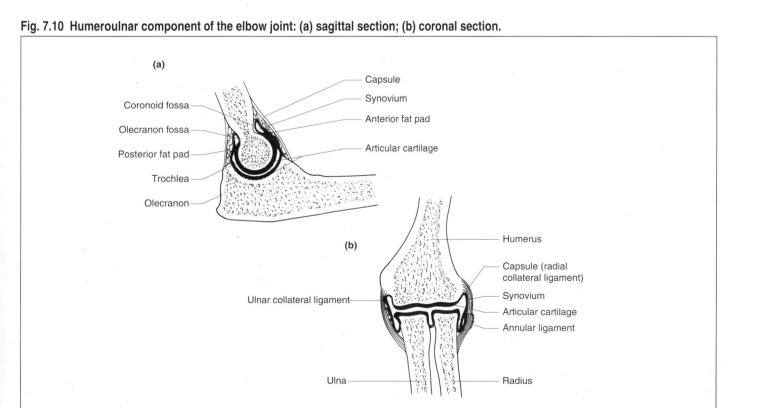

the radius and ulna but more proximally on the humerus to include the olecranon, coranoid and radial fossae within the joint.

Ligaments

These are:

- The radial and ulnar collateral ligaments, which are lateral and medial thickenings of the capsule; and
- The annular ligament, which surrounds the head of the radius and rotates within it.

RADIOLOGICAL FEATURES OF THE ELBOW JOINT

Plain radiographs (see Fig. 7.5)

The capsule of the elbow joint is lax anteriorly and posteriorly so that *effusion* within the joint causes distension of the capsule anteriorly and posteriorly. Fat pads anterior and posterior to the joint are displaced away from the joint by an effusion and become visible as linear lucencies that are separated by soft-tissue densities from the bones on a lateral radiograph.

Arthrography

Arthrography of the elbow joint is achieved by injection of contrast medium between the radial head and the capitellum. The synovial cavity of the joint is outlined and seen to extend proximal to the articular surfaces on the humerus with a configuration on AP views that has been likened to rabbit ears and called the 'Bugs Bunny' sign. On lateral views, a coranoid recess is seen anterior to the lower humerus and an olecranon recess posteriorly.

Distally the synovial cavity is seen to extend anterior to the radius as the preradial recess. This is indented where the annular ligament of the radius surrounds it.

THE INFERIOR RADIOULNAR JOINT (Fig. 7.11)

Type

The inferior radioulnar joint is a synovial pivot joint.

Articular surfaces

These are the head of the ulna and the ulnar notch of the lower end of the radius and the upper surface of the articular disc (the triangular cartilage). This is triangular, with

Fig. 7.11 Joints of the wrist.

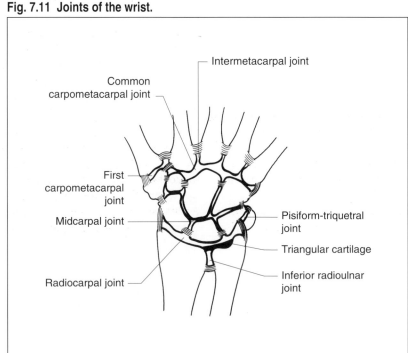

Intermetacarpal joint

Common carpometacarpal joint

First carpometacarpal joint

Midcarpal joint

Radiocarpal joint

Pisiform-triquetral joint

Triangular cartilage

Inferior radioulnar joint

its apex attached to the styloid process of the ulna and the base to the ulnar notch of the radius. It separates the inferior radioulnar and radiocarpal joints.

Capsule

This is slightly thickened anteriorly and posteriorly. It is lax superiorly and extends upwards as a pouch, the recessus sacciformis, in front of the lower part of the interosseus membrane.

THE RADIOCARPAL JOINT (see **Fig. 7.11**)

Type

This is a synovial joint.

Articular surfaces

These are the distal radius and distal surface of the triangular cartilage and the proximal surfaces of the scaphoid, lunate bone and triquetral bones.

Capsule

This is attached around the articular surfaces, except where it extends proximally as the palmar radial recess over the proximal radius to a variable degree.

Ligaments

These are the:

- Palmar and dorsal radiocarpal ligaments;
- Palmar ulnocarpal ligament; and
- Ulnar and radial collateral ligaments.

THE INTERCARPAL JOINTS (see **Fig. 7.11**)

A *midcarpal joint* is found between the between the proximal and distal rows of carpal bones. This is separated from the radiocarpal and the carpometacarpal joints by interosseus ligaments between carpal bones.

The *carpometacarpal joint of the thumb* between the trapezium and the metacarpal of the thumb is separate from the other carpometacarpal joints.

The *carpometacarpal joint of the medial four metacarpals* has a single synovial cavity and is also continuous with the *intermetacarpal joints* of the bases of these bones.

RADIOLOGICAL FEATURES OF THE JOINTS OF THE WRIST AND HAND

Plain radiographs

The normal alignment of the joints of the wrist and hand are visible on PA, lateral and oblique radiographs. Damage to any of the interosseus ligaments can cause displacement of one or more bones.

Arthrography

Arthrography of the radiocarpal or intercarpal or carpometacarpal joints may be achieved by injecting the appropriate space with contrast medium. The synovial cavity extends proximally anterior to the radius as the volar-radial recess. The prestyloid recess is medial to the ulnar styloid process.

The inferior radioulnar, the radiocarpal, the midcarpal and carpometacarpal joints are not usually connected to one another. Studies of arthrograms on cadavers have, however, shown communication between the radiocarpal and inferior radioulnar joint in up to 35% of subjects, between the radiocarpal and midcarpal joints up to 47% and between the pisiformtriquetral joint and the radiocarpal joint in more than 50%. The incidence of these communications increases with age and with force of injection and probably reflects degenerative change.

Magnetic resonance imaging

Bones, intra-articular and periarticular structures can be imaged in several planes. Coronal and sagittal images are used to study the distal radioulnar and the radiocarpal joints. The triangular fibrocartilage is seen to be thin centrally. Its thickened lateral borders may be called the dorsal and ventral radioulnar ligaments.

The carpal tunnel imaged in the axial plane shows the arching carpal bones and the transverse carpal ligament. The deep and superficial digital flexor tendons and the median nerve are seen within the tunnel.

Alignment of carpal bones and the volar and dorsal radiocarpal ligaments are seen on sagittal views. Most important and most frequently identified of these ligaments are the radioscapholunate and radioscaphocapitate ligaments on the palmar surface. Coronal images show the short intercarpal ligaments and intercarpal joints.

THE MUSCLES OF THE UPPER LIMB

Modalities such as CT (**Figs 7.12** and **7.13**) and especially MRI have made imaging of the muscles of the limbs possible. A knowledge of the origin, course and insertion of these muscles is less important in radiology than an understanding of their positions relative to one another in cross-section. A brief description of cross-sectional layout of muscle compartments is therefore appropriate. Muscles related with the shoulder joint have been described in that section (see p. 244).

In *the upper arm* (**Fig. 7.14**), the deltoid muscle covers the upper lateral aspect of the humerus. The flexors of the shoulder — the coracobrachialis and biceps muscles — lie anterior to the humerus in its upper third, while the flexors of the elbow — brachialis and biceps muscles — lie anterior to the lower part of the humerus. Extensors of the elbow joint — the triceps muscle with its long, lateral and medial heads — lie posterior to the humerus.

The neurovascular bundle of brachial artery, basilic vein and median nerve lie superficially, medial to the humerus. The radial nerve and profunda brachii artery lie deeply close to the humerus, at first medially then pass-

Fig. 7.12 CT scan: axial section through the upper arm.

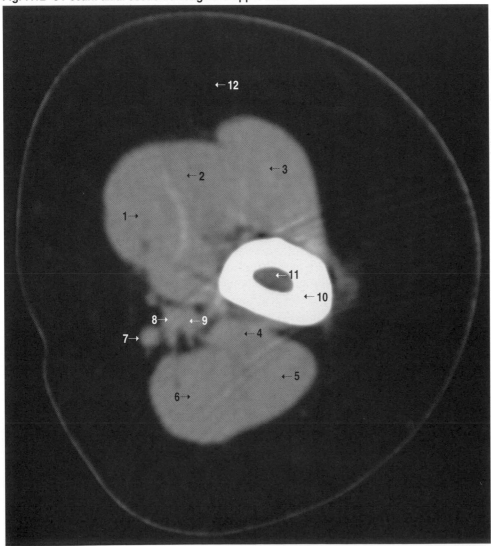

1. Biceps muscle — short head (flexor of the elbow)
2. Biceps muscle — long head (flexor of the elbow)
3. Brachialis muscle (flexor of the elbow)
4. Triceps muscle medial head (extensor of the elbow)
5. Triceps muscle lateral head (extensor of the elbow)
6. Triceps muscle long head (extensor of the elbow)
7. Basilic vein (neurovascular bundle)
8. Brachial artery (neurovascular bundle)
9. Median nerve (neurovascular bundle)
10. Cortex of humeral shaft
11. Medullary cavity
12. Subcutaneous fat in anterior aspect of the upper arm

ing posteriorly close to the lateral side.

In *the forearm* (**Fig. 7.15**) the interosseus membrane unites the radius and ulna and separates anterior and posterior compartments. Anteriorly lie the flexors of the wrist and fingers, flexor digitorum superficialis and profundus. Posteriorly are the extensors of the wrist and fingers and the abductor of the thumb — extensor carpi ulnaris, digitorum and pollicis longus and abductor pollicis longus. The muscles abducting the wrist, flexor carpi radialis and extensor carpi radialis longus and brevis, lie superficially on the radial side and those that adduct the wrist, flexor carpi ulnaris and extensor carpi ulnaris lie on the ulnar side.

The interosseus nerves and arteries lie close to the interosseus membrane. The radial nerve and vessels and the ulnar nerve and vessels lie anteriorly on each side, while the median nerve lies in the midline between the superficial and deep flexor muscles.

The individual muscles may be difficult to distinguish on *axial CT* because of the lack of fat in the forearm. MRI is the superior method in this respect and has the added advantage of allowing direct imaging in many planes.

Fig. 7.13 CT scan: axial section through forearm. The scan was obtained with the palm facing up. Extensive fat allows easier visualization of the muscle groups. The flexors are anterior and the extensors posterior.

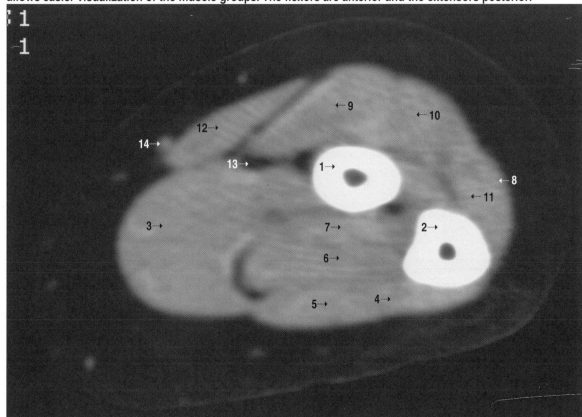

1. Radius
2. Ulna
3. Extensor carpi radialis muscle (longus and brevis)
4. Extensor carpi ulnaris muscle
5. Extensor digitorum muscle
6. Extensor pollicis longus muscle
7. Abductor pollicis longus muscle
8. Flexor carpi ulnaris muscle
9. Flexor carpi radialis muscle
10. Flexor digitorum superficialis muscle
11. Flexor digitorum profundus muscle
12. Brachioradialis muscle
13. Position of radial artery and vein
14. Cephalic vein

Fig. 7.14 Axial section through the upper arm showing muscle compartments: (a) upper humeral level; (b) mid-humeral level.

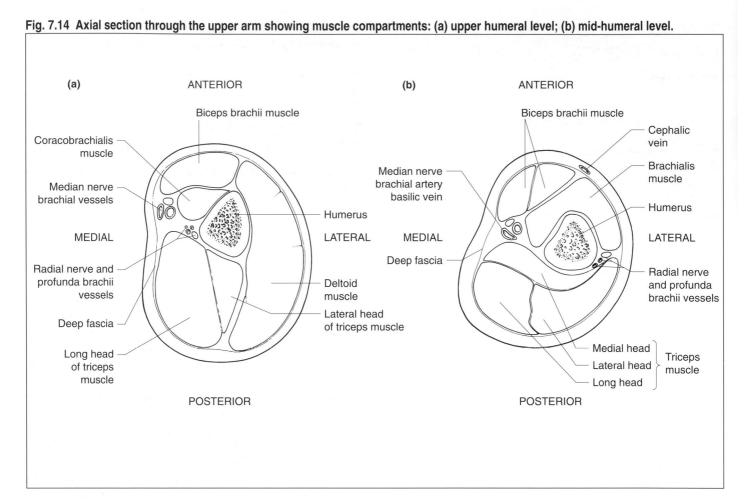

Fig. 7.15 Axial section through the lower arm showing muscle compartments.

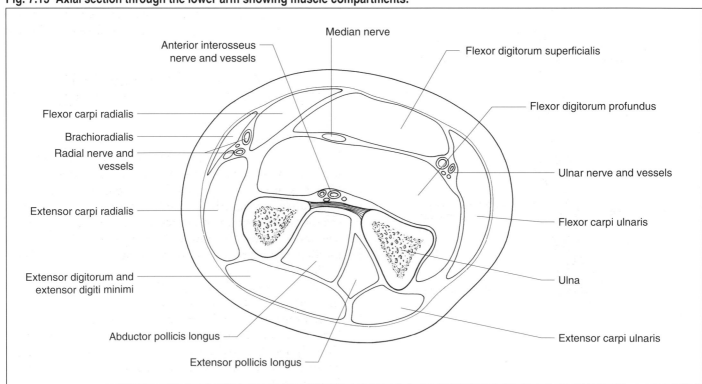

THE ARTERIAL SUPPLY OF THE UPPER LIMB (Fig. 7.16; see Figs 1.42 and 1.43)

The upper limb receives it supply from *the subclavian artery.* This has four branches, namely:

- The vertebral artery;
- The thyrocervical trunk, which supplies the inferior thyroid, suprascapular and transverse cervical arteries;
- The internal thoracic artery; and
- The costocervical trunk which divides into the superior intercostal and the deep cervical arteries.

The subclavian artery becomes *the axillary artery* at the outer border of the first rib. The axillary artery lies with the brachial plexus and the axillary vein. It supplies six arteries to the chest wall and the shoulder:

- The superior thoracic artery;
- The acromiothoracic trunk;
- The lateral thoracic artery;
- The subscapular artery; and
- The anterior and posterior circumflex humeral arteries.

The *brachial artery* begins at the lower border of teres major. Its branches are:

- The profunda brachii artery;
- The nutrient artery to the humerus;
- The muscular branches; and
- The branches to the elbow joint.

At the level of the radial head (but sometimes much more proximally) the brachial artery divides into the radial and ulnar arteries. The *radial artery* passes on the lateral side of the forearm to the wrist, where it gives a branch to the superficial palmar arch and then passes via the floor of the anatomical snuff-box to the dorsum of the hand. It passes between the first and second metacarpals to form the *deep palmar arch.*

The *ulnar artery* is larger and deeper than the radial artery. It gives rise to the *common interosseus artery,* which in turn divides into the anterior and posterior interosseus arteries, the latter passes over the top of the interosseus membrane to supply the muscles of the dorsum of the forearm. Close to the wrist the ulnar artery becomes superficial and having crossed the wrist it becomes the *superficial palmar arch* and sends a branch to the deep palmar arch.

RADIOLOGICAL FEATURES OF THE ARTERIAL SUPPLY OF THE UPPER LIMB

Arteriography (see Fig. 1.42)

Arteriography of the aorta or of its coronary or other branches can be achieved via the arteries of the upper limb. Percutaneous puncture of the axillary artery carries the risks of brachial plexus damage either directly or by haematoma formation. The brachial artery, although smaller, is easier to puncture because of its superficial location over a bone. Damage to the nearby median nerve may occur, as may embolism distally to the radial or ulnar arteries.

Arteriography of the upper limb is achieved usually via the aortic arch by a femoral approach. The vessels and their branches already described are seen. Direct puncture of the subclavian, axillary or brachial arteries is occasionally used, particularly for interventional work such as embolization of arteriovenous malformations of the forearm or hand.

Fig. 7.16 Arteries of the upper limb.

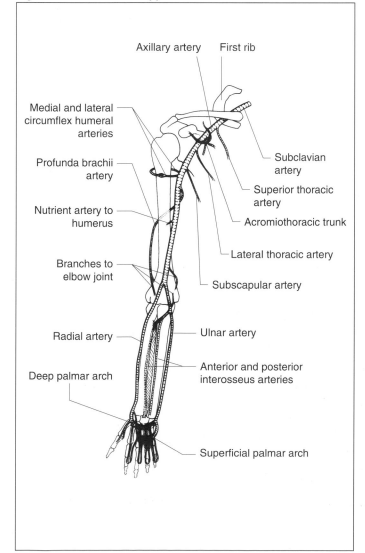

Axillary artery   First rib

Medial and lateral circumflex humeral arteries

Profunda brachii artery

Subclavian artery

Superior thoracic artery

Acromiothoracic trunk

Nutrient artery to humerus

Lateral thoracic artery

Branches to elbow joint

Subscapular artery

Radial artery

Ulnar artery

Anterior and posterior interosseus arteries

Deep palmar arch

Superficial palmar arch

THE VEINS OF THE UPPER LIMB (Fig. 7.17)

Superficial and deep veins drain blood from the upper limb. The *superficial veins* commence in the hand, where smaller veins unite to form three veins — the cephalic and basilic veins from the dorsum and median vein from the palm.

The *cephalic vein* ascends from the radial side of the dorsum of the hand. It winds around the forearm towards the elbow. Here it gives the *median cubital vein* to join the basilic vein and it then continues on the lateral side of the biceps muscle. At the shoulder it passes medially, pierces the clavipectoral fascia to become deep and joins the axillary vein.

The *basilic vein* has a similar course on the medial side of the forearm and elbow. At mid-humeral level it passes deeply and joins the brachial vein to become the axillary vein.

The *median vein of the forearm* passes from the palm along the volar aspect of the forearm to join either the basilic or cephalic veins at the elbow.

The *deep veins* of the upper limb are usually paired *venae comitantes*, which accompany the arteries. The axillary veins are usually double, whereas the subclavian vein is usually single.

RADIOLOGICAL FEATURES OF THE VEINS OF THE UPPER LIMB

Venography

Venography of the upper limb is achieved by injection of the superficial veins of the dorsum of the hand. To visualize the deep veins, films are taken with and without inflation of a tourniquet on the arm above the elbow.

Superior venacavography is achieved by simultaneous injection of veins of both arms. If thrombosis of the superior vena cava (SVC) is suspected and extension into the axillary veins is a possibility then cannulation of the basilic veins is preferable to cannulation of the cephalic veins, since the latter bypass the proximal part of the axillary veins.

Intravenous injection of contrast or radionuclides in dynamic studies

Blood flow in the cephalic vein may be held up at the site where it passes through the clavipectoral fascia. This makes this vein less suitable than the basilic vein for intravenous injection of contrast or radionuclides in dynamic studies.

Fig. 7.17 Superficial veins of the upper limb.

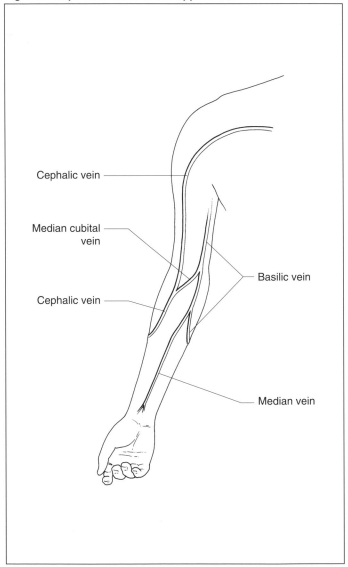

Cephalic vein

Median cubital vein

Cephalic vein

Basilic vein

Median vein

CHAPTER 8 *THE LOWER LIMB*

The bones

The joints

The muscles

The arteries

The veins

THE BONES OF THE LOWER LIMB

THE FEMUR (Fig. 8.1; see Fig. 6.1)

The femur is the longest and the strongest bone of the body. It has a head, neck, shaft and an expanded lower end.

The head is more than half of a sphere and is directed upwards, medially and forwards. It is intra-articular and covered with cartilage apart from a central pit called the fovea, where the ligamentum teres is attached. The blood supply of the femoral head is derived from three sources as follows:

- Vessels in the cancellous bone from the shaft;
- Vessels in the capsule of the hip joint, which reach the head in synovial folds along the neck; and a
- Negligible supply via the fovea from vessels in the ligamentum teres.

The neck of the femur is about 5 cm long and forms an angle of 127° with the shaft. It is also anteverted, that is, it is directed anteriorly at an angle of about 10° with the sagittal plane. Its junction with the shaft is marked superiorly by the greater trochanter and inferiorly and slightly posteriorly by the lesser trochanter. Between these, anteriorly, is a ridge called the intertrochanteric line, and posteriorly a more prominent intertrochanteric crest. The capsule of the hip joint is attached to the intertrochanteric line anteriorly but at the junction of the medial two-thirds and the lateral third of the neck posteriorly.

The shaft of the femur is inclined medially so that, while the heads of the femurs are separated by the pelvis, the lower ends at the knees almost touch. It also has a forwards convexity. The shaft is cylindrical with a prominent ridge posteriorly, the linea aspera. This ridge splits inferiorly into medial and lateral supracondylar lines, with the popliteal surface between them. The medial supracondylar line ends in the adductor tubercle.

The lower end of the femur is expanded into two prominent condyles united anteriorly as the patellar surface, but separated posteriorly by a deep intercondylar notch. The most prominent part of each condyle is called the medial and lateral epicondyle. Above the articular surface on the lateral side is a small depression that marks the origin of the popliteus muscle.

RADIOLOGICAL FEATURES OF THE FEMUR (see Fig. 6.1)

Plain radiographs

A *line along the upper margin of the neck* of the femur transects the femoral head in AP and lateral radiographs. This alignment is changed when the epiphysis is slipped.

A *line along the inferior margin of the neck* of the femur forms a continuous arc with the superior and medial margin of the obturatur foramen of the pelvis. This line, known as *Shenton's line* (see **Fig. 8.6**), is disrupted in congenital dislocation of the hip.

On an AP radiograph, *a line between the lowermost part of each condyle,* while parallel to the upper tibia, lies at an angle of 81° to the shaft of the femur. This amount of genu valgum is normal.

Radiography

The neck of the femur is *anteverted* approximately 10°. In *AP radiography of the neck,* therefore, the leg must be internally rotated 10° to position the neck of the femur parallel to the film.

In a *lateral view of the neck,* a film and grid placed vertically and pressed into the patients side must be positioned at an angle of 127° to the shaft of the femur because of the angulation of neck to the shaft.

Views of the intercondylar fossa (tunnel views) are taken with the knee flexed at an angle of about 135° with a vertical beam and with a beam angled at 70° to the lower leg.

Sesamoid bones

A sesamoid bone called the *fabella* is frequently seen in the lateral head of the gastrocnemius muscle. On radiographs, this is projected on the posterior aspect of the lateral femoral condyle.

Blood supply of the head of the femur

The head of the femur receives its blood supply mainly via the neck as described above. Thus fracture of the neck, especially *subcapital fracture,* disrupts this blood supply and results in ischaemic necrosis of the head in 80% of cases.

Ossification of the femur

The primary centre in the shaft appears in the seventh fetal week. A secondary centre is present in the lower femur at birth (this is a reliable indicator that the fetus is full-term) and another appears in the head between 6 months and 1 year of age. Secondary centres appear in the greater trochanter at 4 years and in the lesser trochanter at 8 years of age. All fuse at 18–20 years of age.

Fig. 8.1 Femur: anterior and posterior views.

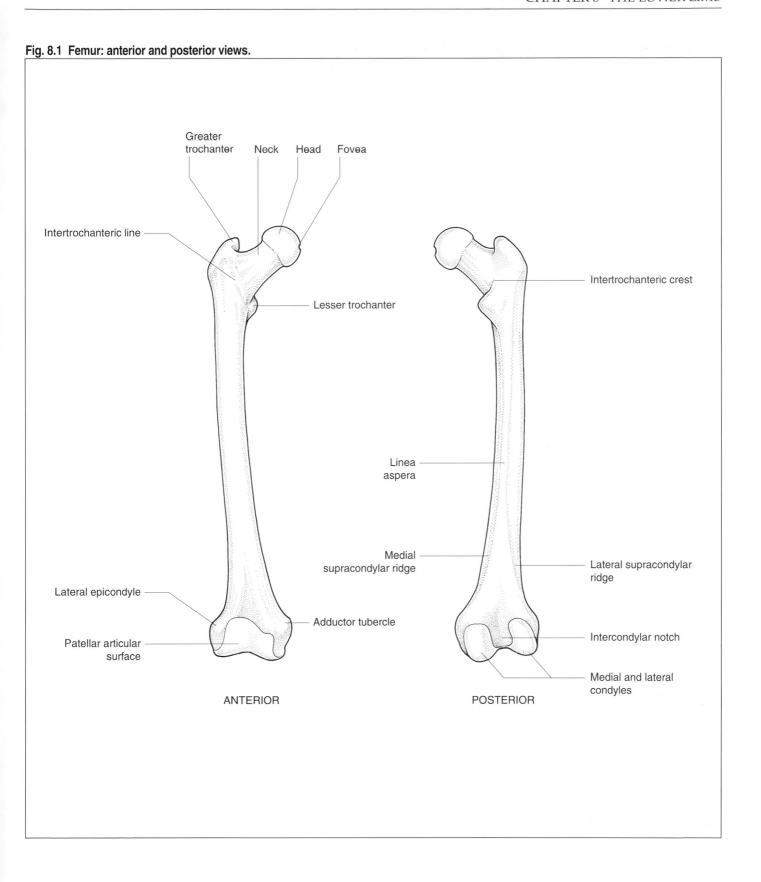

Greater trochanter

Neck

Head

Fovea

Intertrochanteric line

Lesser trochanter

Intertrochanteric crest

Linea aspera

Medial supracondylar ridge

Lateral supracondylar ridge

Lateral epicondyle

Adductor tubercle

Patellar articular surface

Intercondylar notch

Medial and lateral condyles

ANTERIOR

POSTERIOR

Fig. 8.2 Tibia and fibula: (a) anterior view; (b) posterior view.

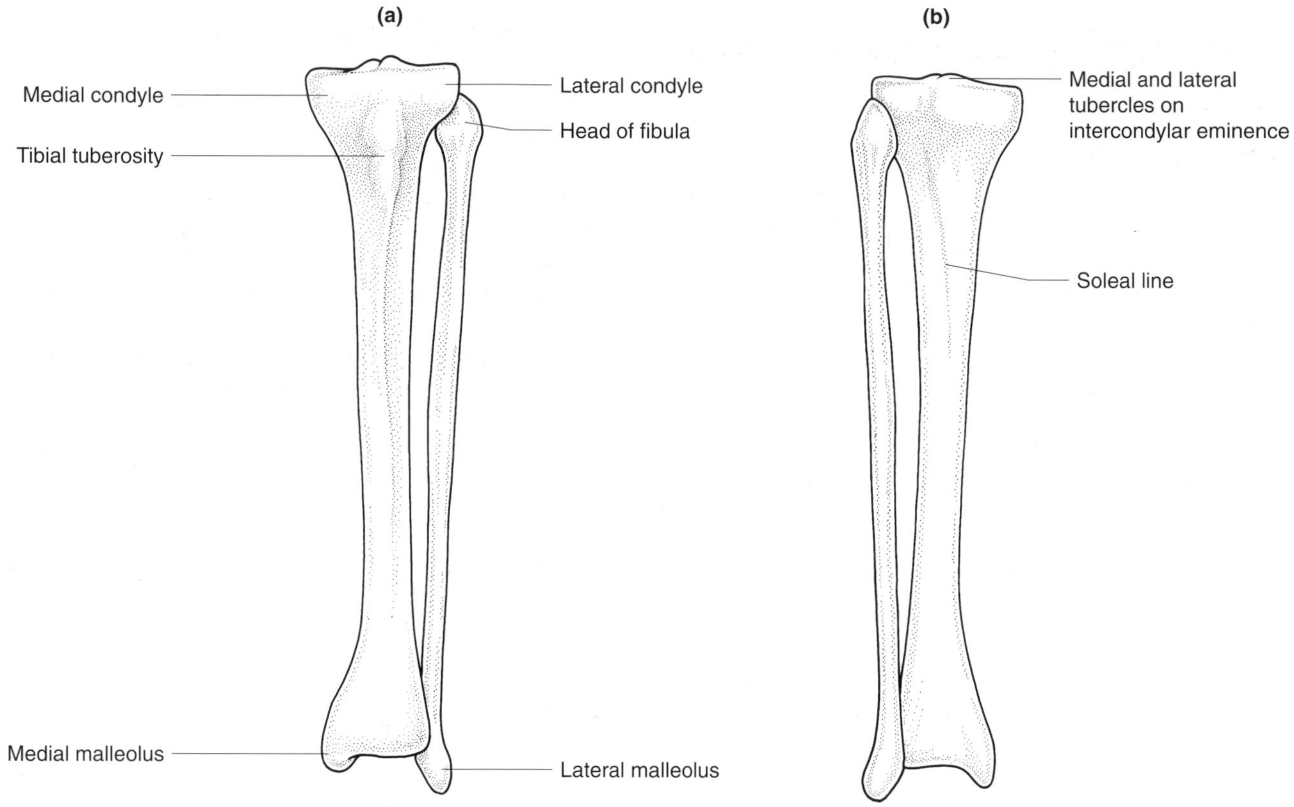

(a)

(b)

Medial condyle

Tibial tuberosity

Lateral condyle

Head of fibula

Medial and lateral tubercles on intercondylar eminence

Soleal line

Medial malleolus

Lateral malleolus

THE PATELLA

This small bone is a sesamoid bone in the quadriceps tendon that continues at its apex as the ligamentum patellae. Its posterior surface is covered with articular cartilage and is entirely within the knee joint, and its anterior surface is covered by the prepatellar bursa.

RADIOLOGICAL FEATURES OF THE PATELLA

Plain radiographs
The outer surface of the patella as seen on *tangential (skyline) views* is irregular due to entry of nutrient vessels here.

Occasionally, the upper outer segment of the patella is separate from the remainder of the bone. Such a patella is called a *bipartite patella* and must be recognized as normal and not fractured.

Dislocation of the patella
Lateral dislocation of the patella is less common than medial dislocation because the lateral condyle of the femur is more prominent than the medial condyle. The vastus medialis muscle inserted into its medial border also resists lateral dislocation.

Fracture of the patella
Transverse fracture of the patella is associated with separation of the fragments by the pull of the quadriceps muscle. *Comminuted fractures* as a result of direct trauma, on the other hand, usually leave the extensor expansion intact and, unlike transverse fractures, do not need open repair.

Ossification
This begins at 3 years and is complete at puberty.

THE TIBIA (Fig. 8.2)

The upper end of the tibia is expanded as the tibial plateau. This has an articular surface with a large medial and smaller lateral condyle, which articulate with the condyles of the femur. Between the condyles is the intercondylar eminence or the tibial spine, which has medial and lateral projections — the medial and lateral intercondylar tubercles.

Anteriorly, at the upper end of the shaft of the tibia is the tibial tubercle into which the ligamentum patellae is inserted. The anteromedial surface of the shaft of the tibia is subcutaneous. The posterior surface of the shaft has a prominent oblique ridge — the soleal line.

The lower end of the tibia has the medial malleolus medially and the fibular notch for the inferior tibiofibular joint laterally. Its inferior surface is flattened and articulates with the talus in the ankle joint.

THE FIBULA (see **Fig. 8.2**)

Apart from its role in the ankle joint, the fibula is mainly a site of origin of muscles and has no weight-bearing function. It has a head with a styloid process into which the biceps femoris is inserted, a neck, a narrow shaft and a lower end expanded as the lateral malleolus. Proximal and distal tibiofibular joints unite it with the tibia and it articulates with the talus in the ankle joint.

The lateral malleolus is more distal than the medial malleolus. The calcaneofibular ligament is attached to its tip. This is often damaged in inversion injuries.

The fibula is proportionately thicker in children than in adults.

RADIOLOGICAL FEATURES OF THE TIBIA AND FIBULA

Plain radiographs
The *tibial tuberosity* is very variable in appearance, particularly during the growth period. Asymmetry and irregularity on radiographs may be quite normal.

Some irregularity of the tibia at the upper part of the *interosseus border* may simulate a periosteal reaction here.

Ossification of the tibia
The primary ossification centre for the shaft of the tibia appears in the seventh fetal week. A secondary ossification centre is present in the upper end at birth and in the lower end at 2 years. The upper centre fuses with the shaft at 20 years, the lower sooner at 18 years.

Ossification of the fibula
Ossification of the primary centre in the shaft begins in the eighth fetal week, in the lower secondary centre in the first year and the upper at 3 years. The lower epiphysis fuses with the shaft at 16 years and the upper at 18 years.

THE BONES OF THE FOOT (Figs 8.3 and 8.4)

In addition to metatarsals and phalanges, there are seven tarsal bones in the foot. These are the talus, calcaneus, navicular, cuboid and three cuneiform bones. Of these, the talus and calcaneus are most important radiologically.

The talus

The long axis of the talus points forwards and medially so that its anterior end is medial to the calcaneus. The talus has a:

- *Body* between the malleoli, with a superior articular surface called the trochlear surface;
- *Neck* grooved inferiorly as the sulcus tali, which, with the sulcus calcanei, forms the sinus tarsi;
- *Head* anteriorly that articulates with the navicular; and
- *Posterior process*, which is sometimes separate as the os trigonum.

The *inferior surface* of the talus (see also the subtalar joint) has a large facet posteriorly for articulation with the calcaneus. Separated from this by the sinus tarsi are three facets, separated by ridges, as follows:

- The middle talocalcaneal facet for the sustentaculum tali of the calcaneus;
- A facet for the plantar ligament; and
- The anterior talocalcaneal articular surface.

These, in turn, are continuous with the talonavicular facet on the head of the talus.

The calcaneus

This is the biggest tarsal bone. It lies under the talus with its long axis pointing forward and laterally. It is irregularly cuboidal in shape with a shelf-like process anteromedially to support the talus — known as the sustentaculum tali. Its upper surface has three facets for the talus (the middle one is on the superior surface of the sustentaculum tali), which correspond with the facets under the talus.

The plantar surface has a large calcaneal tuberosity posteriorly, which has medial and lateral tubercles. There is a small peroneal tubercle on the lateral surface.

The arches of the foot

The longitudinal arch is more pronounced medially. It has two components:

- The medial arch formed by the calcaneus, the talus, the medial three cuneiforms and the first three metatarsal bones; and
- The lateral arch formed by the calcaneus, the cuboid and the fourth and fifth metatarsals.

A series of transverse arches are formed and are most marked at the distal part of the tarsal bones and the proximal end of the metatarsals. Each foot has one half of the full transverse arch.

The arches are maintained by the shape of the bones of the foot, the ligaments and muscles, particularly of the plantar surface.

Fig. 8.3 Bones of the foot: dorsal view.

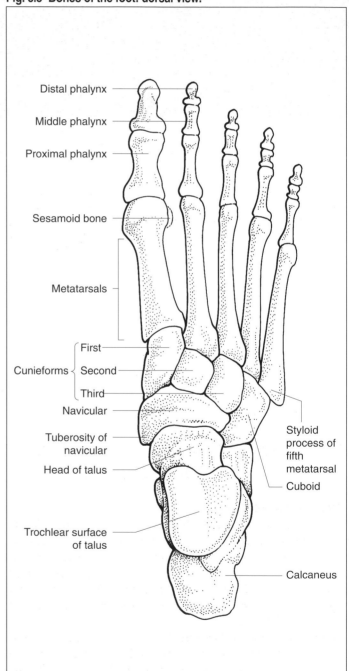

Fig. 8.4 Oblique radiograph of the foot.

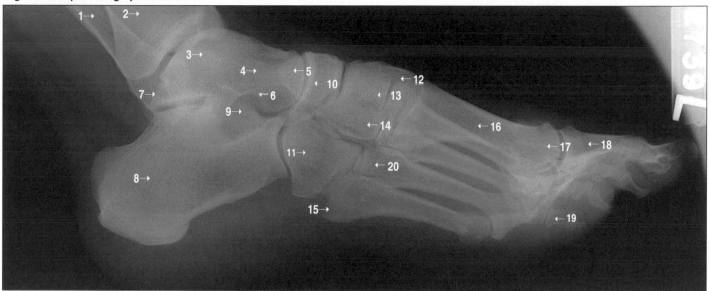

1. Fibula
2. Tibia
3. Talus
4. Neck of talus
5. Head of talus
6. Sinus tarsi
7. Posterior process of talus
8. Calcaneum
9. Sustentaculum tali
10. Navicular
11. Cuboid
12. Medial cuneiform (superimposed)
13. Intermediate cuneiform (superimposed)
14. Lateral cuneiform (superimposed)
15. Styloid process of fifth metatarsal
16. Shaft of first metatarsal
17. Head of first metatarsal
18. Proximal phalanx, first metatarsal
19. Distal phalanx, fifth metatarsal
20. Base of fourth metatarsal

RADIOLOGICAL FEATURES OF THE BONES OF THE FOOT (Fig. 8.5)

Plain radiographs

Boehler's critical angle of the calcaneus (see **Fig. 8.5a**) is the angle between a line drawn from the posterior end to the anterior end of its superior articular facet and a second line from the latter point to the posterosuperior border of the calcaneus. It is normally 30–35° with an angle less than 28° occurring with significant structural damage to the bone.

Heel-pad thickness (see **Fig. 8.5a**) is measured on a lateral radiograph of the calcaneus between the calcaneal tuberosity posteroinferiorly and the skin surface. Normal thicknesses are 21 mm in the female and 23 mm in the male.

On a lateral radiograph of the foot *in children* greater than 5 years old, the *long axis of the talus* points along the shaft of the first metatarsal. In the younger child, the talus is more vertical and its long axis points below the first metatarsal (see **Fig. 8.5b,c**).

The peroneus brevis tendon is attached to *the styloid process of the base of the fifth metatarsal.* The oblique epiphyseal line here should not be confused with a fracture of the styloid process, which is usually transverse (see **Fig. 8.5d,e**).

On a lateral radiograph, *the angle of the longitudinal arch of the foot* is measured between a line along the inferior border of the os calcis and a line along the inferior border of the fifth metatarsal. This angle normally measures 150–170°.

Fig. 8.5 Radiological features of the bones of the foot: (a) Boehler's calcaneal angle and heel pad thickness; (b and c) orientation of the talus in a child; (d and e) styloid process of the fifth metatarsal: epiphyseal line and fracture; (f and g) sesamoids bones of the foot.

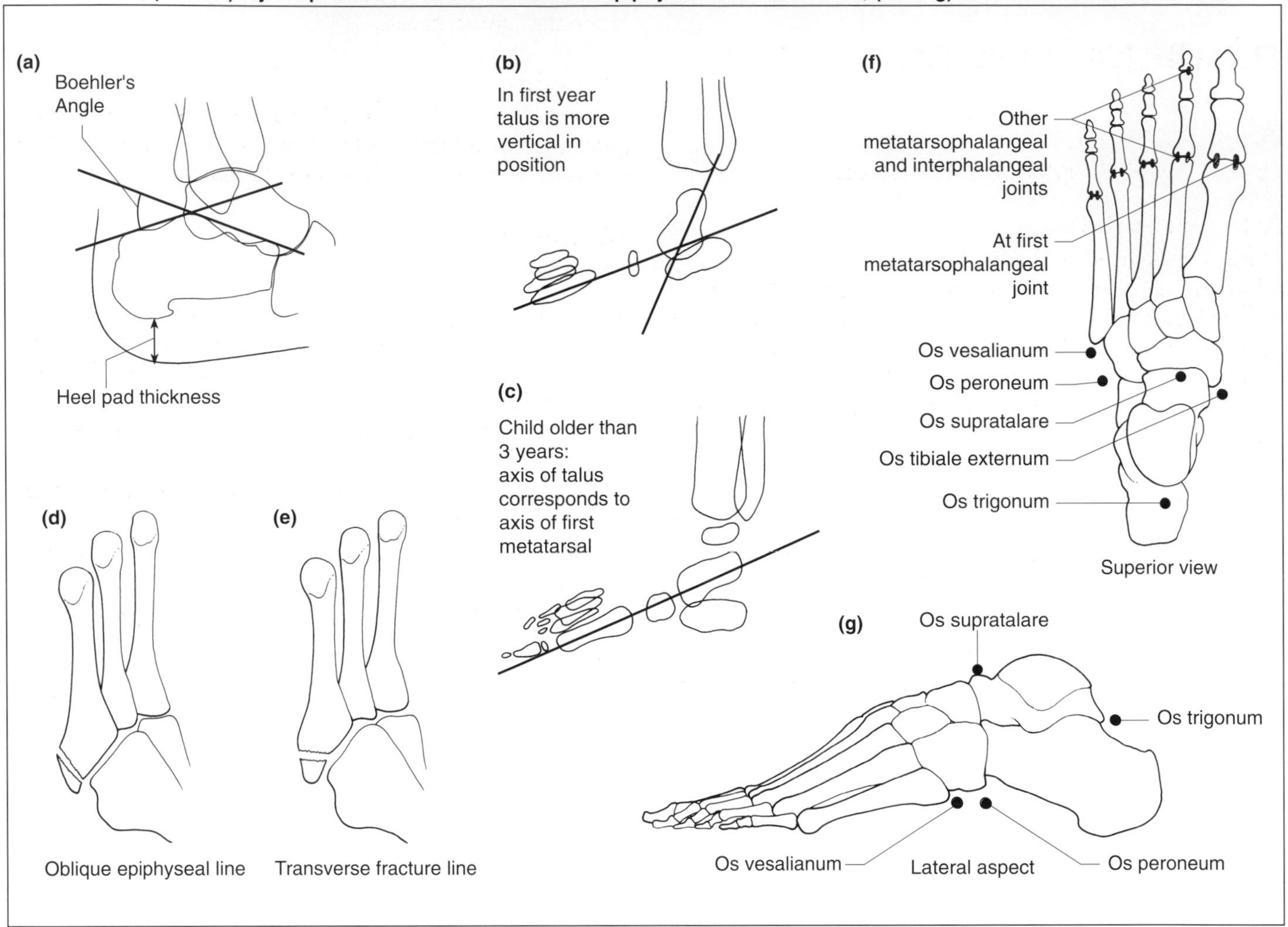

(a) Boehler's Angle

Heel pad thickness

(b) In first year talus is more vertical in position

(c) Child older than 3 years: axis of talus corresponds to axis of first metatarsal

(d) Oblique epiphyseal line

(e) Transverse fracture line

(f) Other metatarsophalangeal and interphalangeal joints

At first metatarsophalangeal joint

Os vesalianum
Os peroneum
Os supratalare
Os tibiale externum
Os trigonum

Superior view

(g) Os supratalare

Os trigonum

Os vesalianum — Lateral aspect — Os peroneum

Sesamoid bones

The commonest sesamoid bones seen in foot radiographs (see **Fig. 8.5f,g**) are:

■ Two sesamoids are found in the tendon of flexor hallucis brevis at the base of the metatarso-phalangeal joint of the hallux. These may be bipartite;
■ Sesamoid bones are often found at other metatarso-phalangeal joints or at the interphalangeal joints of the first and second toes;
■ Os trigonum posterior to the talus;
■ Os vesalianum at the base of the fifth metatarsal;
■ Os perineum between the cuboid and the base of the fifth metatarsal; and
■ Os tibiale externum medial to the tuberosity of the navicular.

Ossification of the bones of the foot

Except for the calcaneus, the tarsal bones ossify from one centre each — the calcaneum and talus ossify in the sixth fetal month and the cuboid is ossified at birth; the cuneiforms and navicular ossify between 1 and 3 years of age.

The *secondary centre of the calcaneus* ossifies in the posterior aspect of the bone at 5 years and its density may be very irregular in the normal foot. It fuses at puberty.

The *navicular* may ossify from many ossification centres. This should not be confused with fragmentation of osteochondrosis or with fracture. Similarly, the *epiphysis at the base of the proximal phalynx of the hallux* may be bipartite in the normal foot.

THE JOINTS OF THE LOWER LIMB

THE HIP JOINT (Fig. 8.6)

Type
The hip joint is a synovial ball-and-socket joint.

Articular surfaces
These are the head of the femur except the fovea, which is a horseshoe-shaped articular surface on the acetabulum. The articular surface is deepened by a fibrocartilaginous ring, the acetabular labrum. The acetabulum has a central nonarticular area for a fat pad and the ligamentum teres and an inferior notch bridged by the transverse acetabular ligament, from which this ligament arises.

Capsule
This is attached to the edge of the acetabulum and its labrum and the transverse acetabular ligament; at the femoral neck it is attached to the trochanters and the intertrochanteric line anteriorly; posteriorly it is attached more proximally on the neck at the junction of its medial two-thirds and its lateral third. From its insertion on the femoral neck, the capsular fibres are reflected back along the neck as the retinacula along which blood vessels reach the femoral head.

Synovium
Synovium lines the capsule and occasionally bulges out anteriorly as a bursa in front of the psoas muscle where this muscle passes in front of the hip joint.

Ligaments
These are as follows:

- Iliofemoral ligament ('Y'-shaped ligament of Bigelow) is an anterior thickening of the capsule between the anteroinferior iliac spine and the neck of the femur to the intertrochanteric line;
- The ischiofemoral ligament is a posterior thickening of the capsule;
- The pubofemoral ligament is a thickening of the capsule inferiorly;
- The transverse acetabular ligament bridges the acetabular notch; and
- The ligamentum teres between the central nonarticular part of the acetabulum and the fovea of the head of the femur.

Fig. 8.6 Hip joint: coronal section.

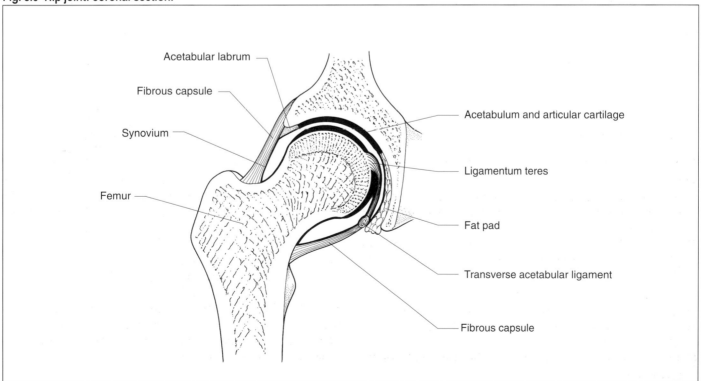

RADIOLOGICAL FEATURES OF THE HIP JOINT

Plain radiographs

On radiographs of the hip joint *pads of fat* seen as linear lucencies outline the capsule of the hip joint and closely applied muscle. Bulging of these is an early sign of joint effusion.

A small *accessory ossicle* is sometimes seen at the superior margin of the acetabulum and should not be confused with a fracture here.

Similarly, irregularity of the superior margin of the acetabulum in children is a normal variant.

In assessment of radiographs of the hip in *infants* (**Fig. 8.7**), the following lines and angles are as described:

- The **Y line** between the unossified centre of each acetabulum, that is, the 'Y'-shaped cartilage between the pubis, ischium and ilium;
- The **acetabular angle,** normally 15–35°;
- The **iliac angle,** normally 65–97°;
- **Shenton's line** along the inferior margin of the femoral neck and along the superior and lateral margins of the obturator foramen of the pelvis should form a continuous arc; and
- Lines along the femoral shafts in **Von Rosen's view** (legs abducted at least 45° and internally rotated) should meet in the midline at the lumbosacral junction.

Arthrography

Arthrography of the hip joint is achieved by injection of contrast anteriorly just below the head of the femur. The synovial cavity, as described above, is outlined. The gap between the articular cartilage covering the bone is smooth and narrow. The ligamentum teres is seen as filling defect within the joint and the transverse ligament of the acetabulum is seen as a defect near the inferior part of the acetabulum. The labrum is visible as a triangular filling defect around the acetabular rim. A superior acetabular recess is found external to the labrum superiorly. An inferior articular recess is seen at the base of the femoral head.

The synovial cavity is seen to extend along the neck of the femur as described above and superior and inferior recesses of the neck are seen in the synovial cavity at the upper and lower ends of the intertrochanteric line.

Ultrasound of the infant hip (Fig. 8.8)

This is useful since visualization of the, as yet unossified, femoral head is possible. The ossified parts of the acetabulum including its roof and the shaft of the femur are seen as echoic areas, while the cartilage of the acetabulum (the triradiate cartilage) and the head of the femur are hypoechoic. The labrum is also visible at the edge of the acetabulum.

Computed tomography of the hip joint

This is particularly useful for visualization in the transverse plane in injuries of the acetabulum. The soft tissues of the pelvis deep to the joint — the obturator internus muscle and the urinary bladder — are also visible.

Fig. 8.7 The infant hip: lines and angles.

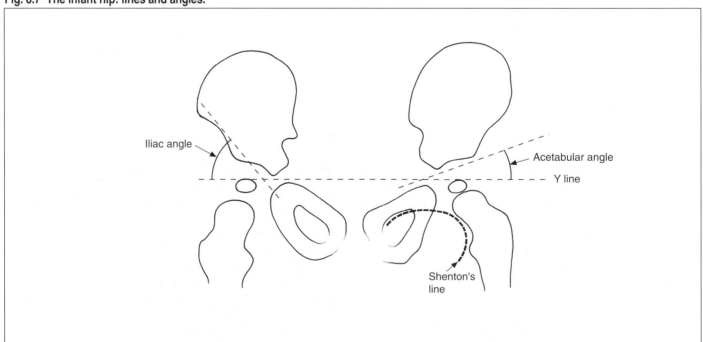

Fig. 8.8 Ultrasound scan of infant hip: coronal view in standard plane.

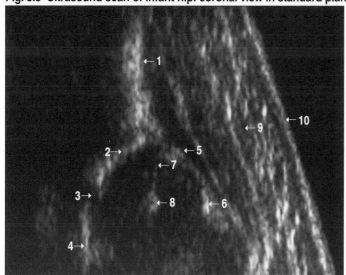

1. Iliac wing
2. Acetabulum (iliac part)
3. Triradiate cartilage
4. Acetabulum (ischial part)
5. Labrum of acetabulum
6. Lower limit of joint capsule as it merges with femoral neck (echogenic focus)
7. Cartilage of femoral head
8. Ossific nucleus of femoral head
9. Gluteal muscles
10. Skin

Magnetic resonance imaging of the hip

MRI is used primarily in the diagnosis of osteonecrosis of the hip. Coronal views are useful and both hips can be viewed simultaneously. The subarticular bone is particularly important in early diagnosis in this condition. A prominent fovea may be misleading but this is usually bilaterally symmetrical. The epiphyseal line, if present, is seen as a low-intensity signal. Bands of low signal intensity from the dome of the femoral head to the medial femoral neck are normal stress trabeculations.

THE KNEE JOINT (Fig. 8.9)

Type

The knee joint is a synovial hinge joint.

Articular surfaces

These are the condyles and the patellar surfaces of the femur; the tibial articular surfaces on the tibial plateau, and the deep surface of the patella.

Capsule

This is attached at the margins of the articular surface, except superiorly where the joint cavity communicates with the suprapatellar bursa (between quadriceps femoris muscle and the femur) and posteriorly where it communicates with the bursa under the medial head of gastrocnemius. Occasionally the joint cavity is also continuous with the bursa under the lateral head of the gastrocnemius muscle or under semimembranosus. The capsule is perforated by the popliteus muscle posteriorly.

Synovium

The synovium lines the capsule and its associated bursae. A fat pad in the joint deep to the ligamentum patellae is called the infrapatellar fat pad. The synovium covering this fat pad is projected into the joint as two alar folds.

Ligaments

These are as follows:

- Medial (tibial) collateral ligament may be separated from the capsule by a bursa;
- Lateral collateral ligament attached to the fibula and always clear of the capsule;
- Ligamentum patellae and medial and lateral patellar retinaculae; and
- Oblique popliteal ligament posteriorly.

Internal structures (Fig. 8.10)

Anterior and posterior cruciate ligaments arise from the anterior and posterior parts of the intercondylar area of the tibia, and are named by their tibial origin. They are inserted into the inner aspect of the lateral and medial femoral condyles respectively. The anterior cruciate ligament resists hyperextension of the knee and the posterior cruciate resists hyperflexion.

The medial and lateral menisci (or semilunar cartilages) are two crescentic structures, triangular in cross-section, which deepen slightly the articular surface of the tibia. Each is attached peripherally to the tibia and to the capsule (the left is less well attached). The upper and lower surfaces of the menisci are free. Each is described as having an anterior and posterior horn attached to the intercondylar area of the tibia.

The medial meniscus is bigger, less curved and thinner. Its posterior horn is thick (14 mm) but it thins progressively to the anterior horn, which is 6 mm thick.

The lateral meniscus is smaller, more curved (nearly circular rather than semicircular) and of more uniform

Fig. 8.9 Knee joint: sagittal section.

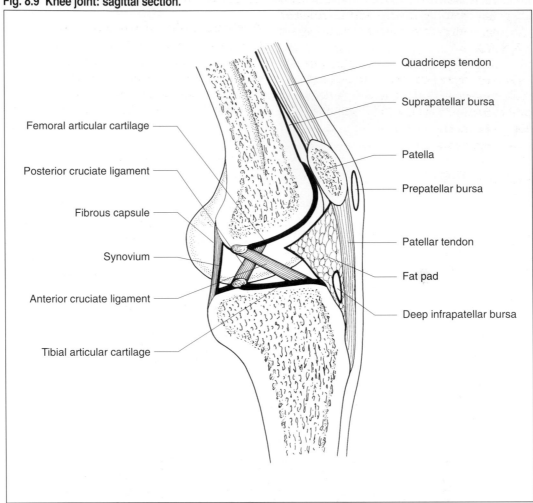

Quadriceps tendon

Suprapatellar bursa

Patella

Prepatellar bursa

Patellar tendon

Fat pad

Deep infrapatellar bursa

Femoral articular cartilage

Posterior cruciate ligament

Fibrous capsule

Synovium

Anterior cruciate ligament

Tibial articular cartilage

Fig. 8.10 Upper end of the tibia: axial section showing menisci and attachments of the cruciate ligaments.

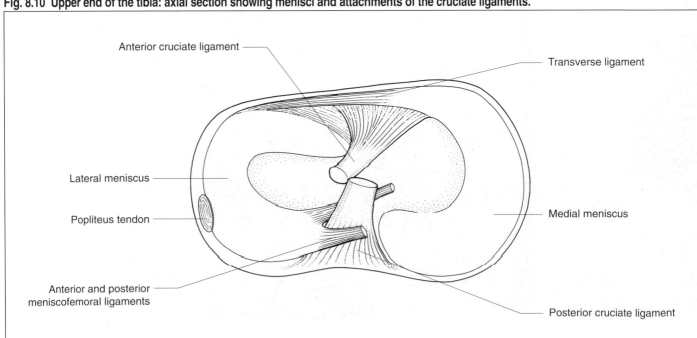

Anterior cruciate ligament

Transverse ligament

Lateral meniscus

Medial meniscus

Popliteus tendon

Anterior and posterior meniscofemoral ligaments

Posterior cruciate ligament

thickness (10 mm). The lateral meniscus is less well attached to the capsule than the medial and is grooved posterolaterally by the tendon of popliteus, which passes between it and the capsule.

The transverse ligament passes between the anterior horns of the menisci. The meniscofemoral ligament passes between the posterior horn of the lateral ligament and the medial femoral condyle. This latter ligament has anterior and posterior parts that pass in front of and behind the posterior cruciate ligament.

RADIOLOGICAL FEATURES OF THE KNEE JOINT

Plain radiographs of the knee joint (Fig. 8.11)

Subcutaneous and intra-articular fat (the infrapatellar fat pad) outline some of the soft tissues around the joint. The ligamentum patellae is made visible this way.

The suprapatellar bursa is best seen on radiographs when distended with fluid. It is then seen as a soft-tissue density above the patella.

Arthrography of the knee joint

Contrast medium and air are introduced into the joint deep to the patella and allow visualization of the synovial cavity of the joint as described above including the suprapatellar bursa and some or all of the associated bursae that may be connected with the joint cavity.

Occasionally, a posterior pouch from the synovium is seen to extend into the popliteal fossa. If such a diverticulum becomes inflamed or its neck becomes obstructed it is referred to as a *Baker's cyst.*

The *menisci* are seen as filling defects, triangular in cross-section, whose upper and lower surfaces are outlined by contrast. Their bases are attached to the capsule (some contrast may pass lateral to the lateral meniscus, which is less firmly attached to the capsule). The tendon of popliteus is seen to groove the lateral meniscus posterolaterally.

A *discoid meniscus* is a variant that extends far into the joint space.

Fig. 8.11 Knee: (a) AP radiograph; (b) lateral radiograph.

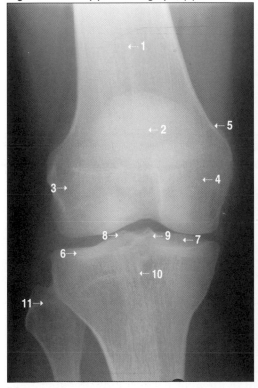

(a)

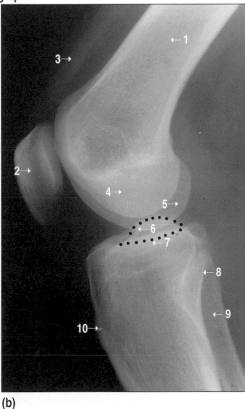

(b)

(a) AP view of knee
1. Femur
2. Patella
3. Lateral epicondyle
4. Medial epicondyle
5. Adductor tubercle
6. Lateral tibial plateau
7. Medial tibial plateau
8. Lateral tibial spine (intercondylar eminence)
9. Medial tibial spine (intercondylar eminence)
10. Fused growth plate, proximial tibia
11. Head of fibula

(b) Lateral view of knee
1. Distal femur
2. Patella
3. Quadriceps tendon
4. Epicondyles (superimposed)
5. Femoral condyle
6. Tibial spines (superimposed)
7. Tibial plateaux (superimposed)
8. Head of fibula
9. Neck of fibula
10. Tibial tuberosity

Fig. 8.12 MRI scan of the knee: sagittal section, T1-weighted image.

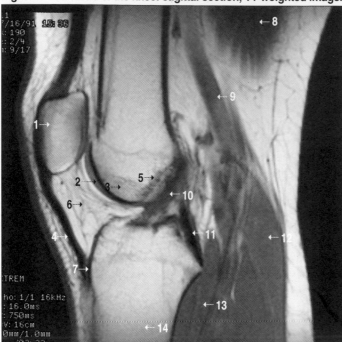

1. Patella
2. Articular cartilage
3. Lateral femoral condyle
4. Patellar ligament
5. Intercondylar notch
6. Infrapatellar fat pad
7. Tibial tuberosity
8. Semimembranosis muscle
9. Popliteal vessel
10. Anterior cruciate ligament
11. Posterior cruciate ligament
12. Gastrocnemius muscle
13. Popliteus muscle
14. Tibia

Magnetic resonance imaging of the knee (Fig. 8.12)

MRI is used in the evaluation of internal derangements of the knee. Sagittal sections are used for viewing the menisci and cruciate ligaments. The anterior cruciate ligament is seen as a straight band between tibia and femur, while the posterior ligament is gently curved in the relaxed, extended and slightly externally rotated knee. The triangular sections of the menisci are seen. Normal structures such as the popliteus tendon and the meniscofemoral ligament (fibres from the posterior ends of the menisci to the femoral condyles) and the inter-meniscal ligament between the anterior horns must not be confused with separated fragments.

Axial sections are used to image the patellofemoral joint and coronal sections for the collateral ligaments.

THE TIBIOFIBULAR JOINTS

The proximal tibiofibular joint is a synovial plane joint that is strengthened anteriorly and posteriorly by ligaments. The distal tibiofibular joint is a syndesmosis, which is united by an interosseus ligament that is continuous above with the interosseus membrane. The interosseus membrane acts as an accessory ligament to both joints.

THE ANKLE JOINT (Fig. 8.13)

Type

The ankle joint is a synovial hinge joint.

Articular surfaces

These are:

■ The lower tibia and the inner surface of the medial malleolus;
■ The medial surface of the lateral malleolus of the fibula; and
■ The trochlear surface of the head of the talus.

The articular surface of the talus is broader anteriorly than posteriorly. This makes the ankle more stable in dorsiflexion (i.e. standing) and more mobile in plantar flexion.

Capsule

This is attached to the margins of the articular surfaces, except where it extends distally to the neck of the talus.

Synovium

This lines the capsule and frequently passes up between the lower end of the tibia and the fibula.

Ligaments

The capsule of the ankle joint is thickened with ligaments medially and laterally but is weak anteriorly and posteriorly.

The *deltoid ligament* is a triangular ligament on the medial aspect of the ankle. It is attached to the apex of the medial malleolus and inferiorly to the medial aspect of the talus, the sustentaculum tali of the calcaneus and the tuberosity of the navicular.

Laterally, the ankle is strengthened by three ligaments:

■ The *posterior talofibular ligament,* which passes medially from the lowest part of the malleolar fossa of the fibula to the posterior process of the talus;
■ The *calcaneofibular ligament,* which passes from the apex of the lateral malleolus to the calcaneus; and
■ The *anterior talofibular ligament,* which passes anteromedially from the lateral malleolus to the lateral aspect of the neck of the talus.

RADIOLOGICAL FEATURES OF THE ANKLE JOINT

Plain radiographs

On AP radiographs of the ankle joint the tibiotalar surfaces are seen to be parallel to each other and perpendicular to the shaft of the tibia. The articular surfaces of the malleoli on each side are symmetrical about a line through the shaft of the tibia, each making an equal angle with the inferior surface of the tibia.

Fig. 8.13 Ankle: (a) medial view — deltoid ligament; (b) lateral view.

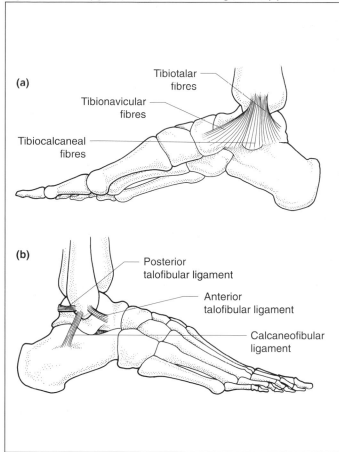

(a)

Tibiotalar fibres

Tibionavicular fibres

Tibiocalcaneal fibres

(b)

Posterior talofibular ligament

Anterior talofibular ligament

Calcaneofibular ligament

The *medial and lateral ligaments of the ankle joint* are not visible on plain radiographs but their integrity can be deduced from normal joint alignment in standard views and, where appropriate, stress views. Where the distance between the medial malleolus and the talus is increased then disruption of the deltoid ligament can be diagnosed, and where there is increased distance between the lateral malleolus and the talus without bony injury this is due to disruption of the lateral ligaments. In general loss of parallelism of the articular surface is significant.

The term **trimalleolar fracture** is sometimes used although there are only two malleoli. The third 'malleolus' is the posterior lip of the tibial articular surface.

Arthrography

The synovial cavity is outlined by injection of contrast and integrity of the medial and lateral ligaments can be assessed. The normal articular surfaces are seen to be smooth and parallel. Recesses of the synovial cavity are sometimes prominent anterior and posterior to the tibia and anterior to the inferior tibiofibular joint.

Filling of the synovium around the tendons of flexor hallucis longus or flexor digitorum longus is also considered normal — both are filled in 20% of arthrograms. The posterior subtalar joint is filled in 10% of normal studies. All other extravasations are abnormal.

Computed tomography

This can be combined with arthrography to assess the bony components of the ankle joint.

Magnetic resonance imaging

This technique is particularly useful for soft tissues, especially ligaments and tendons. The achilles tendon can be seen inserting into the posterior aspect of the calcaneus, separated from the posterior surface of the tibia by a fat pad. The cartilage surface of the articulating bones can be visualized directly, as can the deltoid and talofibular ligaments. Tendons of tibialis anterior, extensor hallucis longus, extensor digitorum longus and peroneus tertius muscles pass deep to the flexor reticunaculum on the posterior aspect of the joint, while the tendons of peroneus longus and brevis pass beneath the peroneal retinaculum on the lateral aspect of the ankle.

THE SUBTALAR JOINT

This synovial joint is responsible for inversion and eversion of the ankle. It has two parts each with its own capsule and synovial cavity as follows:

- The *talocalcaneal joint* between the posterior facet on the inferior surface of the talus and the corresponding facet on the calcaneus;
- The *talocalcaneo-navicular joint* has four contiguous parts (see also the inferior surface of the talus):
- Between the inferior surface of the talus and
  — the sustentaculum tali of the calcaneus
  — the plantar calcaneonavicular ligament and
  — the anterior talocalcaneal facet; and
- Between the head of the talus and the navicular bone.

RADIOLOGICAL FEATURES OF THE SUBTALAR JOINT

Plain radiography

In radiography of the subtalar joint, oblique views of the ankle with the foot internally rotated 45° are used. Films are exposed with tube angulations of 10°, 20°, 30° and 40° for complete visualization of the complex articular surfaces.

Computed tomography

The three components of the talocalcaneal joint, the posterior, the sustenaculum tali and the anterior components, can be seen by coronal imaging with CT.

Magnetic resonance imaging

In addition to bones, MRI can identify muscles. peroneal muscles, that contribute to the stability of the joint as well as ligaments such as:

- The interosseus talocalcaneal ligament;
- The plantar calcaneonavicular 'spring' ligament from the sustenaculum tali to the navicular;
- The short plantar ligament from the calcaneus to the cuboid; and
- The long plantar ligament from the calcaneus to the base of the metacarpals.

OTHER JOINTS OF THE FOOT

The intertarsal, tarsometatarsal, metatarsophalangeal and interphalangeal joints of the foot are synovial joints, each with its own capsule and synovial cavity.

THE MUSCLES OF THE LOWER LIMB

A knowledge of the origin, course and insertion of muscles is less important in radiology than an understanding of the relative position of muscle groups as seen on cross-sectional imaging modalities such as CT and MRI (**Figs 8.14** and **8.15**). A brief description of cross-sectional layout of muscles is therefore appropriate.

In the upper thigh (**Fig. 8.16**) muscles that flex the hip and extend the knee are found anteriorly, that is, the quadriceps femoris muscle made up of the rectus femoris and vastus lateralis, medialis and intermedius muscles. Sartorius, a thin flat strap muscle with similar action, is

also found superficially in the anterior compartment.

The adductor muscles are found medially. These are, from anterior to posterior, the adductor longus, brevis and magnus muscles, with the adductor gracilis lying superficially.

Posteriorly lie the extensors of the hip, the glutei and the flexors of the knee — the hamstrings, that is the biceps femoris, semimembranosus and semitendinosus muscles.

The femoral artery, vein and nerve lie superficially between the anterior and adductor compartments, with the profunda femoris vessels lying deeply close to the femur in the same plane.

At **mid-thigh level** (**Fig. 8.17**), the same general arrangement of muscles and neurovascular bundles is found. The rectus femoris and vasti anteriorly more nearly surround the femur here, and the adductors come to lie posteromedially. The biceps, semitendinosus and semimembranosus lie posterolaterally.

The femoral vessels lie in the adductor canal deep to the sartorius muscle and between the anterior and adductor compartments. The profunda vessels lie almost posterior to the femur also between these compartments. The sciatic nerve lies between the muscles of the adductor compartment and the hamstring muscles.

In the **lower leg** (**Fig. 8.18**), the tibia lies anteromedially subcutaneously. The fibula lies laterally and is more centrally placed. The interosseus membrane between these separates anterior and posterior compartments.

Anterior to the interosseus membrane lie the extensors (dorsiflexors) of the ankle and toes: tibialis anterior and

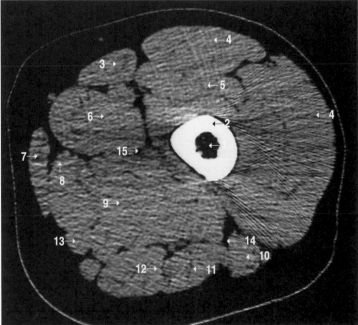

Fig. 8.14 Axial CTscan of thigh.

1. Medullary cavity of femur
2. Cortex of femur
3. Rectus femoris muscle
4. Vastus lateralis muscle
5. Vastus intermedius muscle
6. Vastus medialis muscle
7. Sartorius muscle
8. Superificial femoral vessels in adductor canal
9. Adductor magnus
10. Biceps femoris muscle (long head)
11. Semitendinosus muscle
12. Semimembranosus muscle
13. Gracilis muscle
14. Position of sciatic nerve
15. Deep femoral vessels

Fig. 8.15 Axial CT scan of calf.

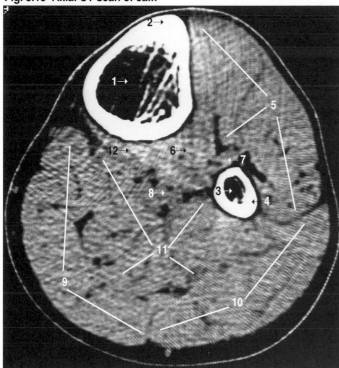

extensor digitorum longus. Peroneus brevis is also part of this group (it extends the ankle in addition to everting the ankle) and is found below the lower third of the fibula.

Posterior to the interosseus membrane lie the flexors (plantar flexors) of the ankle and toes. A deep group include tibialis posterior and, in the lower two-thirds, flexor digitorum and flexor hallucis longus muscles. More superficially lie the soleus, and the gastrocnemius muscle with its medial and lateral heads. These latter two muscles unite inferiorly to form the calcaneal (Achilles) tendon.

1. Medulla of tibia
2. Cortex of tibia
3. Medulla of fibula
4. Cortex of fibula
5. Muscles of anterior tibial compartment
6. Tibialis posterior muscle
7. Anterior tibial artery, vein and nerve
8. Posterior tibial artery, vein and nerve
9. Medial head of gastrocnemius muscle
10. Lateral head of gastrocnemius muscle
11. Soleus muscle
12. Popliteus muscle

Fig. 8.16 Axial section of upper thigh.

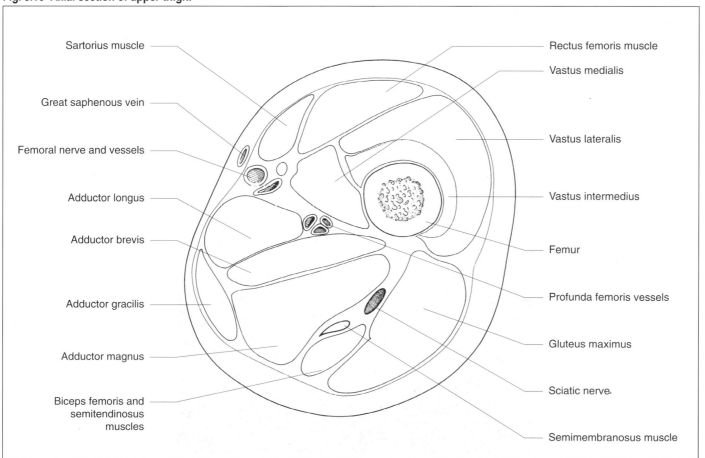

Sartorius muscle

Great saphenous vein

Femoral nerve and vessels

Adductor longus

Adductor brevis

Adductor gracilis

Adductor magnus

Biceps femoris and semitendinosus muscles

Rectus femoris muscle

Vastus medialis

Vastus lateralis

Vastus intermedius

Femur

Profunda femoris vessels

Gluteus maximus

Sciatic nerve

Semimembranosus muscle

Fig. 8.17 Axial section of mid-thigh.

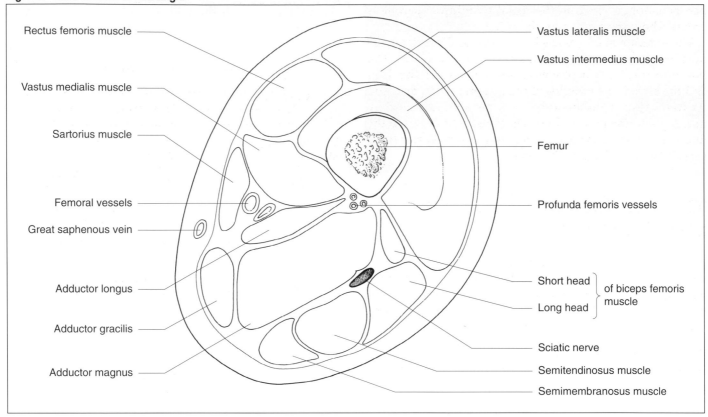

Rectus femoris muscle

Vastus medialis muscle

Sartorius muscle

Femoral vessels

Great saphenous vein

Adductor longus

Adductor gracilis

Adductor magnus

Vastus lateralis muscle

Vastus intermedius muscle

Femur

Profunda femoris vessels

Short head ⎫ of biceps femoris
Long head ⎭ muscle

Sciatic nerve

Semitendinosus muscle

Semimembranosus muscle

Fig. 8.18 Axial section of mid-calf.

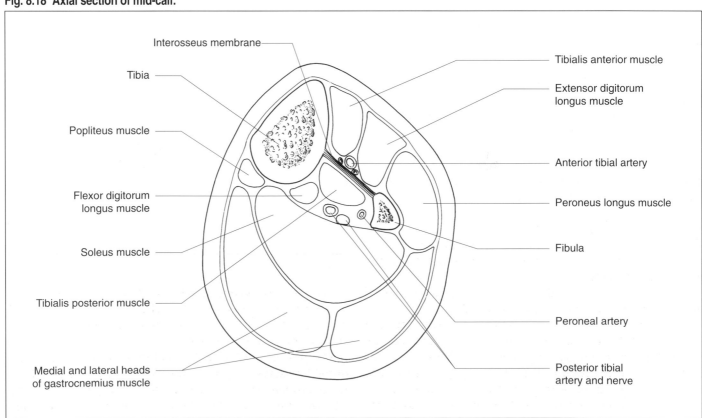

Interosseus membrane

Tibia

Popliteus muscle

Flexor digitorum longus muscle

Soleus muscle

Tibialis posterior muscle

Medial and lateral heads of gastrocnemius muscle

Tibialis anterior muscle

Extensor digitorum longus muscle

Anterior tibial artery

Peroneus longus muscle

Fibula

Peroneal artery

Posterior tibial artery and nerve

A lateral compartment contains two peroneal muscles: peroneus longus and, in the distal two-thirds, peroneus brevis. These are everters of the ankle.

The anterior tibial vessels lie anterior to the interosseus membrane deep to the muscles of this compartment. The posterior tibial and peroneal vessels lie between the deep and the superficial muscles of the posterior compartment. At first close together, these vessels separate as they descend and the peroneal vessels come to lie closer to the fibula in the same muscle plane, while the posterior tibial vessels become closer to the tibia.

THE ARTERIES OF THE LOWER LIMB (Figs 8.19–8.21)

The external iliac artery becomes the *common femoral artery* where it crosses under the inguinal ligament midway between the anterior superior iliac spine and the pubic symphysis. The common femoral artery has three superficial branches at this point, namely:

- The superficial circumflex iliac artery;
- The superficial inferior epigastric artery; and
- The superficial pudendal artery.

The *profunda femoris artery*, its biggest branch, arises 5 cm distal to the inguinal ligament and has six branches as follows:

- Medial and lateral circumflex femoral arteries; and
- Four perforating arteries.

Medial and lateral circumflex femoral arteries

These arteries form a ring around the upper femur. The lateral circumflex femoral artery has an ascending branch that anastomoses with a branch of the superior gluteal artery and it also sends a descending branch to the knee. Thus it can provide a route of collateral supply capable of bypassing an obstructed common femoral artery or an obstructed superficial femoral artery.

Four perforating arteries

These supply the muscles of the thigh (the last of these is the continuation of the profunda) and surround the femur on angiography.

The femoral artery continues as the *superficial femoral artery* and has few branches in the thigh. It passes in the adductor canal between vastus medialis, the adductors and sartorius. At the junction of the upper two-thirds and the lower thirds of the femur it passes through the adductor hiatus close to the femur and into the popliteal fossa to become the popliteal artery. Just before it does this it supplies a descending branch to the genicular anastomosis.

Fig. 8.19 Arteries of the lower limb as seen on angiography.

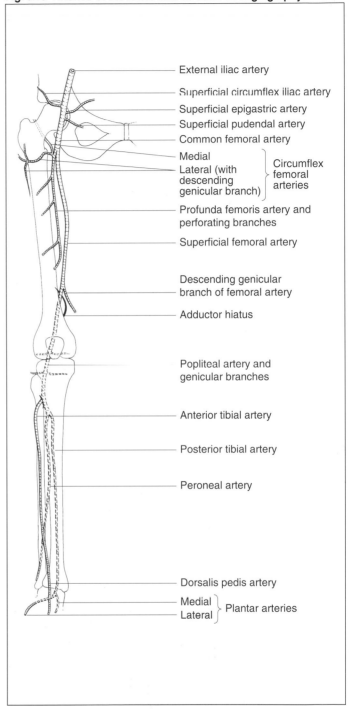

External iliac artery
Superficial circumflex iliac artery
Superficial epigastric artery
Superficial pudendal artery
Common femoral artery
Medial
Lateral (with descending genicular branch) } Circumflex femoral arteries
Profunda femoris artery and perforating branches
Superficial femoral artery
Descending genicular branch of femoral artery
Adductor hiatus
Popliteal artery and genicular branches
Anterior tibial artery
Posterior tibial artery
Peroneal artery
Dorsalis pedis artery
Medial } Plantar arteries
Lateral

The *popliteal artery* (see **Fig. 8.21**) supplies branches to the genicular anastomosis, branches to the knee joint and divides at the lower border of the knee joint into anterior and posterior tibial arteries.

The *posterior tibial artery* is the larger of the two terminal branches. Its proximal part is sometimes called the *tibioperoneal trunk*. It gives rise to the peroneal artery 2.5 cm from its origin. The posterior tibial artery then passes between the superficial and deep muscles of the posterior compartment of the lower leg. As it descends it becomes more medial.

The posterior tibial artery supplies branches to the genicular anastomosis, to the muscles, the skin and the tibia. At the ankle it supplies a medial malleolar branch to the ankle anastomosis and then passes posterior to the medial malleolus (half way between the tip of the malleolus and the midline posteriorly) to divide into the medial and lateral plantar arteries, the principal supply to the foot.

The *peroneal artery* as it descends, comes to lie close to the medial aspect of the posterior of the fibula. It runs behind the distal tibiofibular joint and ends as calcaneal branches supplying the superior and lateral aspects of that bone. Its other branches are the:

■ Muscular branches;
■ Nutrient artery to the fibula;
■ Perforating branch, which perforates the interosseus membrane about 5 cm above the lateral malleolus and descends anteriorly to supply branches to the tarsus; and a
■ Communicating branch, which joins a similar branch from the posterior tibial artery as part of the circle of vessels around the ankle.

The *anterior tibial artery*, after it arises from the popliteal artery, passes above the upper margin of the interosseus membrane and descends anterior to this membrane until it becomes superficial at the ankle midway between the malleoli.

This continues as the *dorsalis pedis artery*, which, having supplied the arcuate artery for the metatarsal and digital arteries, passes between the first and second metatarsals to join the plantar arch.

RADIOLOGICAL FEATURES OF THE ARTERIES OF THE LOWER LIMB

Arteriography of the lower limb (see Figs 8.19–8.21)

This is performed by catheterization of the femoral artery or, in special circumstances, by translumbar aortography or even by approaching the aortic arch from one of the upper limb arteries.

In arteriography, the femoral artery is projected over the lower part of the head of the femur. The superficial femoral artery has a vertical course, while the shaft of the femur lies obliquely. The artery, as a result, is medial to the upper shaft but posterior to the lower shaft as it approaches the popliteal fossa. The profunda femoris artery lies closer to the femur and is also distinguished from the superficial femoral artery by its numerous branches — the superficial femoral artery has no signifi-

Fig. 8.20 Femoral artery angiogram.

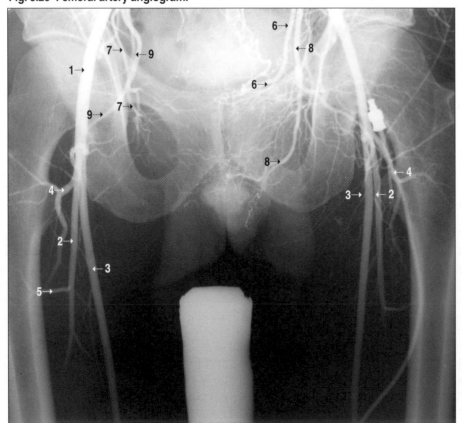

1. Common femoral artery
2. Profunda femoris artery
3. Superficial femoral artery
4. Lateral circumflex femoral artery
5. Perforating artery
6. Superior vesical artery
7. Obturator artery
8. Internal pudenal artery
9. Inferior gluteal artery

Fig. 8.21 Femoral angiogram: popliteal arteries.

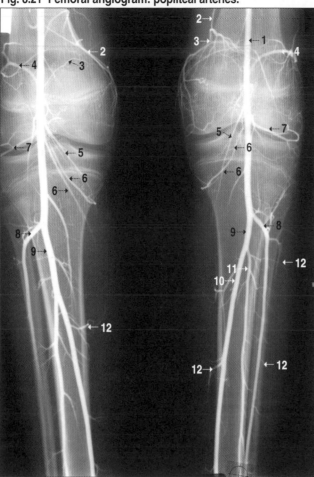

1. Popliteal artery
2. Descending genicular artery
3. Medial superior genicular artery
4. Lateral superior gencicular artery
5. Middle genicular artery
6. Medial inferior genicular artery
7. Lateral inferior genicular artery
8. Anterior tibial artery
9. Tibioperoneal trunk
10. Posterior tibial artery
11. Peroneal artery
12. Muscular branches

cant branch in the thigh. The origin and proximal part of the profunda tend to overlie the superficial femoral artery in AP views and are best seen in oblique views.

The division of the popliteal into anterior and posterior tibial arteries (called the trifurcation because the posterior tibial artery soon gives rise to the peroneal artery) lies over the proximal tibiofibular joint. The anterior tibial artery arises at an angle, while the posterior tibial (the tibioperoneal trunk) is a more direct continuation of the popliteal artery.

The three main vessels of the lower leg lie over and between the shafts of the tibia and fibula. Slight internal rotation of the foot helps to project the tibia away from the fibula and allow the vessels to be seen between them.

The dorsalis pedis artery is best seen on lateral views of the foot and the medial and lateral plantar arteries and the plantar arch are seen on dorsiplantar views of the foot.

Ultrasound

These arteries can be imaged using ultrasound and doppler ultrasound, especially where they are superficial, that is, the common femoral artery in the inguinal region, the popliteal artery in the popliteal fossa and the dorsalis pedis on the dorsum of the foot.

Collateral arteries

Complete occlusion of a major artery in the leg does not always lead to loss of arterial supply to the limb because of the establishment of collateral supply via alternative routes. Thus occlusion of the common femoral artery can be overcome via branches of the superior and inferior gluteal arteries, which anastomose with branches of the lateral circumflex branch of the profunda femoris artery. Obstruction of flow in the superficial femoral artery can be bypassed by descending branches of the lateral circumflex artery and of the perforating branches of the profunda artery anastomosing with branches of the distal superficial femoral artery and of the popliteal artery in the genicular anastomosis.

The anastomosis between all the anterior tibial, posterior tibial and peroneal arteries around the ankle joint allows any artery reaching the ankle to supply the foot.

THE VEINS OF THE LOWER LIMB (Fig. 8.22)

Venous blood is drained from the lower limb by a system of deep and superficial veins. The normal direction of flow is from superficial to deep veins. Valves are more numerous in the superficial than in the deep system, and more numerous distally than proximally. The valves and the deep fascia of the lower limb help to propel the blood towards the heart.

The **superficial veins** are the long and short saphenous veins. The *long saphenous vein* starts on the medial side of the dorsum of the foot and passes anterior to the medial malleolus. It ascends vertically so that it lies posterior to the medial side of the knee and anterior to the upper thigh, where it receives the anterior femoral cutaneous vein on the anterior surface of the thigh. The long saphenous vein drains into the femoral vein via the saphenous opening in the deep fascia in the lower part of the inguinal triangle.

The *short saphenous vein* begins on the lateral side of the dorsum of the foot and passes posterior to the lateral malleolus. It ascends on the back of the calf and pierces the deep fascia over the popliteal fossa to enter the popliteal vein.

The *deep veins* of the lower limb accompany the arteries as described above. They are usually paired, although more than two veins may accompany one artery.

Perforating (communicating) veins carry blood from superficial veins to the deep veins and are variable in site and number. At least two occur in the medial aspect of the lower leg above the ankle. Perforating veins are also found in the medial aspect of the lower thigh.

RADIOLOGICAL FEATURES OF THE VEINS OF THE LOWER LIMB

Venography

Venography of the lower limb is usually performed in cases of suspected thrombosis of the deep veins and is achieved by injection of contrast medium into the veins on the dorsum of the foot. If a tourniquet is applied to the leg just proximal to the first perforating veins then contrast passes into the deep veins and not into the superficial veins. If both superficial and deep veins are filled these are easily distinguished by their different anatomy as already described.

Retrograde venography is performed by injecting contrast into the femoral vein. Retrograde flow of contrast, and especially flow from deep to superficial veins, only occurs if valves are defective.

Ultrasound

Flow of blood in the veins of the leg can be detected by *doppler ultrasound.* Deep veins tend to occur in pairs. Care must be taken in the interpretation of normal flow in the deep veins since the absence of thrombus in a deep vein may be accompanied by thrombus in another vein running in parallel with the patent vein.

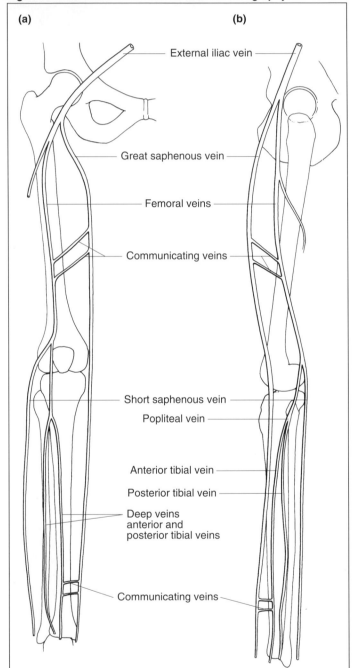

Fig. 8.22 Veins of the lower limb as seen on venography.

(a)

(b)

External iliac vein

Great saphenous vein

Femoral veins

Communicating veins

Short saphenous vein

Popliteal vein

Anterior tibial vein

Posterior tibial vein

Deep veins anterior and posterior tibial veins

Communicating veins

CHAPTER 9 *THE BREAST*

General anatomy of the breast
Radiology of the breast
Age changes in the breast

THE BREAST

The breast **(Fig. 9.1)** overlies the second to sixth ribs on the anterior chest wall. It is hemispherical with an axillary tail and consists of fat and a variable amount of glandular tissue. It is entirely invested by the fascia of the chest wall, which splits into anterior and posterior layers to envelop it. The fascia forms septa called Coopers ligaments, which attach the breast to the skin anteriorly and to the fascia of pectoralis posteriorly. They also run through the breast, providing a supportive framework between the two fascial layers. The pigmented nipple projects from the anterior surface of the breast. It is surrounded by the pigmented areola and its position is variable.

The internal architecture of the breast is arranged into 15–20 lobes, each of which is drained by a single major lactiferous duct that opens onto the nipple. Each lobe is made up of several lobules, which drain via a branching arrangement of ducts to the single lobar duct. Each lobule

Fig. 9.1 The breast: sagittal section.

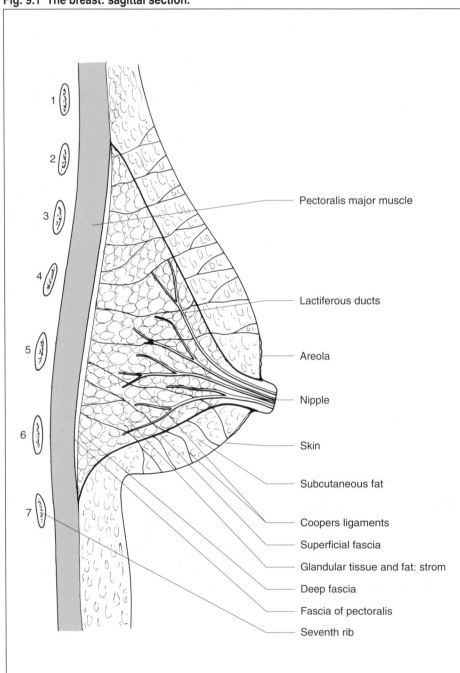

Pectoralis major muscle

Lactiferous ducts

Areola

Nipple

Skin

Subcutaneous fat

Coopers ligaments

Superficial fascia

Glandular tissue and fat: strom

Deep fascia

Fascia of pectoralis

Seventh rib

in turn drains several acini — these are blind saccules into which milk is secreted during lactation. The glandular tissue of the acini and the ductal tissue draining them comprise the breast parenchyma. The fat surrounding the parenchymal structures and the fibrotic framework of the breast constitute the stroma. The relative abundance of parenchyma and stroma varies according to age, parity and other factors.

BLOOD SUPPLY

The blood supply to the breast is composed of the following:

- Branches of the internal mammary (thoracic) artery pierce the intercostal spaces and traverse pectoralis muscle to supply the breast;
- The lateral thoracic branch of the axillary artery; and
- Perforating branches of the anterior intercostal arteries.

Venous drainage accompanies the arteries to the axillary and subclavian veins and the azygous system.

LYMPHATIC DRAINAGE

The lateral aspect of the breast drains to the axillary groups of nodes. The medial side of the breast drains to the internal thoracic chain.

RADIOLOGY OF THE BREAST

MAMMOGRAPHY

This technique uses a low-energy X-ray beam to maximize differences in soft tissue density and demonstrate the internal architecture of the breast. Compression of the breast, a short exposure time and the use of high-quality screen-film equipment improve image quality.

XEROMAMMOGRAPHY

In xeromammography the X-rays discharge a charged selenium-coated metal plate. During processing, charged blue-toner particles stick to the latent image on the selenium plate. This gives a blue-white image of the breast parenchyma. Xeromammography causes 'edge-enhancement', that is, it accentuates the margins of structures in the breast causing them to stand out from the fat. Compression of the breast is not required for xeromammography and the chest wall may also be included on the lateral film.

ULTRASOUND

Ultrasound of the breast may be performed by direct contact scanning or through a water bath. The subcutaneous fat appears anechoic. Linear reflections of Coopers ligaments are sometimes seen traversing the fat. In young women with glandular breasts, the parenchyma is of homogenously high echogenicity. With increasing age the pattern is less homogenous, with increasing deposits of fat showing as anechoic areas. The lactiferous ducts may be seen as small tubular anechoic structures radiating from the nipple. Deep to the breast, an anechoic area of retromammary fat is seen anterior to the echogenic pectoralis muscle.

MAGNETIC RESONANCE IMAGING

This technique is preformed with the breast suspended in a surface coil. With MRI the breast and chest wall may be demonstrated; skin, subcutaneous fat, connective tissue, parenchyma and vessels are also shown. Connective tissue is of low signal intensity and fat has the highest signal intensity. Parenchymal tissue varies in appearance, as with mammography, according to the subject's age and hormonal status.

MAMMOGRAPHIC PATTERNS

Depending on the parenchymal pattern, that is, the relative composition of ductal, fatty and fibrotic or glandular tissue, the following may be seen on the mammogram. The ducts radiate out from the nipple, tapering gradually and are visualized because of the fibrotic tissue that surrounds them. They appear as serpiginous structures and are best seen in the upper outer quadrant. When fat predominates the ducts are visualized easily. When fibrotic and glandular tissue predominate, the ducts are difficult to see. Blood vessels may be distinguished from ducts since they run more haphazardly through the breast and have a more uniform calibre, whereas ducts increase in calibre as they converge onto the nipple.

AGE CHANGES IN THE BREAST

During adolescence the growing breast becomes increasingly glandular. During pregnancy and breast-feeding the number of acini increases with glandular tissue predominating. When lactation stops, the glandular tissue involutes so that the breast is even less glandular than it was prior to pregnancy. Thus the breast of a parous woman is less glandular than the breast of a nulliparous woman of the same age. Apart from the situation during pregnancy and lactation, parenchymal atrophy starts in early adulthood and is accelerated at the menopause, with diminishing amounts of glandular tissue and an increasing amount of fat.

FURTHER READING

GENERAL READING

The following include some of the anatomy 'bibles', such as Gray's Anatomy and Grant's Atlas, as well as some excellent atlases of sectional anatomy. The larger radiology textbooks such as those by Taveras and Ferruci, Grainger and Allison and Sutton all contain excellent sections on normal anatomy in most chapters, the one by Taveras and Ferruci being the most extensive.

Anderson JE 1983 Grant's Atlas of Anatomy, 8th edn. Williams and Wilkins, Baltimore.

Dean MRE 1987 Basic Anatomy and Physiology for Radiographers, 2nd edn. Blackwell Scientific Publications, Oxford.

Ellis H 1976 Clinical Anatomy — A Revision and Applied Anatomy for Clinical Studentss, 6th edn. Blackwell Scientific Publications, Oxford.

Ellis H, Logan B and Dixon A 1991 Human Cross-Sectional Anatomy: Atlas of Body Sections and CT images. Butterworth-Heinemann, Oxford.

Grainger, RG and Allison, DJ 1992 Diagnostic Radiology — An Anglo-American Textbook of Imaging, 2nd edn. Churchill Livingstone, Edinburgh.

Haaga JR and Alfidi RJ 1988 Computerised Tomography of the Whole Body, 2nd edn. CV Mosby, St Louis.

Keats TE 1988 Atlas of Normal Roentgen Variants, 4th edn. Medical Publishers, New York.

Keats TE 1992 An Atlas of Normal Roentgen Variants that may Simulate Disease, 5th edn. Mosby Year Book, St Louis.

Lee JKT, Sagel SS and Stanley RJ 1989 Computed Body Tomography with MRI Correlation, 2nd edn. Raven Press, New York.

Lufkin RB 1990 The MRI Manual. Mosby Year Book, St Louis.

Lyons EA 1990 Practical Color Atlas of Sectional Anatomy. Rowen Press.

McGrath P and Mills P 1985 Atlas of Sectional Anatomy: Head, Neck and Trunk, 2nd edn. S. Karger.

McMinn RMH 1990 Last's Anatomy — Regional and Applied, 8th edn. Churchill Livingstone, Edinburgh.

Meschan I 1975 An Atlas of Anatomy Basic to Radiology. WB Saunders, Philadelphia.

Morley P, Donald G and Saunders R 1983 Ultrasound Sectional Anatomy. Churchill Livingstone, Edinburgh.

Romanes GJ 1981 Cunningham's Textbook of Anatomy, 12th edn. Oxford University Press, Oxford.

Silverman D 1987 Caffey's Paediatric X-ray Diagnosis, 8th edn. Year Book Medical Publishers, Chicago.

Simon G and Hamilton WJ 1978 X-ray Anatomy. Butterworths, London.

Sutton D 1987 A Textbook of Radiology and Imaging, 4th edn. Churchill Livingstone, Edinburgh.

Taveras, JM and Ferruci, JT 1991 Radiology — Diagnosis, Imaging, Intervention. JB Lippincott, Philadelphia.

Wegener OH 1983 Whole Body Computerized Tomography. S. Karger.

Weir J and Abrahams P 1986 An Atlas of Radiological Anatomy. 2nd edn. Churchill Livingstone, London.

Williams PL, Warwick R, Dyson M and Bannister LH (eds) 1989 Gray's Anatomy, 37th edn. Longmans, London.

CNS, HEAD AND NECK

Cremin BJ, Chilton SJ and Peacock WJ 1983 Anatomical landmarks in anterior fontanelle ultrasonography. *British Journal of Radiology* **56**: 517–526.

Hammerschlag SB, Hesselink JR and Weber AL 1983 Computed Tomography of the Eye and Orbit. Appleton Lange.

Phelps PD and Lloyd GS 1990 Radiology of the Ear, 2nd edn. Springer, Berlin.

Schnitzlein HN and Murtagh FR 1985 Imaging anatomy of the head and spine. In: A Photographic Colour Atlas of MRI, CT, Gross and Microscopic Anatomy in Axial, Coronal and Sagittal Planes. Urban and Schwarzenberg.

Valvassori GE, Potter GD, Hanafee WN, Carter BL and Buckingham RA 1984 Radiology of the Ear, Nose and Throat. WB Saunders, Philadelphia.

Wilson M 1963 The Anatomic Foundation of Neuroradiology of the Brain. Little Brown, Boston.

CHEST

Felson B 1973 Chest Roentogenology. WB Saunders, Philadelphia.

Fraser RG Pare JAP Pare PD Fraser RS G Genereux P 1990 Diagnosis of Diseases of the Chest. Vol. I, Chapter 1. The Normal Chest. WB Saunders, Philadelphia.

Nadich DP, Zerhouni EA and Siegelmann SS 1990 CT/MR of the Thorax, 2nd edn. Raven Press, New York.

ABDOMEN, PELVIS AND GASTROINTESTINAL TRACT

Couinaud C 1957 Le Foie. Masson et Cie, Paris.

Feldberg MAM 1983 Computed Tomography of the Retroperitoneum: An Anatomical and Pathological Atlas with Emphasis on the Fascial Planes. Martinus Nijhoff, Dordrecht.

Gelfand DW 1984 Gastrointestinal Radiology: Performing and Interpreting Fluoroscopic Examinations. Churchill Livingstone, London.

Healey JE and Schroy PC 1953 Anatomy of the biliary ducts within the liver. *Archives of Surgery* **66**: 599–616.

Herlinger H, Lunderquist A and Wallace S (eds) 1983 Clinical Radiology of the Liver. Marcell Dekker, New York.

Margulis AR and Burhenne HJ 1989 Alimentary Tract Radiology, 4th edn. CV Mosby, Philadelphia.

Margulis AR and Burhenne HJ 1989 Alimentary Tract Radiology. CV Mosby, St Louis.

Marks WM and Cullen PW 1981 Gastroesophageal region: Source of confusion on CT. *American Journal of Radiology* **136**: 359–362.

Meyers MA 1986 Computed Tomography of the Gastrointestinal Tract. Springer, Berlin.

Meyers MA 1982 Dynamic Radiology of the Abdomen: Normal and Pathologic Anatomy, 2nd edn. Springer, Berlin.

Whalen JP 1976 Radiology of the Abdomen — Anatomic Basis. Lea and Febiger, Philadelphia.

SPINE AND LIMBS

Forrester DM and Braun JC 1987 Radiology of Joint Diseases, 3rd edn. WB Saunders, Philadelphia.

Freiberger RH and Kaye JJ 1979 Arthrography. Appleton-Century-Crofts.

Guerra J Jr *et al.* 1978 The adult hip, an anatomic study, Part II: The soft-tissue landmarks. *Radiology* **128**: 11–20.

Keck C. 1960 Discography, techniques and interpretation. *Archives of Surgery* **80**: 580–585.

McCulloch JA and Waddell G 1978 Lateral lumbar discography. *British Journal of Radiology* **51**: 498–502.

Resnick D 1989 Bone and Joint Imaging. WB Saunders, Philadelphia.

MAMMOGRAPHY

Tabar L and Dean PB 1985 Teaching Atlas of Mammography, 2nd edn. Georg Thieme.

ANGIOGRAPHY

Herbert L Abrams 1982 Coronary Angiography. Little Brown, Boston.

Herbert L Abrams 1983 Abrams Angiography: Vascular and Interventional Radiology, 3rd edn. Little Brown, Boston.

INDEX

A

Abdomen   147-204
  see individual subsections
Abdominal aorta   192-3, 204
  branches of   192
  computed tomography   192-3
  magnetic resonance imaging   193
  radiology   192-3
  ultrasound   192
Abdominal wall   148, 201-4
Accessory fissures   118
Acromioclavicular joint   243
Adenoids   31
Adrenal glands   190-2, 202
  anatomy   190-1
  arterial supply   191
  arteriography   192
  computed tomography   191
  magnetic resonance imaging   192
  radiology   191
  ultrasound   192
  variants   191
  venography   192
  venous drainage   191
Alar ligament   95
Ambient cisterns   66-7
Ampulla
  of uterine tubes   228
  of Vater   174
Anal canal   213
  blood supply   213
  lymph drainage   213
Angiography
  adrenal   192
  aortic arch   40
  bronchial   104, 123
  cardiac   131
  carotid   41, 76
  cerebral   76
  coeliac   156
  colonic   167
  coronary   131
  duodenal   159
  hepatic   171
  iliac   216
  lower limb   272
  mesenteric   194, 195
  pancreatic   179
  pulmonary   123
  renal   189
  spinal   104
  upper limb   251
  vertebral   74

Ankle joint
  anatomy   266
  arthrography   267
  plain radiographs   266-7
  radiology   266-7
Annulus fibosis   97
Anterior descending artery   129
Anterior jugular vein   41
Anterior junction line   143
Aorta   132-3, 140
  abdominal   192
  arch   132
  ascending   132
  isthmus   133
  thoracic   132
  see also Abdominal aorta
Aortic valve   128
Aortopulmonary mediastinal stripe   143
Aortopulmonary window   140, 143
Apical ligament   95
Appendices epiploicae   162
Appendix   162
  barium-enema examination   162
  position of   162
  radiology   162
  ultrasound   162
Aqueduct   9
  cerebral   63
Arachnoid mater   68, 100
Arteries
  anterior tibial   273
  aorta   132, 140, 192
  arteria radicularis magna (artery of
    Adamkiewicz)   101
  ascending pharyngeal   39
  axillary   251
  basilar   75
  brachial   251
  bronchial   115, 119
  caroticotympanic   71
  central retinal   20
  cerebellar   75
  cerebral, anterior   73
    middle   73
    posterior   78
  carotid, common   38
    external   38
    internal   38, 73
  choroidal, anterior   73
    posterior   75
  circle of Willis   76
  coeliac   192, 194
  communicating, anterior   73
    posterior   71

  coronary, left   129
    right   128
  deep palmar arch   251
  dorsalis pedis   272
  facial   39
  femoral, common   271
    deep (profunda femoris)   271
    superficial   271
  frontopolar   73
  gastric and gastroepiploic   152,
    158
  hepatic   170
  iliac, common   214
    external   215
    internal   214
  lingual   39
  marginal   165
  maxillary   39
  meningeal, accessory   40;
    middle   8, 40
  meningohypophyseal   71
  mesenteric, inferior   165, 195
    superior   164, 194
  middle temporal   8
  occipital   39
  ophthalmic   20, 71
  pancreas, of   178
  peroneal   271
  phrenic   110
  popliteal   271
  pulmonary   118, 134
  posterior tibial   271
  profunda femoris   271
  pterygoid   7
  radial   251
  radicular   101
  radiculomedullary   101
  renal   185, 189
  splenic   180
  striate   73
  subclavian   43, 134, 251
  superficial palmar arch   251
  superior thyroid   39
  superficial temporal   39
  tibioperoneal trunk   271
  ulnar   251
  vertebrobasilar   43, 73
Arteria radicularis magna   101
Arthrography
  ankle   267
  discography   97
  elbow   246
  facet   95
  hip   262

knee 265
shoulder 245
temporomandibular joint 16
wrist 247
Arteriography *see* Angiography
Arthrography
ankle 267
elbow 246
hip 262
shoulder 245
temporomandibular joint 16
wrist 247
Atlantoaxial joint 95
Atlas 86-7
Atrioventricular bundle of His 131
Atrioventricular node 131
Atrium
right 126
left 128
Auditory cortex 47
Axis 87
Azygo-oesophageal line 143
Azygous fissure 118
Azygous system 138-9

B

Basal ganglia
anatomy 52-3
computed tomography 53
magnetic resonance imaging 53
radiology 53
ultrasound examination of the
neonatal brain 53
Bile ducts 174
ultrasound 174
Biliary system
anatomy 172-5
computed tomography 175
contrast examinations 175
radiology 175
scintigraphy 175
ultrasound 175
Bladder 217-18
blood supply 218
contrast studies 218
cross-sectional imaging 218
lymph drainage 218
peritoneal reflections 218
plain films 218
radiology 218
rupture 218
Boehler's angle 259
Brachiocephalic veins 41, 134

Brain *see* CNS
Brainstem 58-61
anatomy 58
anterior surface 54
Breast 275-7
age changes 277
anatomy 276-7
blood supply 277
lymphatic drainage 277
magnetic resonance imaging
277
mammography 277
radiology 277
ultrasound 277
xeromammography 277
Broad ligament 229
Bronchi
anatomy 115
angiography 104, 123
arteries 115, 119-20
blood supply 115
bronchial tree 116
bronchography 122
computed tomography 123
isotope ventilation-perfusion
scanning 123
lateral chest radiograph 122
PA chest radiograph 120-1
magnetic resonance imaging
123
PA chest radiograph 120
plain tomography 122
radiology 120-3
veins 115, 120
Bronchopulmonary segments 118

C

Caecum 161
Calcaneus 258
Canals of Lambert 118
Cardiac chambers 126-8
Cardiac valves 126-8
Cardiac veins 130
Carina 115
Carotid canal 71
Carotid vessels 38-41, 71
anatomy 38-40
angiography 41, 76-7
computed tomography 41
magnetic resonance imaging 41
radiology 41
ultrasound 41

Carpal angle 243
Carpal bones 242
ossification 242
radiography 242
radiology 242
Carpal tunnel 242
Cartilages
arytenoid 31
corniculate 32
costal 106
cricoid 31
of knee 263
semilunar 263
thyroid 31
Caudate lobe 168, 170
venous drainage 172
Caudate nucleus 52, 53
Cavernous sinuses 56
coronal section 55
Cavum
septi pellucidae 65
vergae 65
Central nervous system (CNS)
45-84
arterial supply 70-7
angiography 76-7
computed tomography 77
magnetic resonance imaging 77
plain radiographs 76
radiology 76-7
cross-sectional anatomy
82-4
radionuclide cerebral
angiogram 77
ultrasound 77
venous drainage 77
Cerebellomedullary cistern 66
Cerebellum 60-1
arterial supply 61
computed tomography 61
function of 61
radiology 61
venous drainage 61
Cerebral aqueduct 63
Cerebral arteries, distribution 70
Cerebral cortex 46
anatomy 46-9
computed tomography 49
radiology 49
Cerebral hemispheres 46-51, 60
medial surface 70
superolateral surface 70
types of fibres 49
white matter of 49-52

Cerebral veins 77-81
  angiography 80
  contrast-enhanced computed
        tomography 80-1
  deep veins 78
  radiology 80-1
  radionucleotide brain scans 81
  skull radiography 80
  superficial veins 78
Cerebrospinal fluid (CSF) 62
  production and flow 67-8
  magnetic resonance imaging 68
  radiology 67-8
    radionuclide cisternography 68
    skull radiographs 68
Cervical myelography 67
Cervical spinal cord, myelographic
      appearance 102
Cervical spine
  magnetic resonance imaging 94
  radiography 92
Cervical vertebrae 86-7
Cervix 226
Chilaiditis syndrome 166
Choroid plexus of the lateral ventricle
      62
Cisterna chyli 198
Cisterna magna 66
Cisterns 66-7
  see Subarachnoid cisterns
        and individual cisterns
Claustrum 53
Clavicle 237-8
  chest radiography 238
  ossification 238
  radiology 238
CNS 45–104
Coccyx 88, 206
Coeliac artery 194
Coeliac trunk, angiography 156
Colon 162-7, 204
  angiography 167
  arterial supply 164-5
  development of 166
  double-contrast barium-enema
        examination 166
  lymphatic drainage 166
  peritoneal attachments 162-3
  radiology 166
  relations of 163
  venous drainage 165
Commissures
  anterior 63
  habenular 49

of fornix 57
posterior 51
Conjuntivae 20
Conus medullaris 48
Cornea 25
Corona radiata 51
Coronary angiography 129, 131
Coronary arteries 128-30
Coronary veins 130
Corpus callosum 49
Costal cartilages 106
Cranial fossae 6
Cruciform ligament 95
Cribriform plate 5
Crista galli 5
Crura of diaphragm 109

D

Deep palmar arch 251
Denticulate ligament 100
Diaphragm 109
  anatomy 109-10, 201, 202
  blood supply 110
  computed tomography 110
  curvature of the dome 110
  lateral chest radiograph 110
  magnetic resonance imaging 110
  nerve supply 110
  openings in 109
  PA chest radiograph 110
  radiology 110, 201, 202
  structures piercing 110
  ultrasound 110
Disc see also Distal radioulnar joint;
        temporomandibular joint;
        intervertebral disc
Ductus arteriosus 132
Ductus venosum 168
Duodenum 157-9, 204
  anatomy 157-8
  angiography 159
  arterial supply 158
  barium studies 158
  computed tomography 159
  lymphatic drainage 158
  radiology 158-9
  ultrasound 159
  venous drainage 158
Dura mater 68, 100

E

Ear 24-6
  anatomy 24-5

computed tomography 25
internal auditory meati 26
coronal section 24
cross-sectional anatomy 25
external ear 24
inner ear 25
internal auditory meatus 25
magnetic resonance imaging 26
middle ear 24
plain films 25
plain tomography 25
radiology 25
Ejaculatory ducts 221
Elbow joint 245-6
  arthrography 246
  plain radiographs 246
  radiology 246
Endocrine glands 37
Endomyelography 104
Endoscopic retrograde cholangio-
        pancreatography (ERCP) 179
Eparterial bronchus 115
Epididymis 224
  blood supply 224
Epidurography 104
Epiglottis 32
Ethmoid sinuses 12
Eye
  computed tomography 23
  internal anatomy and coverings
        21
  magnetic resonance imaging 23
  plain films 22
  radiology 22
  ultrasound 22

F

Facial bones 10
Fallopian tubes 228
  blood supply 228
  lymph drainage 228
Falx
  cerebri 68
  cerebelli 68
Fasciae
  conal 185
  perinephric 185
  pararenal 185
Femur 254
  blood supply of head 254
  ossification 254
  radiography 254
  radiology 254

Filum terminale 98
Fibula 257
  ossification 257
  radiology 257
Fissures, pulmonary
  accessory 118
  azygous 118
  computed tomography 123
  inferior accessory 118
  interlobar 118
  lateral chest radiograph 121-2
  left transverse 118
  oblique (major) 118
  PA chest radiograph 120
Foot
  arches 258
  bones 258-60
    ossification 260
    plain radiographs 259-60
    radiology 259-60
Foramina
  epiploic 199
  interventricular 62, 67
  intervertebral 86
  jugular 8
  lacerum 8
  magnum 8
  obturator 206, 207
  optic 11
  ovale, of base of skull 78
       of heart 126
  rotundum 8
  sacral 88
  spinosum 7, 8
  transversarium 8
Forearm, muscles 249
Fornix 57
Fossae
  coranoid 238
  cranial
    anterior 6
    middle 6
    posterior 6
  glenoid 236, 243
  infrabulbar 219
  ischiorectal 210
  navicular 219
  olecranon 238
  piriform 30
  pituitary 6, 7, 8
  radial 240
  Rosenmueller, of 27
  rhomboid 237
  temporomandibular 14

Fourth ventricle 63-4
Frontal lobe 46
Frontal sinuses 12

G

Gall bladder 172-4
  arterial supply 173
  relations of 173
  venous drainage 174
Genital organs
  female 225
  male 221
Glands see individual glands
Glenohumeral joint 243
Globus pallidus 53
Great vessels 132-4
  radiology 134
Grey matter, subcortical 52-3

H

Habenular commissure 49-51
Hand
  arthrography 247
  magnetic resonance imaging 247
  plain radiographs 247
  radiology 247
Head and neck 1-44
Heart 125-32
  angiocardiography 131
  chest radiography 131
  computed tomography 132
  conducting system 131
  echocardiography 131
  fluoroscopy 131
  gross anatomy and orientation
       125
  magnetic resonance imaging 132
  nuclear medicine studies 131-2
  radiology 131
  SPECT 131-2
Heel-pad thickness 259
Hepatic arteriography 171
Hepatic artery embolization 171
Hepatic scintigraphy 172
Hepatic venography 172
Hilar angle 121
Hilar point 121
Hip joint 261-3
  anatomy 261
  arthrography 262
  computed tomography 262
  magnetic resonance imaging 263

  plain radiographs 262
  radiology 262
  ultrasound of infant hip 262
Hippocampus 57
Humerus 238-9
  ossification 239
  plain radiographs 239
  radiology 239
Humour
  aqueous 21
  vitreous 21
Hyoid bone 32
Hyparterial bronchus 115
Hypophysis cerebri see Pituitary
       gland
Hypothalamus 54
  anatomy 54-5
  magnetic resonance imaging 55
  radiology   55
Hypotonic duodenography 158
Hysterosalpingography 231

I

Ileocaecal valve 161
  barium-enema examinations 161
  computed tomography 161
  radiology 161
Ileum 160
Iliac vessels
  computed tomography 216
  magnetic resonance imaging 216
  radiology 216
  ultrasound 216
Incus 24
Inferior accessory fissure 118
Inferior radioulnar joint 246-7
Inferior vena cava 193, 204
  anatomy 195-6
  cavography 196
  chest radiography 196
  computed tomography 196
  embryology 196
  magnetic resonance imaging 196
  radiology 196
  tributaries of 195
  ultrasound 196
  variants 196
Infraorbital artery 40
Infratemporal fossa, axial section 29
Inguinal ligament 148
Insula (of Reil) 49
Internal capsule 51
  axial section 84

Internal carotid artery 38, 71-3
Internal iliac artery 214-15
Internal jugular vein 41
Interpeduncular cisterns 66
Intervertebral discs
    computed tomography 97
    discography 97
    magnetic resonance imaging 97
    plain radiography 97
    radiology 97
Intestine
    small intestine 158
    jejunum 160
    ilium 160
    caecum 160
    colon 162
    rectum 213

J

Jaw *see also* Mandible; Maxilla
Jejunum 160, 204
Joints
    acromioclavicular 243
    ankle 266
    atlantoaxial 95
    atlanto-occipital 95
    carpal 247
    elbow 245
    facet, of vertebra 95
    glenohumeral 243
    of hand 247
    hip 261
    inferior radioulnar 246
    intercarpal 247
    intervertebral 95
    knee 263
    neurocentral 95
    sacroiliac 95
    shoulder 243
    sternoclavicular 243
    subtalar 267
    temporomandibular 16
    tibiofibular 266
    radiocarpal 247
    wrist 247
Jugular arch 41

K

Kidneys 184-9
    anatomy 184-6
    arteriography 189
    blood supply 185
    computed tomography 187
    development of 18
    developmental abnormalities and
        variants 186
    fascial spaces 185-6
    internal structure 184
    interventional procedures 189
    intravenous urography 187
    magnetic resonance imaging
        187-9
    radiology 186-9, 204
    relations of 184
    scintigraphy 189
    ultrasound 187
    venous drainage 185
Knee joint 263-6
    anatomy 263-5
    arthrography 265
    magnetic resonance imaging
        266
    plain radiographs 265
    radiology 265-6

L

Lacrimal apparatus 23
Lacrimal duct 11
Lacrimal gland
    computed tomography 23
    dacrocystography 23
    magnetic resonance imaging 23
    radiology 23
Large intestine 162
Laryngopharynx 30
Larynx 31-5
    anatomy 31-2
    axial section 33
    computed tomography 34, 35
    coronal section 32
    cross-sectional anatomy 33
    glottic level 33
    infraglottic level 33
    lateral views 35
    magnetic resonance imaging 35
    plain radiography 33
    radiology 33
    sagittal section showing cartilages
        32
    soft-tissue view 30
    supraglottic level 33
    tomography 35
    xeroradiography 35
Lens 21
Ligaments
    alar 95
    annular 246
    apical 95
    broad 227
    calcaneofibular 266
    coliateral
        fibular 263
        of elbow 246
        of knee 263
        of radiocarpal 247
        tibial 263
    coracocromial 244
    coracohumeral 244
    coronary of liver 200
    costoclavicular 243
    cruciate
        of atlantoaxial 95
        of knee 263
    deltoid 266
    denticulate 100
    dorsal of wrist 247
    falciform 168
    gastrosplenic 180
    glenohumeral 244
    iliofemoral 261
    iliolumbar 95
    inguinal 148, 207
    interosseus
        of leg 266
        of wrist 267
    interspinous 97
    intertransverse 97
    ischiofemoral 261
    lienorenal 180
    longitudinal 96
    medial of ankle 266
    meniscofemoral 265
    oblique popliteal 263
    of Trietz 157
    ovarian 229
    parametrial 227
    patellar 263
    pubofemoral 261
    pubocervical 227
    puboprostatic 218, 221
    pulmonary 113
    radiocarpal 247
    round 227
    sacroiliac 207
    sacrospinous 207
    sacrotuberous 207
    supraspinous 96
    suspensory of ovary 229
    talofibular 266
    tibiofibular 226
    transverse acetabular 261
    transverse humeral 244

transverse, of atlantoaxial joint   95
triangular of liver   200
uterosacral   227
umbilical, median, medial and
      lateral   149
vocal   31
ligamenta flava   97
ligamentum arteriosum   132
ligamentum teres
   of hip   261
   of liver   168
ligamentum nuchae   96
Lentiform nucleus   52
Limbic lobe
   anatomy   57
   components of   57
   magnetic resonance imaging   57
   radiology   57
ultrasound examination of the
      neonatal brain   57
Liver   167-72, 201-4
   anatomy   167-9
   arterial supply   170
   computed tomography   170, 175
   lobes   168
   lymphatic drainage   170
   magnetic resonance imaging   171
   peritoneal attachments   200
   radiology   170-2
   segmental anatomy   169
   ultrasound   171
   venous drainage   170
Lower limb   253-74
   arteries   271
      arteriography   272-3
      collateral arteries   273
      computed tomography   272
      magnetic resonance imaging
         272
      radiology   272-3
      ultrasound   273, 274
   bones   254-60
   joints   261-3
   muscles   268-9
   veins   274
      radiology   274
   venography   274
Lower urinary tract   217-20
Lumbar puncture for myelography
      97, 102
Lumbar spinal cord, myelographic
      appearance   103
Lumbar spine, radiography   93
Lumbar vertebrae   88

Lung   118-23
   bronchography   122
   isotope ventilation-perfusion
         scanning   123
   magnetic resonance imaging   123
   PA chest radiograph   120
   plain tomography   122
   radiology   120-3
Lung anatomy   118-20
Lung roots   120
Lymph nodes
   see individual areas drained

M

Malleus   24
Mandible
   anatomy   14
   arthrography   16
   orthopantomography   16
   plain films   16
   radiology   16
Marginal artery   165
Mastoid   6
Maxillary artery   39-40
Maxillary sinuses   12-13
Maxillary vein   41
Meatus
   external auditory   24
   internal auditory   25
Meckl's diverticulum   160
Medial epicondyle, avulsion of   239
Mediastinal contours
         frontal chest radiograph   139-40
         lateral chest radiograph   140
Mediastinal divisions   124
Mediastinal lines   140-3
   anterior junctional   143
   aortopulmonary mediastinal stripe
         143
   paraspinal   143
   pleuro-oesophageal   143
   posterior tracheal   143
   right paratracheal   143
Mediastinum   124
   anatomy   144
   chest radiography   139-46
   cross-sectional anatomy   143-6
   lymphatics   138
   nerves of   139
   posterior   135
Medulla oblongata
   anatomy   59
   blood supply   59

cervical myelography   59
computed tomography   59
cranial nerves   59
external features   59
magnetic resonance imaging   59
radiology   59
Membrana tectorla   95
Meninges
   anatomy   68-9
   arterial supply   69
   computed tomography   69
   nerve supply   69
   radiography   69
   radiology   69
Menisci
   of knee   263
   of temporomandibular joint   16
   of wrist   247
Metacarpal index   243
Metacarpal sign   243
Metacarpals   242-3
   ossification   243
   radiology   243
Midbrain
   axial section   83
   blood supply   58
   computed tomography   58
   cranial nerves   58
   external features   58
   internal features   58
   magnetic resonance imaging   58
   radiology   58
Motor cortex   46
Muscles
   anterior abdominal wall, of   148
   ciliary, of eye   21
   diaphragm   109
   extrinsic ocular   20
   intercostal   106
   lower limb, of   268
   nasopharynx, of   27
   pelvic floor, of   209
   pelvis, of   207
   posterior abdominal wall, of   201
   tongue, of   16
   upper limb, of   248
Myelography, lumbar puncture for
      97, 102

N

Nasal cavity
   anatomy   12-13
   computed tomography   13

plain films   13
radiology   13
Nasal sinuses
  see individual paranasal sinuses
Nasopharynx
  anatomy   27
  axial section   28
    computed tomography   28
    cross-sectional anatomy   30
  spaces related to   28
Neck   *see* Head and neck
Neck vessels   38-44
  anatomy   38-40
  radiology   43
Neonatal head, ultrasound   52
Nerves
  brachial plexus   251
  cranial   58, 59
  femoral   268
  median   248
  optic   21
  phrenic   139
  radial   248, 249
  spinal   98
  sympathetic   139
  ulnar   249
  vagus   59, 139, 154
Nucleus polyposis   97

O

Oblique (major) fissure   118
Occipital association cortex   49
Occipital lobe   47-9
Oesophagus   135-7
  anatomy   135
  barium studies   137
  blood supply   135
  cross-sectional imaging   137
  lymph drainage   135
  plain films   137
  radiology   137
Optic nerve   21
Oral cavity
  anatomy   16
  radiology   17
Orbit
  anatomy   20
  computed tomography   23
  contents of   20-1
  magnetic resonance imaging   23
  plain films   22
  radiology   22
  ultrasound   22

Oropharynx   30
Ovaries   229
  blood supply   229
  lymph drainage   229
  ultrasound   229

P

Palate   16
Pancreas   176-9, 203, 204
  anatomy   176-8
  angiography   179
  arterial supply   178
  computed tomography   179
  development of   177
  ducts   176
  ERCP   179
  hypotonic duodenography   179
  lymphatic drainage   178
  radiology   178-9
  ultrasound   179
  variations in anatomy   177
  venography   179
  venous drainage   178
Pancreatic ducts   176
Pancreaticobiliary tree, ERCP study
    173
Para-aortic nodes   197-8
Paranasal sinuses
  anatomy   12-13
  computed tomography   13
  plain films   13
  radiology   13
  see also individual sinuses
Paraspinal lines   143
Parathyroid glands   37
    computed tomography   37
    cross-sectional imaging   37
    nuclear medicine studies   37
    radiology   37
Parietal association cortex   47
Parietal lobe   47
Parietal pleura   113
Parotid duct   17
Parotid gland   17
Patella   257
  dislocation   257
  fracture   257
  plain radiographs   257
  radiology   257
Pedicles of vertebra   86
Peduncles
  cerebellum   60
  cerebral   58

Pelvic floor   209-11
  anatomy   209-11
  computed tomography   211
  magnetic resonance imaging   211
  radiology   211
Pelvic muscles   207
Pelvis   205-34
  anatomy   206-7
  arteries   214-16
  blood vessels   214-16
  cross-sectional imaging   209
    lower sacral level
      female   234
      male   233
  lymphatics   216
    cross-sectional imaging   216
  lymphangiography   216
    radiology   216
  mid-sacral level, male/female   232
  nerves   217
  plain films   208-9
  radiology   208-9
Penis   225
  cavernosography   225
  magnetic resonance imaging   225
  radiology   225
  ultrasound   225
Pericallosal cistern   67
Pericardium   125-6
Perineum
  female   234
  male   234
Peritoneal spaces   199-201
  anatomy   199-200
  computed tomography   201
  radiology   201
  ultrasound   201
Peritoneum   199, 200
Phalanges   242-3
  ossification   243
  radiology   243
Pharyngography   31
Pharynx
  and related spaces   26
  computed tomography   31
  coronal images   31
  cross-sectional imaging   31
  magnetic resonance imaging   31
  plain films   31
  radiology   31
  soft-tissue view   30
Phlebography, epidural   104
Phrenic nerves   139
Pia mater   69, 100

Pineal gland 55
  radiology 55
Pituitary gland
  anatomy 55-6
  blood supply 56
  computed tomography 56
  coronal section 55
  magnetic resonance imaging 56
  radiology 56
Pleura
  anatomy 113
  computed tomography 113
  plain films 113
  radiology 113
Pleuro-oesophageal line 143
Pneumoencephalography 65, 67
Pons 58-9
  axial section 82
  blood supply 59
  computed tomography 59
  cranial nerves 58
  external features 58
  magnetic resonance imaging 59
  radiology 59
Pontine cistern 66
Pores of Kohn 118
Portal vein 170, 175, 182-3
  ultrasound 174
Portal venography 172
Portal venous system 182-3
  computed tomography 183
  portography 183
  radiology 183
  ultrasound 183
Portosystemic anastomoses 183
Posterior abdominal wall 159
  veins of 196-7
  azygous and ascending lumbar
      venography 196
  contrast-enhanced computed
      tomography 196-7
  radiology 196-7
Posterior commissure 51
Posterior fossa
  axial section 82
  veins of 80
Posterior junction line 143
Posterior tracheal stripe 143
Preaortic nodes 197
Prefrontal area 46
Premotor cortex 46
Projection fibres 51
  computed tomography 51
  magnetic resonance imaging 51

plain films 51
  radiology 51
Properitoneal fat 149
Prostate gland 221
  blood supply 221
  cross-sectional imaging 222
  radiology 222
  ultrasound 222
Psoas muscle 184
Pubic symphysis 206
Pulmonary angiography 123
Pulmonary arteries 118, 134
  lateral chest radiograph 122
Pulmonary ligament 113
Pulmonary vasculature 121
  computed tomography 123
Pulmonary veins 119
  lateral chest radiograph 122
Pyloric canal 151

Q

Quadrigeminal cistern 66

R

Radial artery 251
Radicular arteries 101
Radiculomedullary arteries 101
Radiocarpal joint 247
Radius 240-1
  ossification 241
  plain radiographs 241
  radiology 241
Rectum 213
  barium enema 213
  computed tomography 213
  magnetic resonance imaging 213
  plain films 213
  radiology 213
Rectus sheath 148
Recurrent laryngeal nerves 139
Renal venography 189
Renal vessels 204
Reproductive organs, male 221-5
Reproductive tract, female 225-31
  computed tomography 230
  cross-sectional imaging 231
  magnetic resonance imaging 230
  radiology 229-31
  ultrasound 229-30
Retina 21
Retroaortic nodes 198
Retroperitoneum, fascial spaces 186

Ribs 106
Right atrium 126
Right ventricle 126-8
Rotator cuff, shoulder 244
Ruptured anterior urethra, contrast
      urethrography 149

S

Sacrum 88, 206
Salivary glands
  anatomy 17
  cross-sectional imaging 18
  radiology 18
  sialography 18
  ultrasound 18
Scaphoid 242
Scapula 236
  isotope bone scan 237
  ossification 237
  plain radiographs 236-7
  radiology 236-7
Scrotum
  blood supply 224
  fluid collections in 224
  lymph drainage 224
Seminal vesicles 221
  blood supply 221
  cross-sectional imaging 222
  lymph drainage 221
  radiology 222
  ultrasound 222
Sensory cortex 47
Sesamoid bones 243, 254, 260
Shoulder joint 243-5
  arthrography with or without
      computed tomography 245
  magnetic resonance imaging 245
  plain radiographs 244-5
  radiology 244
Sigmoid colon
  barium enema 213
  blood supply 212
  computed tomography 213
  lymph drainage 213
  magnetic resonance imaging 213
  plain films 213
  radiology 213
Sinoatrial node 131
Situs inversus 121
Skull
  anatomy 2
  calcification 9
  growing 9

neonatal 9
plain films 51
radiography 55, 56, 64-5, 68, 69, 80
sutures 2, 3, 9
Skull base
  anatomy 5
  bones 5-6
  cross-sectional imaging 9
  foramina of 8
  plain films 8-9
  radiology 8-9
Skull vault
  anatomy 2
  cross-sectional imaging 9
  plain films 8-9
  radiology 8-9
Small intestine 159-61
  anatomy 159-60
  arterial supply 160
  barium studies 160
  computed tomography 161
  radiology 160-1
  venous drainage 160
Spermatic cord 224
  blood supply 224
Sphenoid sinuses 12
Spinal angiography 98, 104
Spinal canal 93
Spinal column 85-104
  magnetic resonance imaging 94
  ligaments of 97
Spinal cord 98-100
  blood supply 101-4
  radiology 102-4
  computed tomography 103-4
  cross-section of 99
Spinal column
  ligaments of
    computed tomography 97
    lumbar puncture for myelography
      97
  magnetic resonance imaging 97
  radiology 97
  magnetic resonance imaging 104
  myelographic technique 102
  radiology 102-4
  venous drainage 101
Spinal meninges
  anatomy 100
  radiology 102-4
Spleen
  anatomical variants 181
  anatomy 180-1
  blood supply 180
  computed tomography 181

magnetic resonance imaging 181
  portography 181
  radiology 181, 202, 204
  scintigraphy 181
  ultrasound 181
Splenic vein 182
Splenoportography 183
Stapes 24
Stensen's duct 17
Sternoclavicular joint 243
Sternum 108
  computed tomography 108
  ossification 108
  plain films 108
  radiology 108
Stomach 151-6
  anatomy 151-4
  anterior relations 151
  arterial supply 152
  computed tomography 155
  double-contrast barium-meal
    examination 154
  lymph drainage 154
  posterior relations 152
  radiology 154-6
  vagal supply 154
  venous drainage 153-4
Subarachnoid cisterns
  anatomy 66-7
  cervical myelography 67
  computed tomography 67
  magnetic resonance imaging 67
  radiology 67
Subarachnoid haemorrhage 69
Subclavian arteries 43-4, 134, 251
  angiography 44
Subclavian veins 44
  venography 44
Subdural haematoma 69
Sublingual gland 18
Submandibular gland 18
Subphrenic spaces 222
Subtalar joint 267
  computed tomography 267
  magnetic resonance imaging 267
  plain radiography 267
  radiology 267
Superior vena cava 134
Superior venacavography 252
Supernumerary bones 242
Suprarenal gland see Adrenal
    glands
Sustenaculum tali 258
Suprasellar cisterns 67
Sympathetic trunk 139

T

Taeniae coli 162
Talus 258
Teeth
  nomenclature and anatomy 15
  orthopantomography 16
  plain films 16
  radiology 16
Temporal association cortex 47
Temporal lobe 47
  axial section 82
Temporomandibular joint, anatomy
    14
Tendons of extensors of fingers 243
Testis 223
  blood supply 224
  lymph drainage 224
  magnetic resonance imaging 225
  radiology 224-5
  ultrasound 224-5
Thalamus
  anatomy 54
  axial section 84
  computed tomography 55
  radiology 55
  ultrasound examination of the
    neonatal brain 55
Thoracic cage
  anatomy 106
  radiology 106-8
Thoracic duct 138
Thoracic spinal cord, myelographic
    appearance 102
Thoracic spine, radiography 92
Thoracic vertebrae 87-8
Thorax 105-46
  computed tomography 127
Thymus 138
Thyroid gland 35-7
  anatomy 35
  axial section 36, 37
  blood supply 35-6
  computed tomography 37
  cross-sectional anatomy 35
  ectopic tissue 36
  lymph drainage 35-6
  magnetic resonance imaging 37
  nuclear medicine studies 36
  plain films 36
  radiology 36
  ultrasound 36, 37
Tibia 257
  ossification 257
  plain radiographs 257

radiology 257
Tibiofibular joints 266
Tibioperoneal trunk 271
Trachea
  anatomy 114
  blood supply 114
  lateral chest radiograph 122
  PA chest radiograph 120
  plain tomography 122
Transverse (minor) fissure 118
Tympanic membrane 24

U

Ulna 240-1
  ossification 241
  plain radiographs 241
  radiology 241
Ulnar artery 251
Umbilical ligaments 149
Upper limb 235-52
  arterial supply 251
  arteriography 251
  bones 236-7
  intravenous injection of contrast or
    radionuclides in dynamic
    studies 252
  joints 243-7
  muscles 248-50
  radiology 251
  veins of, radiology 252
  venography 252
Ureter
  anatomy 189-90
  blood supply 189
  computed tomography 190
  development of 190
  developmental abnormalities and
    variants 190
  intravenous pyelography 190
  pelvic 217
  radiology 190
  ultrasound 190
Ureterocoele 190
Urethra
  female 220
  male 218-20
    radiology 220
Uterus 226-7
  blood supply 228
  ligamentous support 227
  normal variants 227
  ultrasound 228, 229

V

Vagina 225-6
  blood supply 226
  lymph drainage 226
  ultrasound 228
Vaginography 231
Vagus nerves 139
Vas deferens 224
Veins
  adrenal 191, 192
  anastomic of brain 78
  ascending lumbar 196
  axillary 251
  azygous 71, 138, 196
  basal 79
  basilic 252
  brachiocephalic 134
  bronchial 175, 120
  cardiac 130
  cephalic 252
  cerebral
    anterior 78
    deep middle 78
    great cerebral vein of Galen 74
    superficial 78
    internal 79
  choroid 178
  femoral 274
  facial 91
  Galen, great vein of 74
  gastric 153
  gonadal 195
  hemiazygous 196
  hepatic 170
  iliac 216
  jugular
    anterior 41
    external 41
    internal 41
  lumbar 71
  lumbar azygous 196
  maxillary 41
  median, of forearm 252
  mesenteric
    inferior 182
    superior 182
  ophthalmic 20
  ovarian 229, 195
  pancreaticoduodenal 182
  perforating, of leg 274
  popliteal 274
  posterior fossa, veins of 80

portal 170, 182, 183
profunda femoris 274
pulmonary 119
renal 185, 189
retromandibular 421
saphenous
  long 274
  short 274
septal 178
splenic 180
subclavian 44
thalamostriate 78
testicular 195
umbilical 168
venae cavae
  inferior 193, 195
  superior 134
vermian 80
vertebral 41, 71
Venography
  adrenal 196
  ascending lumbar 196
  azygous 196
  cavography
    superior 134
    inferior 196
  iliac 216
  lower limb 274
  portal 183
  renal 189
  splenic 181
  upper limb 252
Venous sinuses 77-8
  angiography 80
  contrast-enhanced computed
    tomography 80-1
  radiology 80-1
  radionucleotide brain scans 81
  skull radiography 80
Ventricles 62-5
  anatomy 62-4
  anterior horn 62
  body 62
  computed tomography 65
  magnetic resonance imaging 65
  inferior horn 62
  lateral ventricle 62
  occipital horn 62
  radiology 64-5
  skull radiographs 64-5
  ultrasound scanning of the
    neonatal brain 65
  ventriculography 65

Vermiform appendix   162
Vermis   61
Vertebra
  cervical   86
  coccygeal   88
  lumbar   88
  sacral   88
  thoracic   87
Vertebra prominens   87
Vertebrae   86
  ossification   93
  radiology   91-4
Vertebral body, axial computed
        tomography   93
Vertebral column   86-97
  anatomy   86-8
  blood supply   98

  radiology   98
  spinal angiography   98
joints of   95-6
  computed tomography   96
  disease processes   96-7
  facet (apophyseal joint)
      arthrography   95
  magnetic resonance imaging   96
  plain radiographs   95
  ligaments of   96-7
  radiography   91-2
Vertebral system, angiography   76-7
Vertebral vein   41
Vertebrobasilar system   73-5
Visceral pleura   113
Visual cortex   49
Vocal cords   32

Weigert-Meyer law   190
White matter of the cerebral

W hemispheres   49
Wrist
  arthrography   247
  magnetic resonance imaging   247
  plain radiographs   247
  radiology   247

X

Xiphoid, of sternum   108

Y, Z

Zygoma   10